Essentials of Health Policy and Law

Joel B. Teitelbaum, JD, LLM

The George Washington University
School of Public Health and Health Services
Department of Health Policy
Washington, DC

Sara E. Wilensky, JD, MPP

The George Washington University
School of Public Health and Health Services
Department of Health Policy
Washington, DC

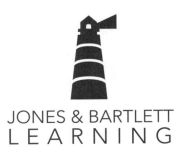

JONES & BARTLETT
LEARNING

World Headquarters

Jones & Bartlett Learning
40 Tall Pine Drive
Sudbury, MA 01776
978-443-5000
info@jblearning.com
www.jblearning.com

Jones & Bartlett Learning
Canada
6339 Ormindale Way
Mississauga, Ontario L5V 1J2
Canada

Jones & Bartlett Learning
International
Barb House, Barb Mews
London W6 7PA
United Kingdom

Jones & Bartlett Learning books and products are available through most bookstores and online booksellers. To contact Jones & Bartlett Learning directly, call 800-832-0034, fax 978-443-8000, or visit our website, www.jblearning.com.

Substantial discounts on bulk quantities of Jones & Bartlett Learning publications are available to corporations, professional associations, and other qualified organizations. For details and specific discount information, contact the special sales department at Jones & Bartlett Learning via the above contact information or send an email to specialsales@jblearning.com.

This publication is designed to provide accurate and authoritative information in regard to the subject matter covered. It is sold with the understanding that the publisher is not engaged in rendering legal, accounting, or other professional service. If legal advice or other expert assistance is required, the service of a competent professional person should be sought.

Library of Congress Cataloging-in-Publication Data
Teitelbaum, Joel Bern.
  Essentials of health policy and law / Joel B. Teitelbaum and Sara E. Wilensky.
     p. ; cm.
  Includes index.
  ISBN-13: 978-0-7637-3442-8
  ISBN-10: 0-7637-3442-X
  1. Medical policy--United States--Textbooks. 2. Medical laws and legislation--United States--Textbooks. I. Wilensky, Sara E. II. Title.
  [DNLM: 1. Health Policy--legislation & jurisprudence--United States. WA 33 AA1 T265e 2007]
  RA395.A3T45 2007
  362.10973--dc22
                            2006037755
  6048

Production Credits
Publisher: Michael Brown
Production Director: Amy Rose
Associate Production Editor: Daniel Stone
Associate Editor: Katey Birtcher
Marketing Manager: Sophie H. Fleck
Manufacturing Buyer: Therese Connell
Cover Design: Kristin E. Ohlin
Composition: Arlene Apone
Photo Research Manager: Kimberly Potvin
Photo Researcher: Christine McKeen
Illustrations: Teresa Smolinski
Printing and Binding: DB Hess
Cover Printing: John P. Pow Company

Printed in the United States of America
14 13 12 11 10   10 9 8 7 6 5 4

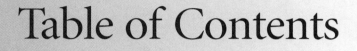

Table of Contents

Part II   Essential Issues in Health Policy and Law

Part III Basic Skills in Health Policy Analysis

Prologue

Health policies and laws are an inescapable and critical component of our everyday lives. The accessibility, cost, and quality of health care; the country's preparedness for disasters; the safety of the food, water, and medications we consume; the right to make individual decisions about one's own health and well-being; and scores of other important issues are at the heart of health policy and law. These policies and laws have a strong and lasting effect on our quality of lives as individuals and on our safety and welfare as a nation.

Professors Joel Teitelbaum and Sara Wilensky do a marvelous job in this text of capturing the breadth of health services and public health policy and law. Their training as policy analysts and lawyers shines through as they systematically describe and analyze the complex field of health policy and law and provide vivid examples to help you make sense of it, too. Equally apparent is their wealth of experience teaching health policy and law at both the undergraduate and graduate levels. Between them, they have designed and taught many health policy and/or law courses, supplemented their teaching of health policy and law by integrating writing and analytic skills into their courses, designed a Bachelor of Science degree program in public health, and received teaching awards for their efforts. Readers of this textbook are the beneficiaries of their experience, enthusiasm, and commitment, as you will see in the pages that follow.

Essentials of Health Policy and Law stands on its own as a text. Even so, the accompanying *Essential Readings in Health Policy and Law* provides abundant illustrations of the development, influence, and consequences of health policies and laws. The carefully selected articles, legal opinions, and public policy documents in the supplemental reader allows students to delve deeper into the topics and issues explored in this book.

I am pleased that *Essentials of Health Policy and Law* is a part of the **Essential Public Health** series. From the earliest stages of the series' development, Professors Teitelbaum and Wilensky have played a central role. They have closely coordinated efforts with other series authors to ensure that the series provides a comprehensive approach with only intended overlap. Many of their approaches to organizing and presenting materials have been widely used in the series. A full list of the available and forthcoming titles in the series can be found at http://www.jbpub.com/essentialpublichealth.

I am confident that you will enjoy reading and greatly benefit from *Essentials of Health Policy and Law*. Whether you are studying public health, public policy, healthcare administration, or one of several other disciplines to which health policy and law is critical, this book is a key component of your education.

Richard Riegelman MD, MPH, PhD
Series Editor

The Essential Public Health Series

Log on to www.jbpub.com/essentialpublichealth for the most current information on availability.

CURRENT AND FORTHCOMING TITLES IN THE *ESSENTIAL PUBLIC HEALTH SERIES*:

Public Health 101: Healthy People–Healthy Populations—Richard Riegelman, MD, MPH, PhD

Epidemiology 101—Robert H. Friis, PhD

Global Health 101, Second Edition—Richard Skolnik, MPA

Case Studies in Global Health: Millions Saved—Ruth Levine, PhD & the What Works Working Group

Essentials of Public Health, Second Edition—Bernard J. Turnock, MD, MPH

Essential Case Studies in Public Health: Putting Public Health into Practice—Katherine Hunting, PhD, MPH & Brenda L. Gleason, MA, MPH

Essentials of Evidence-Based Public Health—Richard Riegelman, MD, MPH, PhD

Essentials of Infectious Disease Epidemiology—Manya Magnus, PhD, MPH

Essential Readings in Infectious Disease Epidemiology—Manya Magnus, PhD, MPH

Essentials of Biostatistics in Public Health, Second Edition—Lisa M. Sullivan, PhD (with Workbook: *Statistical Computations Using Excel*)

Essentials of Public Health Biology: A Guide for the Study of Pathophysiology—Constance Urciolo Battle, MD

Essentials of Environmental Health, Second Edition—Robert H. Friis, PhD

Essentials of Health, Culture, and Diversity—Mark Edberg, PhD

Essentials of Health Behavior: Social and Behavioral Theory in Public Health—Mark Edberg, PhD

Essential Readings in Health Behavior: Theory and Practice—Mark Edberg, PhD

Essentials of Health Policy and Law—Joel B. Teitelbaum, JD, LLM & Sara E. Wilensky, JD, MPP

Essential Readings in Health Policy and Law—Joel B. Teitelbaum, JD, LLM & Sara E. Wilensky, JD, MPP

Essentials of Health Economics—Diane M. Dewar, PhD

Essentials of Global Community Health—Jaime Gofin, MD, MPH & Rosa Gofin, MD, MPH

Essentials of Program Planning and Evaluation—Karen McDonnell, PhD

Essentials of Public Health Communication—Claudia Parvanta, PhD; David E. Nelson, MD, MPH; Sarah A. Parvanta, MPH; & Richard N. Harner, MD

Essentials of Public Health Ethics—Ruth Gaare Bernheim, JD, MPH & James F. Childress, PhD

Essentials of Management and Leadership in Public Health—Robert Burke, PhD & Leonard Friedman, PhD, MPH

Essentials of Public Health Preparedness—Rebecca Katz, PhD, MPH

ABOUT THE EDITOR:

Richard K. Riegelman, MD, MPH, PhD, is Professor of Epidemiology-Biostatistics, Medicine, and Health Policy, and Founding Dean of The George Washington University School of Public Health and Health Services in Washington, DC. He has taken a lead role in developing the Educated Citizen and Public Health initiative which has brought together arts and sciences and public health education associations to implement the Institute of Medicine of the National Academies' recommendation that "…all undergraduates should have access to education in public health." Dr. Riegelman also led the development of George Washington's undergraduate major and minor and currently teaches "Public Health 101" and "Epidemiology 101" to undergraduates.

Preface

Health policy and law are matters of national and local focus and concern. Public opinion polls, media coverage, and policy debates at all levels of government and in private industry attest to the important place that health care and public health hold in the minds of the American public, policymakers, and lawmakers. The constant attention showered on health policy–related topics also highlights their complexity, which stems from multiple factors.

First, like most challenging public policy problems, pressing health policy questions simultaneously implicate politics, law, ethics, and social mores, all of which come with their own set of competing interests and advocates. Second, health policy debates often involve deeply personal matters pertaining to one's quality—or very definition—of life, philosophical questions about whether health care should be a market commodity or a social good, or profound questions about how to appropriately balance population welfare with closely guarded individual freedoms and liberties. Third, it is often not abundantly clear how to begin tackling a particular health policy problem. For example, is it one best handled by the medical care system, the public health system, or both? Which level of government—federal or state—has the authority or ability to take action? Should the problem be handled legislatively or through regulatory channels? The final ingredient that makes health policy problems such a complex stew is the rapid developments often experienced in the areas of healthcare research, medical technology, and public health threats. Generally speaking, this kind of rapid evolution is a confounding problem for the usually slow-moving American policy and lawmaking machinery.

Broadly defined, the goal of health policy is to promote and protect the health of individuals and of populations bound by common circumstances. Because the legal system provides the formal structure through which public policy—including health policy—is debated, effectuated, and interpreted, law is an indispensable component of the study of health policy. Indeed, law is inherent to the expression of public policy: Major changes to policies often demand the creation, amendment, or rescission of laws. As such, students studying policy must learn about the law, legal process, and legal concepts.

The range of topics fairly included under the banner of "health policy and law" is breathtaking. For example, what effect is healthcare spending having on national and state economies? How should finite financial resources be allocated between health care and public health? How can we ensure that the trust funds established to account for Medicare's income and disbursements remain solvent in the future as an enormous group of Baby Boomers becomes eligible for program benefits? What kind of return (in terms of quality of individual care and the overall health of the population) should we expect from the staggering amount of money we collectively spend on health? Should individuals have a legal entitlement to health insurance? How can we best attack extant health disparities based on race, ethnicity, and socioeconomic status? What policies will best protect the privacy of personal health information in an increasingly electronic medical system? Can advanced information technology systems improve the quality of individual and population health? Should the right to have an abortion continue to be protected under the federal Constitution? Should physician assistance in dying be promoted as a laudable social value? Will mapping the human genome lead to discrimination based on underlying health status? How prepared is the country for natural and man-made catastrophes, like pandemic influenza or bioterrorism attacks? What effect will chronic diseases, such as diabetes and obesity-related conditions, have on health care delivery and financing? How can we best harness advancing scientific findings for the benefit of the public's health?

As seen from this partial list of questions, the breadth of issues encountered in the study of health policy and law is virtually limitless, and we do not grapple with all of the preceding questions in this book. We do, however, introduce you to many of the policies and laws that give rise to them, provide an intellectual framework for thinking about how to address them going forward, and direct you to additional relevant readings. Given the prominent role played by policy and law in the health of all Americans, and the fact that the Institute of Medicine recommends that students of public health and other interdisciplinary subjects (for example, public policy or medicine), receive health policy and law training,[1(pp95-98)] the aim of this book is to help you understand the broad context of American health policy and law, the essential issues impacting and flowing out of the health care and public health systems, and how health policies and laws are influenced and formulated. Think of this textbook as an extended manual—introductory, concise, and straightforward—to the seminal issues in U.S. health policy and law, and thus as a jumping off point for discussion, reflection, research, and analysis.

To further assist with those pursuits, this book is accompanied by *Essential Readings in Health Policy and Law* (to be published by Jones and Bartlett Publishers in 2008). It is a compilation of carefully selected readings meant to allow for deeper analysis of issues covered in this textbook, as well as some issues not covered due to space constraints.

Part I of this textbook includes three preparatory chapters. Chapter 1 describes the influential role of policy and law in health care and public health and introduces various conceptual frameworks through which the study of health policy and law can take place. The chapter also illustrates why it is important to include policy and law in the study of health care and public health. However, an advanced exploration of health policy and law in individual and population health necessitates a basic and practical comprehension of policy and law in general, including the policymaking process and the workings of the legal system. Thus, Chapter 2 discusses both the meaning of policy and the policymaking process, including the basic functions, structures, and powers of the legislative and executive branches of government and the respective roles of the federal and state governments in policymaking. Chapter 3 then describes the meaning and sources of law and several key features of the U.S. legal system, including the separation of powers doctrine, federalism, the role of courts, and due process. (Note that Part I assumes students' basic knowledge of the organization of the healthcare system and of the functions of public health agencies. However, for students without this background, *Essential Readings in Health Policy and Law* includes a section covering these and other basic health care and public health topics.)

Part II offers several chapters focusing on key substantive health policy and law issues. Chapters 4 and 5 cover the fundamentals of health insurance and health economics, respectively, and set up a subsequent thematic discussion in Chapters 6–8 concerning gaps in healthcare coverage, coverage reform efforts, and the importance of policy and law to both. Specifically, Chapter 4 describes the function of risk and uncertainty in health insurance, defines the basic elements of health insurance, discusses important health policy issues relating to health insurance, and more; Chapter 5 explains why it is important for health policymakers to be familiar with basic economic concepts; the basic tenets of supply, demand, and markets; and the way in which health insurance affects economic conditions. Chapter 5 also applies economic concepts to health policy problems.

Chapter 6 picks up on the themes of Chapters 4 and 5 and explains how federal and state policymakers have created health insurance programs for individuals and populations who otherwise might go without health insurance coverage. The basic structure, administration, financing, and eligibility rules of the three main U.S. public health insurance programs—Medicaid, the State Children's Health Insurance Program (SCHIP), and Medicare—are discussed, as are key health policy questions relating to each program. Chapter 7 discusses the fact that notwithstanding the private health insurance market and the public programs enacted to address its limitations, there remains in this nation an enormous uninsured population. The chapter describes who is uninsured and why, the ramifications of being uninsured, and how the uninsured receive needed medical care, as well as the reasons why this country has failed to achieve major health reform on a national level. Chapter 8 examines the ways in which the law creates, protects, and restricts individual rights in the contexts of health care and public health, including a discussion of laws (like Medicaid and Medicare) that further aim to level the playing field where access to health care is concerned. The chapter also, however, introduces the "no-duty to treat" principle, which holds that there is no general legal duty on the part of health providers to provide care and which rests at the heart of the legal framework pertaining to healthcare rights and duties. Finally, Chapter 9 reflects on several important policy and legal aspects of health care quality, including the evolution of the standard of care, tort liability for health care providers and insurers, and preventable medical errors.

The book concludes in Part III by teaching the basic skills of health policy analysis. Because the substance of health policy can only be understood as the product of an infinite number of policy choices as to whether and how to intervene in many types of health policy problems, Chapter 10 explains how to structure and write a short health policy analysis. This type of analysis is a tool frequently used by policy analysts when they assess policy options and discuss rationales for their health policy recommendations.

REFERENCES

1. Gebbie K, Rosenstock L, Hernandez LM, eds. *Who Will Keep the Public Healthy?: Educating Public Health Professionals for the 21st Century.* Washington, D.C.: The National Academies Press; 2003.

Acknowledgments

We are grateful to many people who generously contributed their guidance, assistance, and encouragement to us during the writing of this book. At the top of the list is Dr. Richard Riegelman, Founding Dean of The George Washington University School of Public Health and Health Services and Professor of Epidemiology and Biostatistics, Medicine, and Health Policy. The *Essential Public Health* book series was his brainchild, and his stewardship of the project (as Series Editor) made our involvement in it both enriching and enjoyable. We are indebted to him for his guidance and confidence.

We also would like to single out two other colleagues for special thanks. Ruth Katz, Dean of GW's School of Public Health and Health Services and the Walter G. Ross Professor of Health Policy, has been unwavering in her support of our work, including this textbook, and for that we owe her our sincere thanks. Sara Rosenbaum, our Department Chair and the Harold and Jane Hirsh Professor of Health Law and Policy, has been a wonderful mentor, colleague, and friend for many years. We are indebted to her for supporting our decision to undertake the writing of this book and for her efforts in making the end result a stronger product.

We also want to collectively recognize the many students and colleagues who in reviewing specific chapters gave willingly of their time and expertise. Though there are too many to name individually, each played a critical role in bringing this book to fruition, and for that we are most appreciative. This finished product has been greatly enhanced by—in the parlance of the day—their unvarnished advice.

At various times during the writing of this book we were blessed to have the help of five stellar research assistants: V. Nelligan Coogan, Mara B. McDermott, Sarah E. Mutinsky, Dana E. Thomas—all of them members of the Hirsh Health Law and Policy Program, which houses GW's combined law-public health degree and certificate programs—and Ramona Whittington, a candidate for a Master of Public Health degree in Health Policy. Their research assistance and steady supply of good cheer proved invaluable, and we could not have completed this book without them.

Our gratitude extends also to Mike Brown, publisher for Jones and Bartlett, for his encouragement, and to his staff, for their technical expertise.

Finally, we wish to thank those closest to us. Sara gives special thanks to Trish Manha—her life-partner, cheerleader, reviewer, and constant supporter—who made it possible for Sara to complete this book while maintaining her sanity and humor. Sara would also like to thank her mother, Dr. Gail Wilensky, for sharing her knowledge of all things health policy while busy with one or two projects of her own. Joel sends special thanks to Tanya Ehrmann and Jared and Layna Teitelbaum, collectively the source of more affection than he can describe and who at the end of the day are what really matter.

About the Authors

Joel B. Teitelbaum, JD, LLM, is an Associate Professor and the Vice Chair of the Department of Health Policy at The George Washington University (GW) School of Public Health and Health Services in Washington, DC. He is also the Managing Director of the School's Hirsh Health Law and Policy Program.

Professor Teitelbaum has taught graduate courses on healthcare law, healthcare civil rights, public health law, minority health policy, and long-term care law and policy, and an undergraduate survey course on health law. He has authored or co-authored many articles, book chapters, policy papers, and reports on civil rights issues in health care, managed care law and policy, and behavioral healthcare quality. He has directed or managed several health law and policy research projects, including ones sponsored by the District of Columbia Department of Health; the Henry J. Kaiser Family Foundation's Commission on Medicaid and the Uninsured; the Center for Health Care Strategies, Inc.; and the U.S. Substance Abuse and Mental Health Services Administration. In addition, Professor Teitelbaum was co-recipient of the Robert Wood Johnson Foundation Investigator Award in Health Policy Research, which he used to explore the creation of a new framework for applying Title VI of the 1964 Civil Rights Act to the modern healthcare system.

As Vice Chair of the Department of Health Policy, Professor Teitelbaum is responsible for the department's day-to-day academic operations. As Managing Director of the Hirsh Health Law and Policy Program, he oversees a program designed to foster an interdisciplinary approach to the study of health law, health policy, health care, and public health through educational and research opportunities for law students, health professions students, and practicing lawyers.

Professor Teitelbaum serves on the Board of Directors of DePaul University College of Law's Center for the Study of Race and Bioethics, which identifies health care access barriers among minority populations and shapes public policy that will help eliminate those barriers; the Council of Advisors for Physician-Parent Caregivers, Inc., which facilitates communication and collaboration between caregivers and parents of children with special healthcare needs; and the Board of Advisors for Project HEALTH D.C., part of a national student organization addressing socioeconomic, medical, and environmental causes of poor health in low-income children. He is also heavily involved in GW service activities. Among other things, he has served as Chair of the Medical Center Faculty Senate's Executive Committee, Chair of the School of Public Health's Curriculum Committee, Chair of the Department of Health Policy's Curriculum Committee, and Co-Chair of the committee that created and implemented GW's undergraduate Bachelor of Science degree in public health.

Professor Teitelbaum is a member of Delta Omega, the national honor society recognizing excellence in the field of public health; the American Constitution Society for Law and Policy; the American Society of Law, Medicine, and Ethics; the State Bar of Wisconsin; and the Washington Council of Lawyers.

Sara E. Wilensky, JD, MPP, is an Assistant Research Professor of Health Policy at The George Washington University (GW) School of Public Health and Health Services in Washington, DC. She is also the Managing Director of the School's Geiger Gibson Program in Community Health Policy.

Professor Wilensky has taught a health policy analysis course required of all health policy majors in the Master's of Public Health degree program at GW as well as the introductory health policy course required of all undergraduate students majoring in public health. She has been the principal investigator or co-principal investigator on numerous health policy research projects relating to a variety of topics, such as Medicaid coverage, access and financing, community health centers, childhood obesity, HIV preventive services, financing of public hospitals, and data sharing barriers and opportunities between public health and Medicaid agencies.

Professor Wilensky is involved with several GW service activities: She is the chair of the Health Policy department's Student Affairs and Alumni Committee; she has been heavily involved in making GW's Writing in the Disciplines program part of the undergraduate major in public health; and she is the advisor to students receiving a Master's in Public Policy or a Masters in Public Administration with a focus on health policy from GW's School of Public Policy and Public Administration.

As Managing Director of the Geiger Gibson Program in Community Health Policy, Professor Wilensky oversees a program designed to train the next generation of community health leaders and to celebrate the history of health centers nationwide. The program has housed several distinguished visitors with accomplished careers in community health centers, hosted an annual symposium as part of the National Association of Community Health Center Policy and Issues Forum, launched a History Project designed to tell the story of every health center, and conducted research on a variety of health center issues.

Prior to joining GW, Professor Wilensky was a law clerk for federal Judge Harvey Bartle, III in the Eastern District of Pennsylvania, and worked as an associate at the law firm of Cutler and Stanfield, in Denver, Colorado.

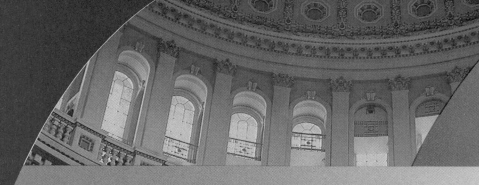

Photo Credits

Cover Image
© Steve Maehl/ShutterStock, Inc.

Chapter 2
Description: The building of the US Senate.
Credit line: © Michael Holcomb/ShutterStock, Inc.

Chapter 3
Description: The building of the US Supreme Court.
Credit line: © Douglas Toombs/ShutterStock, Inc.

Chapter 4
Description: A stethoscope and a set of patient records.
Credit line: © Amy Walters/ShutterStock, Inc.

Chapter 5
Description: Stethoscope on top of paper currency.
Credit line: © IRP/ShutterStock, Inc.

Chapter 6
Description: White pills and pill bottle.
Credit line: © Andy Piatt/ShutterStock, Inc.

Chapter 7
Description: Detail of historic building.
Credit line: © Aaron Kohr/ShutterStock, Inc.

Chapter 8
Description: Liquid being dropped into test tubes.
Credit line: © Cre8tive Images/ShutterStock, Inc.

Chapter 9
Description: Collage of medical images.
Credit line: © Lorelyn Medina/ShutterStock, Inc.

Chapter 10
Description: Detail of business person writing on form.
Credit line: © Liv Friis-larsen/ShutterStock, Inc.

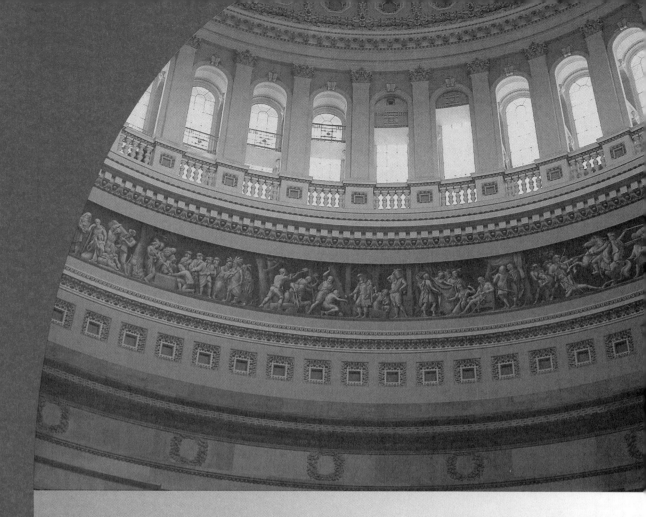

PART I

Overview of Policy and Law in the United States

Part I of this textbook contains three chapters aimed at preparing you for the substantive health policy and law discussions found in Chapters 4–9 and the skills-based discussion of policy analysis in Chapter 10. Chapter 1 describes generally the role of policy and law in health care and public health and introduces conceptual frameworks for studying health policy and law. Chapter 2 describes the meaning of policy and the policymaking process. Finally, Chapter 3 provides an overview of the meaning and sources of law and of several important features of the legal system.

CHAPTER 1

Introduction: Understanding the Role of and Conceptualizing Health Policy and Law

LEARNING OBJECTIVES

By the end of this chapter you will be able to:

- Describe generally the important role played by policy and law in the health of individuals and populations
- Describe three ways to conceptualize health policy and law

INTRODUCTION

In the Preface, we began to sketch the outlines of the overall picture of health policy and law, briefly describing their importance to contemporary society, their complexity, and their breadth. In this chapter, we aim to darken those outlines and fill in the picture a bit, by introducing the role played by policy and law in the health of individuals and populations and by describing three conceptual frameworks with which you can approach the study of health policy and law. In the chapters that follow, we draw the picture in much sharper contrast, providing a measure of clarity in an area that is neither readily discernable—even to those who use and work in the health care and public health systems—nor easily redrawn by those who shape them through policy and law.

The goals of this chapter are to describe why it is important to include policy and law in the study of health care and public health and how you might conceptualize health policy and law when undertaking your studies. To achieve these goals, we first briefly discuss the vast influence of policy and law in health care and public health. You will have a much better feel for the full reach of policy and law into these areas after you read the chapters that lie ahead, but we dedicate a few pages

here to give you a sense of why it is critical to examine policy- and lawmaking as part of your broader health studies. We then describe three ways to conceptualize health policy and law. As you will discover, we have elected to draw on each of the three conceptual frameworks at different points in the book, rather than maintain focus on only one of them.

THE ROLE OF POLICY AND LAW IN HEALTH CARE AND PUBLIC HEALTH

The forceful influence of policy and law in the health of individuals and populations is undeniable. Policy and law have always been fundamental to shaping the practice of individual health care in the United States and to achieving both everyday and landmark public health improvements.

Centuries-old legal principles have, since this country's inception, provided the bedrock on which health care quality laws are built, and today the health care industry is regulated in many different ways. Indeed, federal and state policy and law shape virtually all aspects of the health care system, from structure and organization to service delivery, to financing, and to administrative and judicial oversight. Whether pertaining to the accreditation and certification of individual or institutional health care providers, requirements to provide care under certain circumstances, the creation of public insurance programs, the regulation of private insurance systems, or any of a number of other issues, policy and law drive the health care system to a degree unknown by most people.

In fact, professional digests that survey and report on the subjects of health policy and law typically include in their pages information on topics like the advertising and marketing of health services and products, the impact of health expenditures on federal and state budgets, antitrust concerns, health care contracting, employment issues, patents, taxation, health care discrimination and disparities, consumer protection, bioterrorism, health insurance, prescription drug regulation, assisted suicide, biotechnology, human subject research, patient privacy and confidentiality, organ availability and donation, and more. Choices made by policymakers and decisions handed down through the legal system impact how we undertake, experience, analyze, and research all of these specific aspects of the health care system.

Once you've read the next two preparatory chapters—one on policy and the policymaking process, the other on law and the legal system—and begin to digest the substantive health-specific chapters that follow them, the full force of policy and law in shaping the individual health care system will unfold. For now, simply keep in the back of your mind the fact that policy and law heavily influence the way in which health care is accessed, medicine is practiced, treatments are paid for, and much more.

The role of policy and law in public health is no less important than in individual health care, but the influence of policy and law in the field of public health is less frequently articulated. In fact, policy and law have long played a seminal role in everyday public health activities (think, for example, of food establishment inspections, occupational safety standards, policies related to health services for persons with chronic health conditions such as diabetes, and policies and laws affecting the extent to which public health agencies are able to gauge whether individuals in a community suffer from certain health conditions), as well as in many historic public health accomplishments (water and air purification, reduction in the spread of communicable diseases through compulsory immunization laws, reduction in the number of automobile-related deaths through seatbelt and consumer safety laws, and several others).[a] Public health professionals and students quickly learn to appreciate that combating public health threats requires both vigorous policymaking and adequate legal powers. Additionally, enhanced fears about bioterrorism and new infectious diseases have only increased the public's belief that policy and law are important tools in creating an environment in which people can achieve optimal health and safety.

Of course, policies and laws do not always favor what many people believe to be in the best interests of public health and welfare. A policy or law might, for example, favor the economic interests of a private, for-profit company over the residents of the community in which the company is located.[b] Why? Because one main focus of policy and law in the realm of public health is on locating the appropriate balance between public regulation of private individuals and corporations, and the ability of those same parties to exercise rights that allow them to function free of overly intrusive government intervention. Achieving this balance is not easy for policymakers. Not all interested parties agree on things like the extent to which car makers should alter their operations to reduce environmentally harmful auto emissions, or on the degree to which companies should be limited in advertising cigarettes, or whether gun manufacturers should be held liable in cases where injuries or killings result from the negligent use of their products.

How do policymakers and the legal system reach a satisfactory public health/private right balance? The competing interests at the heart of public health are mainly addressed through two types of policies and laws: those that define the functions and powers of public health agencies, and those that aim to directly protect and promote health.[c] State-level policymakers and public health officials create these types of policies and laws through what are known as their *police powers*. These powers represent the inherent authority of state and local governments to regulate individuals and private business in the name of public health promotion and protection. The importance of police powers cannot be overstated; it is fair to say that they are the most critical aspect of the sovereignty that states retained at the founding of the country, when the colonies agreed to a governmental structure consisting of a strong national government. Furthermore, the reach of police powers should not be underestimated, particularly because they permit public health authorities to coerce private parties to engage in (or refrain from) activities in the name of public health and welfare.[d] However, states do not need to exercise their police powers in order to affect or engage in public health–related policymaking. Because the public's health is impacted by many social, economic, and environmental factors, public health agencies also conduct policy-relevant research, disseminate information aimed at helping people engage in healthy behaviors, and establish collaborative relationships with health care providers and purchasers and with other government policymaking agencies.

Federal policy and law also play a role in public health. For instance, although the word *health* never appears in the U.S. Constitution, the document confers powers on the federal government—to tax and spend, for example—that allow it to engage in public health promotion and disease prevention activities. The power to tax (or establish exemptions from taxation) allows Congress to encourage healthy behaviors, as witnessed by the heavy taxes levied on packages of cigarettes. The power to spend enables Congress to establish executive branch public health agencies and to allocate public health–specific funds to states and localities.

CONCEPTUALIZING HEALTH POLICY AND LAW

You have just read about the importance of taking policy and law into account when studying health care and public health. The next step is to begin thinking about how you might conceptually approach the study of health policy and law.

There are multiple ways to conceptualize the many important topics that fall under the umbrella of health policy and law. We introduce three conceptual frameworks in this section: one premised on the broad topical domains of health policy and law, one based on prevailing historical factors, and one focused on the individuals and entities impacted by a particular policy or legal determination (see Box 1-1).

We draw on these frameworks to various degrees in this book. For example, the topical domain approach of framework 1 is on display in Chapter 8 (individual rights in health care and public health) and Chapter 9 (health care quality policy and law). Framework 2's focus on historical perspectives is highlighted in Chapter 6 (government health insurance programs), Chapter 7 (health reform), and Chapter 8.

Finally, framework 3, which approaches the study of health policy and law from the perspectives of key stakeholders, is drawn on in Chapter 2 (policy and the policymaking process), Chapter 8, and Chapter 9. We turn now to a description of each framework.

The Three Broad Topical Domains of Health Policy and Law

One way to conceptualize health policy and law is as consisting of three large topical domains. One domain is reserved for policy and law concerns in the area of *health care*, another for issues arising in the *public health* arena, and the last for controversies in the field of *bioethics*. As you contemplate these topical domains, bear in mind that they are not individual silos whose contents never spill over into the others. Indeed, this sort of spillage is common (and, as noted in the preface, is one reason why fixing health policy problems can be terribly complicated). We briefly touch on each domain in the following sections.

Health Care Policy and Law

In the most general sense, this domain is concerned with an individual's access to care (e.g., what policies and laws impact an individual's ability to access needed care?), the quality of the care the person received (e.g., was it appropriate, cost-effective, and non-negligent?), and how the person's care is going to be financed (e.g., is the person insured or uninsured?). However, "access," "quality," and "financing" are themselves rather large subdomains with their own sets of complex policy and legal issues, and in fact it is common for students to take semester-long policy and/or law courses focused on just one of these subdomains.

Public Health Policy and Law

The second large topical domain is that of public health policy and law. A central focus here is on why and how the government regulates private individuals and corporations in the name of protecting the health, safety, and welfare of the general public. Imagine, for example, that the federal government was considering a blanket policy decision to vaccinate individuals across the country against the deadly smallpox disease, believing that the decision was in the best interests of national security. Would this decision be desirable from a national policy perspective? Would it be legal? If the program's desirability and legality are not immediately clear, how would you go about analyzing and assessing them? These are the kinds of questions with which public health policy and law practitioners and scholars grapple.

Box 1-1   Three Conceptual Frameworks for Studying Health Policy and Law

Framework 1. Study based on the broad topical domains of:
   a. Health care
   b. Public health
   c. Bioethics

Framework 2. Study based on historically dominant social, political, and economic perspectives:
   a. Professional autonomy
   b. Social contract
   c. Free market

Framework 3. Study based on the perspectives of key stakeholders:
   a. Individuals
   b. The public
   c. Health care professionals
   d. Federal and state governments
   e. Managed care and traditional insurance companies
   f. Employers
   g. The pharmaceutical industry
   h. The research community
   i. Interest groups
   j. Others

Bioethics

Finally, there is the bioethics domain to health policy and law. Strictly speaking, the term *bioethics* is used to describe ethical issues raised in the context of medical practice or biomedical research. More comprehensively, bioethics can be thought of as the point at which public policy, law, individual morals, societal values, and medicine intersect. The bioethics domain houses some of the most explosive questions in health policy, including the morality and legality of abortion, the conflicting values around the meaning of death and the rights of individuals nearing the end of life, and the policy and legal consequences of mapping the human genetic code.

Social, Political, and Economic Historical Context

Dividing the substance of health policy and law into broad topical categories is only one way to conceptualize them. A second way to consider health policy and law is in historical terms, based on the social, political, and economic views that dominate a particular era.[e] Considered this way, health policy and law have been influenced over time by three perspectives, all of which are technically active at any given time but each of which has eclipsed the others during specific periods in terms of political, policy, and legal outcomes. These perspectives are termed *professional autonomy*, *social contract*, and *free market*.[1(pp24–35),2]

Professional Autonomy Perspective

The first perspective, grounded in the notion that the medical profession should have the authority to regulate itself, held sway from approximately 1880 to 1960, making it the most dominant of the three perspectives in terms of both the length of time it held favored status and the actual shaping of health policy and law. This model is premised on the idea that physicians' scientific expertise in medical matters should translate into legal authority to oversee essentially all aspects of delivering health care to individuals. In other words, according to proponents of the physician autonomy model, legal oversight of the practice of medicine should be delegated to the medical profession itself. For the extended period of time over which this perspective remained dominant, policymakers and lawmakers were generally willing to allow physicians to control the terms and amount of health care payments, the standards under which medical licenses would be granted, the types of patients they would treat, the type and amount of information to disclose to patients, and the determination as to whether their colleagues in the medical profession were negligent in the treatment of their patients.

Social Contract Perspective

The second perspective that informs a historical conceptualization of health policy and law is that of the "modestly egalitarian social contract."[3(p2),f] This paradigm overshadowed its competitors, and thus guided policy decision making, from roughly 1960 to 1980, a time notable in U.S. history for social progressiveness, civil rights, and racial inclusion. At the center of this perspective is the belief that complete physician autonomy over the delivery and financing of health care is potentially dangerous in terms of patient care and health care expenditures, and that public policy and law can and sometimes should enforce a "social contract" at the expense of physician control. Put differently, this perspective sees physicians as just one of several stakeholders, including but not limited to patients, employers, and society, that lay claim to important rights and interests in the operation of the health care system. Health policies and laws borne of the social contract era centered on enhancing access to health care (e.g., through the now-called Examination and Treatment for Emergency Medical Conditions and Women in Labor Act), creating new health insurance programs (Medicare and Medicaid were established in 1965), and passing anti-discrimination laws (one of the specific purposes of Title VI of the federal 1964 Civil Rights Act was wiping out health care discrimination based on race).

Free Market Perspective

The final historical perspective—grounded in the twin notions of the freedom of the marketplace and of market competition—became dominant in the 1990s and continues with force today. It contends that the markets for health care services and for health insurance operate best in a deregulated environment, and that commercial competition and consumer empowerment will lead to the most efficient health care system. Regardless of the validity of this claim, this perspective argues that the physician autonomy model is falsely premised on the idea of scientific expertise, when in fact most health care services deemed "necessary" by physicians have never been subjected to rigorous scientific validation (think of the typical treatments for the common cold or flu). It further argues that even the modest version of the social contract that heavily influenced health policy and law during the civil rights generation is overly regulatory. Furthermore, market competition proponents claim that both other models are potentially inflationary, since in the first case self-interest will lead autonomous physicians to drive up the cost of their services, and in the second instance public insurance programs like Medicare would lead individuals to seek unnecessary care.

To tie a couple of these historical perspectives together and examine (albeit in somewhat oversimplified fashion) how evolving social and economic mores have influenced health policy and law, consider the example of Medicaid, the joint federal–state health insurance program for low-income individuals. In 1965, Medicaid (which is described at much greater length in Chapter 6) was born out of the prevailing societal mood that it was an important role of government to expand legal expectations among the poor and needy. In other words, its creation exemplified a social contract perspective, which in the context of health touts the view that individuals and society as a whole are important stakeholders in the health care and public health systems. Medicaid entitled eligible individuals to a set of benefits that, according to courts during the era under consideration, was the type of legal entitlement that could be enforced by beneficiaries when they believed their rights under the program were infringed.

These societal expectations and legal rights and protections withstood early challenges during the 1970s, as the costs associated with providing services under Medicaid resulted in state efforts to roll back program benefits. Then, in the 1980s, Medicaid costs soared higher, as eligibility reforms nearly doubled the program's enrollment and some providers (e.g., community health centers) were awarded enhanced payments for the Medicaid services they provided. Still, the social contract perspective held firm, and the program retained its essential egalitarian features.

As noted earlier, however, the gravitational pull of the social contract theory weakened as the 1980s drew to a close. This, coupled with the fact that Medicaid spending continued to increase in the 1990s, led to an increase in the number of calls to terminate program members' legal entitlement to benefits.[g] Also in the 1990s, federal and state policymakers dramatically increased the role of private managed care companies in both Medicaid and Medicare,[h] an example of the trend toward the free market principles described earlier.

Key Stakeholders

A third way to conceptualize health policy and law issues is in terms of the stakeholders whose interests are impacted by certain policy choices or by the passage or interpretation of a law. For example, imagine that in the context of interpreting a state statute regulating physician licensing, your state's highest court ruled that it was permissible for a physician to not treat a patient even though the doctor had been serving as the patient's family physician. What stakeholders could be impacted by this result? Certainly the patient, and other patients whose treatment may be colored by the court's decision. Obviously the

doctor, and other doctors practicing in the same state, could be impacted by the court's conclusion. What about the state legislature? Perhaps it unintentionally drafted the licensing statute in ambiguous fashion, which led the court to determine that the law conferred no legal responsibility on the physician to respond to a member of a family that was part of the doctor's patient load. Or maybe the legislature is implicated in another way—maybe it drafted the law with such clarity that no other outcome was likely to result, but the citizenry of the state were outraged because its elected officials created public policy out of step with constituents' values. Note how this last example draws in the perspective of another key stakeholder—the broader public.

Of course, patients, health care providers, governments, and the public are not the only key stakeholders in important matters of health policy and law. Managed care and traditional insurance companies, employers, the pharmaceutical industry, the medical device industry, the research community, interest groups, and others all may have a strong interest in various policies or laws under debate.

CONCLUSION

This chapter's descriptions of the roles played by policy and law in the health of individuals and populations, and of the ways to conceptualize health policy and law, were cursory by design; after all, you will explore these roles and conceptual frameworks in more detail in subsequent chapters. But what we hope is apparent to you at this early stage is the fact that the study of policy and law is essential to the study of both health care and public health. Consider the short list of major problems with this country's health system as described in a recent book edited and written by a group of leading scholars[1]: the coverage and financing of health care, health care quality, health disparities, and threats to population health.[3(p10)] All of the responses and fixes to these problems—and to many other health care– and public health–related concerns—will invariably and necessarily involve creative policymaking and rigorous legal reform. This fact is neither surprising nor undesirable: Policy and law have long been used to effectuate positive social change. Since the founding of this country, the fields of health care and public health have experienced this phenomenon, and given the many serious problems playing out in these arenas right now, there is little reason to expect that policy and law will not be two of the primary drivers of health-related reform in the years ahead.

Policy and legal considerations are not only relevant in the context of major health care and public health problems going forward, however—they are critical to the daily functioning of the health system, and to the health and safety of individuals and communities across a range of everyday life events. Take pregnancy and childbirth, for example. Approximately 11,000 births occur each day in this country, and society views pregnancy and childbirth as more or less normal and unremarkable events. In fact, the process of becoming pregnant, accessing and receiving high-quality prenatal health care, and experiencing a successful delivery is crucial not only to the physical, mental, and emotional health and well-being of individuals and families, but also to the long-term economic and social health of the nation. It further implicates a dizzying number of interesting and important policy questions. Consider the following:

- Should there be a legal right to health care in the context of pregnancy and, if so, should that right begin at the point of planning to get pregnant, at the moment of conception, at the point of labor, or at some other point?
- Regardless of legal rights to care, how should the nation finance the cost of pregnancy care? Should individuals and families be expected to save enough money to pay out-of-pocket for what is a predictable event? Should the government help subsidize the cost of prenatal care? If so, in what way? Should care be subsidized at the same rate for everyone, or should subsidy levels be based on financial need?
- Regarding the quality of care, what is known about the type of obstetrical care women should receive, and how do individuals know they are getting that care? Given the importance of this type of care, what policy steps are taken to assure that the care is sound? What should the law's response be when a newborn or pregnant woman is harmed through an act of negligence? When should clinician errors be considered preventable and their commission thus tied to a public policy response? And what should the response be?
- What should the legal and social response be to prospective parents who act in ways risky to the health of a fetus? Should there be no societal response because the prospective parents' actions are purely a matter of individual right? Does it depend on what the actions are?
- Is it important to track pregnancy and birth rates through public health surveillance systems? Why or why not? If it is an important function, should the data tracking be made compulsory or voluntary?
- How well does the public health system control known risks to pregnancies, both in communities and in the workplace?

- Finally, who should answer these questions? The federal government? States? Individuals? Should courts play a role in answering some or all of them? Whose interests are implicated in each question, and how do these stakeholders affect the policymaking process?

There are scores of topics—pregnancy and childbirth among them—that implicate a range of complex health policy questions, and these are the types of questions this textbook and *Essential Readings in Health Policy and Law* prepare you to ask and address. Before you turn your attention to the essential principles, components, and issues of health policy and law, however, you must understand something about policy and law generally. The next two chapters provide grounding in policy and law and supply the basic information needed to study policy and law in a health context. They define policy and law, discuss the political and legal systems, introduce the administrative agencies and functions at the heart of the government's role in health care and public health, and more. With the information from these chapters at your disposal, you will be better equipped to think through some of the threshold questions common to many policy debates, including:

- Which sector—public, private, or not-for-profit (or some combination of them)—should respond to the policy problem?
- If government responds, at what level—federal or state—should the problem be addressed?
- What branch of government is best-suited to address—or more attuned to—the policy issue?
- When the government takes the lead in responding to a policy concern, what is the appropriate role of the private and not-for-profit sectors in also attacking the problem?
- What legal barriers might there be to the type of policy change being contemplated?

Once you have the knowledge to be able to critically assess these types of questions, you will be able to focus more specifically on the application of policy and law to critical issues in health care and public health.

REFERENCES

1. Rosenblatt RE, Law SA, Rosenbaum S. *Law and the American Health Care System.* Westbury, NY: The Foundation Press; 1997.

2. Rosenblatt RE. The four ages of health law. *Health Matrix: J Law-Med.* 2004;14:155.

3. Mechanic D, Rogut LB, Colby DC, Knickman JR, eds. *Policy Challenges in Modern Health Care.* New Brunswick, N.J.: Rutgers University Press; 2005.

ENDNOTES

a. See, e.g., Wendy E. Parmet, "Introduction: The Interdependency of Law and Public Health," in *Law in Public Health Practice*, eds. Richard A. Goodman et al. (Oxford: Oxford University Press, 2003).

b. For an engrossing example of the ways in which law and legal process might stand in the way of effective public health regulation, we recommend Jonathan Harr, *A Civil Action* (New York: Vintage Books, 1995).

c. See, e.g., Larry O. Gostin, Jeffrey P. Koplan, and Frank P. Grad, "The Law and the Public's Health: The Foundations," in *Law in Public Health Practice*, eds. Richard A. Goodman et al. (Oxford: Oxford University Press, 2003).

d. Police powers are discussed in more detail in Chapter 8, which covers individual rights in health care and public health.

e. The particular historical framework we describe here was developed to apply to health care, rather than public health. We do not mean to imply, however, that it is impossible to consider public health from a historical, or evolutionary, vantage point. In fact, it is fair to say that public health practice may be on the verge of entering its third historical phase. Throughout the 19th and most of the 20th centuries, protection of the public's health occurred mainly through direct regulation of private behavior. In the latter stages of the 20th century, strict reliance on regulation gave way to an approach that combined regulation with chronic disease management and public health promotion, an approach that necessitated a more active collaboration between public health agencies and health care providers and purchasers. Now, it appears that public health professionals are adding to this revised practice model another strategic initiative: building collaborative relationships with policymaking agencies whose responsibilities are not directly related to public health—for example, agencies whose primary fields are transportation or agriculture.

f. The authors write that the American social contract lags behind those of other developed countries, and thus use the phrase "modestly egalitarian" in describing it.

g. By 2005, proponents of weakening Medicaid-enrolled persons' entitlement to program benefits had made significant strides: Congress passed a law called the Deficit Reduction Act that, among other things, granted states the ability to redefine the benefits and services to which Medicaid beneficiaries are entitled. This law is discussed in detail in Chapter 6.

h. This topic is also covered in depth in Chapter 6.

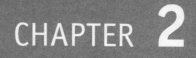

CHAPTER 2

Policy and the Policymaking Process

LEARNING OBJECTIVES

By the end of this chapter you will be able to:

- Describe the concepts of policy and policymaking
- Describe the basic function, structure, and powers of the legislative branch of government
- Describe the basic function, structure, and powers of the executive branch of government
- Explain the role of federal and state governments in the policymaking process
- Explain the role of interest groups in the policymaking process

INTRODUCTION

The first steps for any student of health policy are to understand what policy is generally and to learn about the policymaking process. It is vital to consider policy questions in the particular context in which they arise, both in terms of the general politics of the issue and the values and powers of the policymaker. As you will discover, there is no single definition of policy. Even so, this chapter arms you with the information needed to know what issues to consider when thinking about a public policy problem, how to account for a variety of competing policy views, and what policy options are possible given the political process in the United States.

The chapter first defines what policy is and then moves to a discussion of the policymaking process by examining the roles and powers of the two political branches of government—the legislative and executive branches. (The judicial branch's role in policymaking is discussed in Chapter 3.) As part of this discussion, we introduce you to federal and state agencies that make up the health care and public health bureaucracy. We conclude with a discussion about the roles of interest groups in policymaking and the influence they wield in the policymaking process.

DEFINING POLICY

In this section we consider various aspects of what we mean by the term *policy*. Before delving into the policymaking process, we identify which issues fall within the realm of a public policy decision and, generally, what kinds of decisions might be made by policymakers.

Identifying Public Problems

Scholars have defined policy in many different ways. Consider a few of them:

> Authoritative decisions made in the legislative, executive, or judicial branches of government that are intended to direct or influence the actions, behaviors, and decisions of others.[1(p243)]

> A course of action adopted and pursued by a government, party, statesman, or other individual or organization.[2(p124)]

> Authoritative decisions and guidelines that direct human behavior toward specific goals either in the private or the public sector.[3(p125)]

The differences in these definitions raise several important issues. The first question to consider is whether private actors make policy or whether policymaking is an activity for the government only. The first definition refers only to governmental policymakers, the second definition allows for both public and private policymakers, and the third definition is unclear on this issue. Of course, the government is a key player in any policy field, and it is certainly true that decisions by government entities represent public policy. However, in this text we also focus on private actors who make policy. Decisions by commercial insurance companies, private employers, influential individuals, and others can all be part of health policy. For example, when a major health insurance company decides to cover obesity prevention measures, or when the Bill and Melinda Gates Foundation provides grants to develop crops that are high in essential vitamins and minerals to improve the nutrition of people in developing countries, they are making health policy decisions.

Regardless of whether the policy maker is a public or private figure, it is necessary that the decision being made is an *authoritative* decision. These are decisions made by an individual or group with the power to implement the decision. There are a variety of levels where these kinds of decisions can take place. For example, within government authoritative decisions may be made by the president, cabinet officials, agency heads, members of Congress, governors, state legislatures, public health commissioners, and many others.

But all decisions by public and private individuals or entities are not necessarily policy decisions. The key issue to determining whether a "decision" represents a "policy" is whether the question at hand is an individual concern or a public policy problem. A public policy problem goes beyond the individual sphere and affects the greater community. Whereas an individual might decide to take advantage of employer-sponsored health insurance, a public policy question is whether all employers should be required to offer health insurance to their employees. Whereas an individual might decide to purchase a generic (as opposed to a brand name) drug to save money, a public policy question is whether patients should be induced to buy less expensive generic drugs. When deciding whether something is a public policy decision, the focus is not only on who is making a decision, but also on what kind of decision is being made.

Furthermore, just because a problem is identified as a public policy problem does not necessarily mean the only solution involves government intervention. For example, consider the problem of an influenza vaccine shortage. Although there are government-oriented solutions to this problem, such as expanding public research and development or creating production incentives through tax cuts or subsidies to encourage private manufacturers to produce more vaccine, other solutions may rely solely on private actors. Private companies may

decide to invest in the research and development of new ways to produce vaccines, or to build new plants to increase production capacity, because they believe they can make a profit in the long run. Just as private individuals and entities can make policy decisions for their own benefit, they can also play a central role in solving public policy problems. A lengthier discussion about options for solving public policy problems and arguments for and against government intervention is found in Chapter 5, which covers health economics.

Structuring Policy Options

Considered broadly, there are different ways to approach public policy problems. For example, some policy options are voluntary whereas others are mandatory. It is important to recognize that authoritative decisions do not always *require* others to act or refrain from acting in a certain way. Some of the most important and effective policies are those that provide incentives to others to change their behavior. Indeed, the power of persuasion is very important to public officials, particularly at the federal level, which is limited in its ability to force states and individuals to take certain actions. This stems from the fact that the U.S. Constitution limits Congress and the executive to specific powers and reserves all other powers for the states.[a] However, members of the federal government may use their enumerated powers, such as those to tax and spend, to persuade states and others to act in desired ways.

For example, the Constitution does not give the legislative or executive branches the power to protect the public's health, meaning that the area is primarily within the purview of states to regulate. As a result, Congress and the president cannot require states to create emergency preparedness plans. Yet, Congress may provide incentives to states to do so by offering them federal money in return for state preparedness plans that meet certain criteria established by the federal government.[b]

In addition, it is important to remember that inaction can also be a policy decision. Deciding to do nothing may be a decision to keep a prior decision in place or not to engage in a new issue. For example, a governor could decide against trying to change a restrictive abortion law or a state legislature could choose not to pass a law allowing for small business insurance purchasing pools. Both of these inactions result in important policy decisions that will affect the choices and opportunities available to individuals, advocacy organizations, and others.

This brief discussion about policy has raised several important issues to consider when identifying policy options. The next section provides a detailed discussion of the policymaking process, providing you with the background knowledge necessary to identify and understand the roles and powers of various policymakers.

PUBLIC POLICYMAKING STRUCTURE AND PROCESS

The public policymaking structure refers to the various branches of government and the individuals and entities within each branch that play a role in making and implementing policy decisions. This chapter focuses on two branches of government—the legislative and executive branches—while Chapter 3 discusses the third, the judicial branch. In this section, we review the structure, powers, and constituency of these branches, with a focus on the U.S. House of Representatives, the U.S. Senate, and various commissions and agencies that assist Congress, the president, White House staff, and federal executive branch administrative agencies. In addition to reviewing the policymaking structure, we discuss the processes used by these various individuals and entities for making public policy decisions.

State-Level Policymaking

The federal government does not have a monopoly on policymaking. Indeed, important policy decisions are regularly made at the state level as well, especially in the health care arena. However, because state governments are similar to the federal government in many ways, the policymaking duties and powers that we discuss below can often be applied to a state-level analysis. At the same time, there is a significant amount of variation in how states structure their legislative and executive branches, agencies, and offices, and it is not possible to review the differences that exist among all 50 states. Accordingly, after a brief discussion of state-level policymaking, this chapter focuses primarily on the federal policymaking structure and process.

Like the federal government, each state has three branches of government. State legislatures pass laws, appropriate money within the state, and conduct oversight of state programs and agencies. States also have their own judiciary with trial and appellate courts. The governor is the head of the state executive branch and can set policy, appoint cabinet members, and use state administrative agencies to issue regulations that implement state laws. Although there are limits to a state's power to regulate health care issues, state regulation is an extremely important aspect of health policy. Just a few examples of the health care matters states can regulate include provider licensing, accreditation, some aspects of health insurance, and most public health concerns.

At the same time, it is also important to realize that all state governments are not exactly alike. The governor has more power in some states than others, agencies are combined in different ways among the states, state legislatures may meet annually or biannually, state legislators may be full-time or part-time employees, and so on. Because these differences exist,

it is essential for policy analysts to understand the specific structure of the state in which their client resides.

Furthermore, there are important differences between the federal government and the states. Unlike the federal government, almost all states are required to have a balanced budget, and most states cannot borrow money for operating expenses. These rules mean that states must act to raise revenue or cut programs if they project that their budget will be in deficit by the end of the fiscal year. In addition, about half of the states have tax and expenditure limit rules that restrict tax collection and/or spending and often require legislative supermajorities or voter approval to increase taxes.[4(pp208–209)] As a result, state officials may be more likely than federal officials to make the difficult choice to either limit programs or cut resources from one program to fund another.

As is evident from this brief discussion, state-level policymaking is both a rich area for discussion and a difficult area to make generalizations about because each state is unique. Having highlighted some of the key differences and similarities among the states and between the states and the federal government, we now turn to the legislative and executive branches of the federal government.

The Federal Legislative Branch

Article 1 of the U.S. Constitution makes Congress the lawmaking body of the federal government by granting it "All legislative Powers" and the right to enact "necessary and proper laws" to effectuate its prerogatives.[5] Congressional responsibilities are fulfilled by the two chambers of Congress, the Senate and the House of Representatives ("the House"). The Constitution grants specific powers to Congress, including but not limited to the power to levy taxes, collect revenue, pay debts, provide for the general welfare, regulate interstate and foreign commerce, establish federal courts inferior to the Supreme Court, and declare war.[6] The Senate has the specific power to ratify treaties and confirm nominations of public officials.

The Senate consists of two elected officials from each state, for a total of 100 senators.[c] Each senator is elected in a statewide vote for a six-year term, whereas representatives in the House sit for two-year terms. Due to the lengthy term of its members, the Senate is considered less volatile and more concerned with long-term issues than the House. A senator must be at least 30 years old, a U.S. citizen for at least nine years, and a resident of the state he or she is seeking to represent.[6]

The House includes 435 members[d] allocated proportionally based on the population of the 50 states, with each state guaranteed at least one representative.[e] For example, in 2006 California was allotted 53 representatives while Vermont had only 1. Due to the proportionality rule, members from larger states dominate the House and often hold leadership positions.[4] Members of the House are elected by voters in congressional districts and serve two-year terms. They must be at least 25 years old, a U.S. citizen for at least seven years, and a resident of the state where the election takes place.[8]

Leadership Positions

Leadership roles in Congress are determined by political party affiliation, with the party in the majority gaining many advantages. The vice president of the United States is also the president of the Senate and presides over its proceedings. In the vice president's absence, which is common given the other obligations of the office, the president pro tempore, a mostly ceremonial position, presides over the Senate. In most cases the vice president is not a major player in Senate voting, but with the power to break a tie vote, the vice president wields an important power. The Speaker of the House ("Speaker") presides over that chamber and has the authority to prioritize and schedule bills, refer bills to committees, and name members of joint and conference committees. Other than the vice president's senatorial role, leadership positions in Congress are not elected by the voters, but determined by the members from the party who have been elected to Congress. Other key Congressional leadership positions include:

- **Senate majority leader**—Speaks on behalf of the majority party, schedules floor action and bills, works on committees, directs strategy, and tries to keep the party united.
- **House majority leader**—Works with the Speaker to direct party strategy and set the legislative schedule.
- **House and senate minority leaders**—Speak on behalf of the minority party, direct strategy, and try to maintain party unity; as members of the minority, do not have the legislative duties of the majority leader/Speaker.
- **House and senate majority and minority whips**—Track important legislation, mobilize members to support leadership positions, keep a count of how party members are planning to vote, and generally assist their leaders in managing their party's legislative priorities.

Committees

Committees have been referred to as the "workhorses" of Congress; they are where many key decisions are made and legislative drafting takes place. Given the vast array of issues that Congress contends with in any given legislative session, it is impossible for every member to develop expertise on every issue. Although members vote on bills that cover a wide range of issues, members often concentrate on the areas relevant to the committees on which they serve.

Committees have a variety of important roles, including drafting and amending legislation, educating members on key issues, shepherding the committee's legislation on the floor when it goes before a vote by all the members of one chamber, working with the president, his administration and lobbyists to gain support for a bill, holding hearings, and conducting oversight of executive branch departments, agencies, commissions, and programs within their purview. Committee members often gain expertise in the areas covered by their committees, and other members often rely on their advice when making voting decisions.

Standing committees are generally permanent committees with specified duties and powers. There are 20 standing committees in the House and 21 in the Senate. House committees tend to be larger than those in the Senate, with about 40 members per committee. Some committees have *authorization* jurisdiction, allowing them to create (i.e., authorize) programs and agencies. Other committees have *appropriation* authority, meaning they are responsible for funding (i.e., appropriating) various programs and agencies. Standing committees also have *oversight* authority, meaning they monitor how programs are run and funds are spent. Each chamber of Congress has established specific oversight committees for some programs and issues that cut across committee jurisdiction, as well as committees that review the efficiency and economy of government actions.[9,f]

Not surprisingly, some of the most powerful and popular committees are those that deal with appropriating money. These include:

- **House Ways and Means and Senate Finance committees**—These committees have jurisdiction over legislation concerning taxes, tariffs, and other revenue-generating measures, and over entitlement programs such as Medicare and Social Security. The Constitution requires all taxation and appropriations bills to originate in the House, and House rules require all tax bills to go through the Ways and Means committee.
- **House and Senate Appropriations committees**—These committees have responsibility for writing federal spending bills.
- **House and Senate Budget committees**—These committees are tasked with creating the overall budget plan that helps guide tax and appropriation committee work.
- **House Rules committee**—This committee has jurisdiction over the rules and order of business in the House, including rules for the floor debates, amendments, and voting procedures. All House bills must go to the House Rules committee before reaching the House floor for a vote by all representatives.[g]

Table 2-1 identifies the key health committees and subcommittees and their health-related jurisdictions.

TABLE 2-1 Key Health Committees and Subcommittees

Senate

Committee	*Health-Related Jurisdiction*
Finance Committee: Subcommittee on Health Care	Department of Health and Human Services • Centers for Medicare and Medicaid Services (Medicare, Medicaid, State Children's Health Insurance Program) • Administration for Children and Families Department of the Treasury • Group health plans under the Employee Retirement Income Security Act
Appropriations Committee: Subcommittee on Labor, Health and Human Services, Education and Related Agencies	Department of Health and Human Services • Office of Public Health Service • National Institutes of Health • Centers for Disease Control and Prevention • Health Resources and Services Administration • Substance Abuse and Mental Health Services Administration • Agency for Healthcare Research and Quality Occupational Safety and Health Review Commission Social Security Administration
Appropriations Committee: Subcommittee on Agriculture, Rural Development and Related Services	Department of Health and Human Services Food and Drug Administration
Appropriations Committee: Subcommittee on Interior, Environment and Related Agencies	Department of Health and Human Services • Indian Health Services • Agency for Toxic Substances and Disease Registry
Health, Education, Labor, and Pensions Committee: Subcommittee on Public Health	Bioterrorism and public health preparedness Department of Health and Human Services • Food and Drug Administration • Centers for Disease Control and Prevention • National Institutes of Health • Administration on Aging • Substance Abuse and Mental Health Services Administration • Agency for Healthcare Research and Quality
Committee on Agriculture, Nutrition and Forestry: Subcommittee on Research, Nutrition and General Legislation	• Food stamps • National school lunch program • School breakfast program • Special milk program for children • Special supplemental nutrition program for women, infants and children (WIC)

House

Committee	*Health-Related Jurisdiction*
Committee on Ways and Means: Subcommittee on Health	Social Security Act • Maternal and Child Health block grant • Medicare • Medicaid • Peer review of utilization and quality control of health care organizations

TABLE 2-1 Key Health Committees and Subcommittees *(continued)*

Appropriations Committee: Subcommittee on Labor, Health and Human Services, Education and Related Agencies	Department of Health and Human Services • Office of Public Health Service • National Institutes of Health • Centers for Disease Control and Prevention • Health Resources and Services Administration • Substance Abuse and Mental Health Services Administration • Agency for Healthcare Research and Quality Occupational Safety and Health Review Commission Social Security Administration
Appropriations Committee: Subcommittee on Agriculture, Rural Development and Related Services	Department of Health and Human Services • Food and Drug Administration
Appropriations Committee: Subcommittee on Interior, Environment and Related Agencies	Department of Health and Human Service • Indian Health Services • Agency for Toxic Substances and Disease Registry
Energy and Commerce Committee: Subcommittee on Health	Department of Health and Human Services • Medicaid

Congressional Commissions and Staff Agencies

Although the committee system helps members of Congress focus on particular areas, members often need assistance with in-depth research and policy analysis. Commissions and staff agencies provide members with information they might not otherwise have the time to gather and analyze. There are too many commissions and agencies to list here, but a few key ones include:

- **Congressional Budget Office**—Provides Congress with cost estimates of bills, estimates costs of federal mandates to state and local governments, and forecasts economic trends and spending levels.
- **Government Accountability Office**—An independent, nonpartisan agency that studies how federal tax dollars are spent and advises Congress and executive agencies about more efficient and effective ways to use federal resources.
- **Congressional Research Service**—The public policy research service that conducts nonpartisan, objective research on legislative issues.
- **Medicare Payment Advisory Commission**—An independent federal commission that gives Congress advice on issues relating to the Medicare program, including payment, access to care, and quality of care.

How Laws Are Made

One way that members of Congress indicate their policy preferences is by passing laws that embody their values and the values of their constituents. This is a lengthy process with many steps along the way that could derail a bill (see Figure 2-1).

Before a committee considers a bill, it must be introduced by a member of Congress. Once this occurs, the Speaker refers the bill to one or more committees in the House, and the majority leader does the same in the Senate. The bill may die in committee if there is not sufficient support for it, although there are rarely invoked procedures that allow a bill to be reported to the full chamber even without committee approval. While the bill is in committee, members may hold hearings on it or "mark up" the bill by changing or deleting language in the proposed bill or by adding amendments to it. If a majority of the committee members approves a bill, it goes to the full chamber (House or Senate, depending on where the bill originated).

The full House or Senate then debates the merits of the bill and puts it to a vote. If a majority does not support the bill, it dies on the chamber floor. If a majority supports the bill, it is sent to the other chamber for consideration. The second chamber may pass the exact same bill or a different version of the bill. If the second chamber does not pass any version of the bill, it dies on the

FIGURE 2-1 How a bill becomes a law.

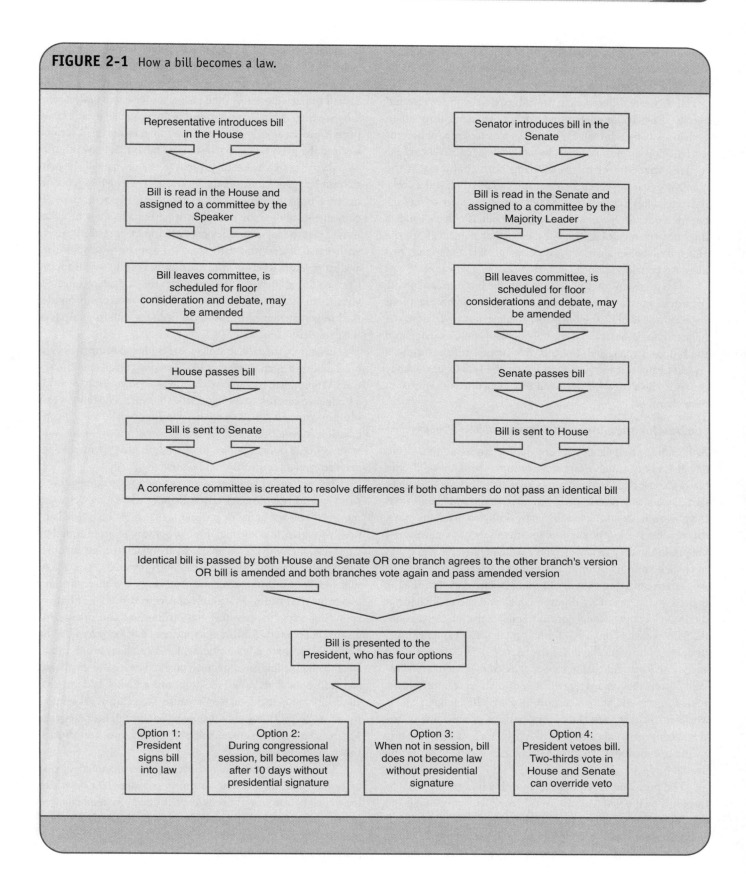

chamber floor and no version of the bill moves forward. If the second chamber passes an identical bill, it goes directly to the president for consideration.

If there are differences in the bills passed by the House and Senate, the two chambers must reach a consensus through an exchange of amendments for the bill to have a chance of becoming law. Consensus building is facilitated by a "conference committee," made up of members from both chambers. If the committee cannot reach a consensus, the bill dies. If the committee reaches a consensus, the bill is sent back to each chamber for a vote on the new version of the bill. If either chamber does not approve of it, the bill dies at that point. If both the House and the Senate pass the new version, it is sent to the president for consideration.

The president may choose to sign the bill into law, or the president may choose to veto the bill. Or, if the president chooses not to sign the bill while Congress is in session, the bill becomes law after 10 days; if Congress is not in session and the bill goes unsigned, the bill dies (this is referred to as a "pocket veto"). If the president vetoes the bill, Congress may override the veto with approval of a two-thirds majority in each chamber.

Congressional Budget and Appropriations Process[10,11]

Although the budget and appropriation processes may sound dry, it is about much more than numbers and charts. If you take a close look at budget documents, they include narratives that discuss why certain programs are being funded and what the government hopes to achieve by doing so. In many ways, this process is a key policy tool for members of Congress and the president; they are able to show which programs and issues have their support through their funding decisions.

Given both the amount of money involved in running the United States (over $2 trillion in 2006) and the various jurisdictions of congressional committees, it is not surprising that the federal budget process is fairly complex. The Congressional Budget and Impoundment Control Act of 1974 ("Budget Act") and subsequent amendments were passed by Congress to create a process that brings together the numerous committees involved in crafting an overall budget plan. The budget process works in concert with the appropriations process, which involves congressional passage of bills from each of the appropriations committees to distribute the funds provided for in the overall budget.

The president is required to submit a budget proposal to Congress by the first Monday in February. This proposal is the administration's request; it is not binding on Congress. Each chamber then passes a *budget resolution*, identifying how the chamber would spend federal money delineated by different categories of spending (e.g., defense, agriculture, transportation). Members from each chamber then meet to develop a single *conference report* reflecting a consensus agreement on the overall budget. Congress then passes a *concurrent budget resolution*, which is binding upon the House and Senate as a blueprint for revenue collection and spending. However, it is not a law and the president is not bound by the budget resolution.

Over the six weeks subsequent to the passage of the concurrent budget resolution, the House and Senate budget committees hold hearings to discuss the budget, and other committees review the budget as it pertains to their jurisdiction. The latter committees provide the budget committees with their "views and estimates" of appropriate spending and/or revenue levels for the upcoming year. In addition, the Congressional Budget Office provides the budget committees with its budget and economic outlook reports and provides the budget and appropriations committees with its analysis of the president's proposal.

In March, the House and Senate budget committees each craft a budget plan during public meetings known as "mark-ups." When the mark-ups are complete, each committee sends a budget resolution to its respective chamber. The budget resolution contains a budget total, spending breakdown, reconciliation instructions, budget enforcement mechanisms, and statements of budget policy. Budget totals are provided as aggregates and as committee allocations.

The federal budget includes two types of spending: *discretionary* and *mandatory*. Discretionary spending refers to money that is set aside for programs that must be funded annually in order to continue. If the programs are not funded by Congress, they will not receive federal dollars to continue their operations. For example, the Head Start program, which provides early childhood education services, is a discretionary program that relies on annual appropriations. Mandatory spending refers to spending on entitlement and other programs that must be funded as a matter of law. For example, the Medicaid program is an entitlement that provides health insurance to eligible low-income individuals. The *authorizing legislation* (the law that created the program) for Medicaid includes eligibility rules and benefits. Because Medicaid is an entitlement program, Congress must provide enough money so the Medicaid agency can meet the obligations found in the authorizing legislation.

The appropriations committees write bills to cover discretionary spending. These committees make their decisions based on the amount of funds available and any *reconciliation instructions*, which direct the appropriate authorizing committee to make changes in the law for mandatory spending programs to meet budgetary goals. Appropriations bills and reconciliation instructions must be signed by the president to become law.

Members of the House and Senate have the opportunity to make changes to the work of the budget committees. Once the House and Senate pass their own versions of the budget resolution, they establish a conference committee to resolve any differences. Once the differences are resolved, each full chamber votes on the compromise budget.

Congress often does not meet Budget Act deadlines (shown in Table 2-2). If the appropriations bills are not passed by every October 1—the beginning of the fiscal year—Congress may pass a *continuing resolution* that allows the government to continue to spend money. If Congress does not pass a continuing resolution or if the president vetoes it, all nonessential activities of federal agencies must stop until additional funds are provided.

Constituents

With the wide array of issues they take on, members of Congress may have an equally wide array of constituents to be concerned about when making policy decisions. Clearly, members are concerned about pleasing the voters who elect them. Even though there may be a variety of policy views to consider, members often prioritize their home constituents. In addition to courting their home-state voters, members often try to court independents or voters from the opposing party in their home state to strengthen their appeal. High approval ratings deter challengers from trying to take an incumbent's congressional seat and allow members of Congress more leeway to pursue their goals and policies.

Although concern for their home-state base may be their first priority, representatives and senators often need to be concerned about supporting their party's position on issues. Today, elected federal politicians are usually affiliated with the Democratic or Republican Party, and voters may be influenced by the party's stance on issues. Also, if the balance of power among the two parties is close in Congress, the parties usually cannot afford to have members defect from their party's positions. Members' concern regarding keeping their party strong is magnified if they hold leadership positions in Congress or are considering running for national office.

Finally, the views of the president may be important for members to consider depending on whether the member and the president share the same party, the particular issue involved, and the president's popularity. Members who are in the same party as the sitting president have incentive to help the president remain popular because they will likely advance many of the same policies. In addition, presidents are often prodigious fundraisers and campaigners who may be able to assist mem-

TABLE 2-2 Federal Budget Process Timeline

First Monday in February	President submits budget proposal to Congress.
March	House completes its budget resolution.
April	Senate completes its budget resolution.
April 15	House and Senate complete concurrent budget resolution.
May	Authorizing committees develop reconciliation language when necessary and report legislation to budget committees. House and Senate develop conference report on reconciliation, which is voted on by each chamber.
June 10	House concludes reporting annual House appropriations bills.
June 15	If necessary, Congress completes reconciliation legislation.
June 30	House completes its appropriations bills.
September 30	Senate completes its appropriations bills. House and Senate complete appropriations conference reports and vote separately on the final bills.
October 1	Fiscal year begins.

Source: Adapted from House Committee on the Budget Majority Caucus, *Basics of the Budget Process*, 107th Cong. Briefing Paper, 2001.

bers during election season. Even when members disagree with the president, the president's power to affect their influence in Congress may be a deterrent to opposing the president. Of course, if the president is exceedingly popular, it is difficult for members of either party to oppose presidential policy goals.

The Federal Executive Branch

Article 2 of the U.S. Constitution establishes the executive branch and vests executive power in the most well-known member of the branch, the president.[12] Of course, the president does not act alone in running the executive branch. Presidents rely on Executive Office agencies and staff such as the Council of Economic Advisors and Office of Management and Budget, as well as policy development offices such as the National Security Council and Domestic Policy Council (see Box 2-1 for a description of one such office).[h] In addition, there are 15 cabinet departments led by individuals selected by the president (subject to Senate confirmation) and additional

Box 2-1 Office of Management and Budget (OMB)

The Office of Management and Budget (OMB) reports directly to the president and plays an important role in policy decisions. OMB is responsible for preparing the presidential budget proposal, which includes reviewing agency requests, coordinating agency requests with presidential priorities, working with Congress to draft appropriation and authorization bills, and working with agencies to make budget cuts when needed. In addition to these budgetary functions, OMB provides an estimate of the cost of regulations, approves agency requests to collect information, plays a role in coordinating domestic policy, and may act as an intermediary politically on behalf of the president. OMB also has an oversight and evaluation function over select federal agencies as a result of the Government Performance and Results Act, which requires agencies to set performance goals and have their performance evaluated.

noncabinet-level agencies, all of which are responsible, among other duties, for interpreting and implementing the laws passed by Congress. All of these advisors identify issues to be addressed and formulate policy options for the president to consider. In theory, all of these parts of the executive branch work in furtherance of the goals set by the president.

The Presidency

The president is the head of the federal executive branch. As powerful as that may sound, the country's founders created three distinct branches of government and limited the president's power in order to ensure that no single individual gained too much control over the nation.[i] As you will see, in some ways the president is very powerful, and in other ways his power is quite limited.

Although there have been third-party candidates for president in the past, generally speaking our country now operates on a two-party system, with Democrats and Republicans as the major parties. Each party selects a candidate for president who represents the party in the election. Presidents (and their vice presidents) are elected through a nationwide vote to serve a four-year term. An individual is limited to serving two four-year terms as president, which may or may not be consecutive.[13,j] To be eligible for election, candidates must be at least 35 years old, a natural born citizen of the United States, and a resident of the country for at least 14 years.

Presidents have many roles. As the unofficial *Chief of State,* the president is seen as the symbol of the country and its citizens.[14(p40)] As the official *Chief Executive Officer,* the president manages the cabinet and executive branch. The president also holds the position of *Commander in Chief of the Armed Forces,* and as such is the top ranking military official in the country. The U.S. Constitution vests the president with other powers, such as the ability to appoint judges to the federal courts, sign treaties with foreign nations, and appoint ambassadors as liaisons to other countries. These powers are all subject to the advice and consent of the Senate.[14(p41)]

AGENDA SETTING. A key tool of the presidency is the ability to put issues on the national agenda and offer a recommended course of action. "[F]raming agendas is what the presidency is all about."[15(p371)] Presidents help set the national agenda because of the role of the president as the country's leader and the amount of media attention given to presidential actions, decisions, and policy recommendations. Unlike many other politicians or interest groups, the president does not have to work hard to receive media coverage. Whether it is the annual State of the Union address, release of the president's budget proposal, a major speech, a press conference, a photo shoot with a foreign leader, or the release of a report, the president's message is continually publicized. In addition, the president's message can be delivered by the vice president, cabinet officers, and party leaders in Congress.

The notion of appealing directly to the country's citizens to focus on a particular issue and to influence legislative debates is referred to as "going public." In going public, presidents try to use support from the American people to gain the attention of Congress and sway policy voting decisions. Because members of Congress are highly concerned about pleasing their constituency to improve their chance for re-election, "the president seeks the aid of a third party—the public—to force other politicians to accept his preferences."[16(p3)]

Sometimes it may be advantageous for the president to place an item on the policy agenda in a less public manner. For example, if a policy is controversial with the general public or if members of the president's party disagree with a proposal, it may be more effective to promote a policy behind the scenes. The president, either directly or through intermediaries, can carefully let members of Congress know which policies are favored. Using combinations of promises of favors and threats to members' interests, the president may be able to influence the outcome of policy debates in Congress even without going public.

In addition to deciding whether to approach Congress publicly or behind the scenes, the president must choose whether to present a preferred policy decision with more or less detail. A policy can be presented broadly through principles or general guidelines or specifically through proposed legislation that is presented to Congress. Each method for conveying the president's goals has pros and cons. If a policy choice is presented in a broad manner, Congress may interpret the policy in a way that the president dislikes. However, if the president presents Congress with a specific proposal or draft legislation, Congressional members may view the president as infringing upon their role as the legislative body and resist working with him.

Whether presidents are successful in placing policy issues on the national agenda and having them resolved in accordance with their preferences depends in part on how much "political capital" a president has available. Political capital is defined as the strength of the president's popularity and of his party, in Congress and in other contexts. Members of Congress are more likely to support a popular president who has the ability to mobilize the public's support, improve members' standing by association with the president and the president's party, and raise money for their campaigns.

Even the most popular president cannot always dictate what issues are on the national agenda, however. Events and decisions outside the president's control often influence what topics most concern the nation. In recent years, the terrorist attacks of September 11, 2001, the subsequent anthrax scare, and the subway and bus bombings in London and Madrid all served to place combating terrorism at the top of the policy and political agenda. The growing concern about an avian flu epidemic has put public health preparedness and vaccine availability on the national agenda. The devastation wrought by Hurricane Katrina has made improved responses to natural disasters a high priority. Thus, even the most popular presidents must be responsive to national and international events that are beyond their control.

PRESIDENTIAL POWERS. As noted earlier, if Congress passes legislation the president dislikes, he has the power to veto it, thereby rejecting the bill. However, the president does not have to actually use the veto to have it be helpful in shaping policy. The president may be able to persuade Congress to change a piece of legislation simply by threatening to veto it, especially if it is a law that is only expected to pass by a slim majority. In general, vetoes are used infrequently, with presidents vetoing only 3% of all legislation since George Washington was president.[14(p43)]

Presidents also have the power to issue executive orders. These are legally binding orders that the president gives to federal administrative agencies under the control of the Executive Office. In general, these orders are used to direct federal agencies and their officials in how they implement specific laws. Executive orders are controversial because under our system of government, Congress, not the executive, is tasked with making laws. In addition, significant policy decisions can be accomplished by using executive orders. For example, an executive order was used by President Truman to integrate the armed forces, by President Eisenhower to desegregate schools, by President Clinton to designate 1.7 million acres in southern Utah as a national monument, and by President George W. Bush to create the federal Office of Homeland Security (which subsequently became a cabinet-level department when Congress established it through legislation).

If Congress believes an executive order is contrary to congressional intent, it has two avenues of recourse. It can amend the law at issue to clarify its intent and effectively stamp out the executive order that is now clearly contrary to the law. (Bear in mind that because the president may veto any bill, in effect it takes a two-thirds majority of Congress to override an executive order.) As an alternative, Congress may challenge the executive order in court, claiming that the president's actions exceed his constitutional powers.

CONSTITUENTS. From this description of the presidency, it is evident that presidents have several layers of constituents to consider when making policy choices. Certainly, the president represents every citizen and the country as a whole as the only nationally elected official (along with the vice president) in the nation. However, the president is also a representative of a particular political party and therefore must consider the views of that party when making policies. The party's views may be evident from the party platform, policies supported by party leadership in Congress, and voters who identify themselves as party members. In addition, the president must keep in mind the foreign policy duties of the office. Depending on the issue, it may be important for the president to take into account the views of other nations or international organizations, such as the United Nations or the World Health Organization.

How does the president decide which policies to pursue? Presidents are driven by multiple goals. They want "their policies to be adopted, they want the policies they put in place to last, and they want to feel they helped solve the problems facing the country."[4(p82)] In addition, presidents often speak of wanting to leave a legacy or ensure their place in history when they leave office.

Given the vast array of constituents that presidents must consider, the president's policy decision-making process involves several layers. As shown in Figure 2-2, presidents consult their agency staff to identify problems, decide which problems are priorities, determine what solutions are available

FIGURE 2-2 Executive agency policymaking.

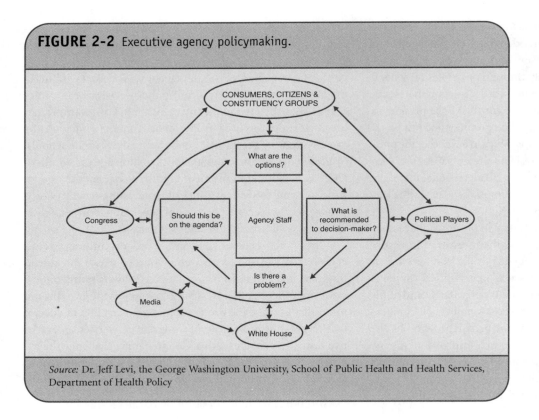

Source: Dr. Jeff Levi, the George Washington University, School of Public Health and Health Services, Department of Health Policy

Structurally, almost all administrative agencies are part of the executive branch, and thus under the power and control of the president.[k] Practically, administrative agencies often work out of the public's eye to implement the laws passed by Congress and the executive orders signed by the president.

Federal agencies fall into two main categories: executive department agencies and independent agencies. Executive department agencies are under the direct control of the president, and department heads serve at the pleasure of the president. These departments include the 15 cabinet-level departments and their subunits. Some of the more well-known executive departments are the Department of Health and Human Services, the Department of Education, the Treasury Department, the Department of State, the Department of Defense, and the newly formed Department of Homeland Security.[l] Independent agency heads are appointed by the president and confirmed by the Senate. They serve a fixed term and may only be removed "for cause," meaning there must be a legitimate reason to fire them. Examples of independent agencies include the Securities and Exchange Commission, the U.S. Postal Service, and the National Labor Relations Board.

Overall, the president fills approximately 2,400 federal jobs.[4(p160)] In general these political appointees have short tenures, lasting an average of two years.[4(p161)] When the administration changes hands after an election, new appointees are usually selected to run the agencies. The daily operations of agencies are run by career civil servants, public employees who do not necessarily come and go with each administration but who often remain at an agency for years, gaining expertise and institutional knowledge about the agencies in which they work. Frequently, there may be tension between the goals of the political appointee and those of the career bureaucrat, who may have the advantage of familiarity with members of Congress and who knows that the political appointee is likely to be replaced in a few years.

to address those problems, and choose the policy option that is the preferred course of action. In addition, the president's staff interacts with members of Congress and other political players to gauge their support for or opposition to various policies. Of course, how the media portrays both problems and potential solutions can be an important ingredient in whether politicians and the general public support the president's initiatives.

In addition, which policies presidents choose to promote may depend in part on when policy decisions are made. First-term presidents must satisfy their constituents if they hope to be re-elected. Although all presidents want to see their favored policies implemented throughout their time in office, second-term presidents may be more willing to support more controversial goals because they cannot run for re-election. Yet, second-term presidents may also be constrained by the desire to keep their party in power, even though another individual will hold the presidential office.

Administrative Agencies

When studying the structure of our government, it is common to review Congress, the presidency, and the court system. Administrative agencies, however, are often overlooked despite the power they wield over the way our country is run.

Administrative agencies can be created by statute, internal department reorganization, or presidential directive.[14(p50)] However they are initially created, agencies must have statutory authority in order to receive appropriations from Congress and act with the force of law. This statutory authority, or enabling statute, outlines the agency's responsibilities and powers.

AGENCY POWERS By necessity, statutes are usually written broadly. Congress does not have the time or expertise to include every detail about how a new program should operate or how a new department will be structured. It is up to the executive branch agency to fill in the details, and it does so by issuing policy statements, developing rules, and promulgating regulations.[m]

For example, in 2001 Congress passed the Medicare, Medicaid, and SCHIP Benefits Improvement and Protection Act, which included a new Medicaid reimbursement system for federally qualified health centers called the Prospective Payment System. Basically, the statute mandated that every health center calculate a baseline per-visit cost that was the average of their 1999 and 2000 costs. Under the act, each year health center reimbursement rates would be determined by the baseline rate plus an inflationary factor called the Medicare Economic Index, adjusted to account for any increase or decrease in a health center's change in scope of service. That was all the statute said. It was up to the Center for Medicare and Medicaid Services (CMS), the federal agency in charge of the Medicaid program, to work out the details. CMS had the choice of issuing regulations, policy notices, information sheets, or the like to flesh out the broadly worded statute.

Many questions were left unresolved by the statute. For example, if the center opened in 2000, how would its baseline be calculated? What if there was an extraordinary event in 1999 or 2000, like a hurricane, that severely damaged a health center; would that affect the baseline calculation? What does a change of scope of service mean? Does it count as a change in scope of service if the health center adds a few dentists to its current dental practice, or would it have to add a new service for the first time in order to trigger the statutory definition? Who determines whether a change in scope of service occurred? The health center? The state Medicaid agency? The regional Medicaid office? CMS? As you can imagine, the list of questions that results from broadly written statutes is almost endless. Agencies are usually the ones that provide the answers.

Promulgating regulations is the most important and powerful role of agencies. Agency regulations have the force of law and must be obeyed just as one obeys a law passed by the legislative branch. Yet, an agency's power to create rules and regulations is not unlimited. The thing being regulated must be within the power of the agency to regulate, as defined by the agency's enabling statute. Sometimes it is not clear whether an agency has acted in an area that is beyond the scope of its authorizing law. In those cases, a court may be the final arbiter of whether the agency acted properly.

In addition, agencies must follow the requirements set forth in the Administrative Procedure Act (APA).[18] The APA contains detailed requirements compelling agencies to issue a notice of their intent to issue a new rule or change an existing rule, and provide for and respond to public comments on the proposed rule. Some agencies are also required to hold hearings and develop rules based on the evidence presented in those hearings.[4(p172)] It is important to know that the APA creates procedural standards that require an agency to follow a particular *process* when promulgating regulations. The APA does not relate to the *substance* of the regulations. As long as an agency follows the necessary notice and comment requirements of the APA, it has wide latitude to issue rules within its scope of power, even if many of the public comments opposed the proposed rules. If an agency does not follow the APA requirements, interested parties may sue the agency in court to force compliance with the law.

CONSTITUENTS. Agency heads, who are not elected, do not have constituents in the same way that the president and members of Congress do. In theory, as members of the executive branch, agency heads should only be concerned with the wishes of the president. In reality, however, that is not always the case. Some presidents have firmer control of their departments than others. If the president gives the departments and agencies broad discretion to make policy decisions, the agencies may have few policy constraints. Practically, however, agency heads want their operation to run smoothly, including having a good working relationship with the individuals or entities regulated by that agency. If an agency antagonizes the people or groups being regulated, they might reach out to their congressional representatives to try to change or limit the agency's personnel or authority. In addition, because Congress appropriates funds to and maintains oversight of many agencies, agency heads are well served by taking Congress's interests into account.

Table 2-3 summarizes the general public policymaking machinery. We next turn our attention to the specific parts of the government bureaucracy that operate in the health arena.

THE HEALTH BUREAUCRACY

The Federal Government

Although several federal agencies have health-related responsibilities, the three most significant health agencies are the Department of Health and Human Services (HHS), the Department of Defense (DOD), and the Department of Veterans Affairs (VA). HHS houses many of the major public

TABLE 2-3 Summary of Public Policymaking Entities

	Congress	President	Administrative Agencies
Main Function	Legislative body	Chief executive of the country	Implement statutes through rulemaking
Main Tools/Powers	Support/oppose legislation Appropriations Oversight	Agenda setting Persuasion Propose solutions Budget proposals Executive orders	Create regulations Provide information
Constituents	Voters in state or district Voters in nation if in leadership role or have national aspirations Party President	Nation (all voters) Public who voted for the president Party Other nations International organizations	President Congress Individuals and entities regulated or served by the agency

health insurance programs and health services that provide care, information, and more to millions of U.S. residents; the DOD and VA operate health insurance programs specifically for military personnel and their families.

Department of Health and Human Services

HHS includes hundreds of programs that cover activities as varied as medical and social science research, preschool education services, substance abuse and prevention services, and health insurance programs, just to name a few. As shown in Figure 2-3, the department has 11 operating divisions: Administration for Children and Families (ACF), Administration on Aging (AoA), Agency for Toxic Substances and Disease Registry (ATSDR), Agency for Healthcare Research and Quality (AHRQ), Centers for Disease Control and Prevention (CDC), Center for Medicare and Medicaid Services (CMS), Food and Drug Administration (FDA), Health Resources Services Administration (HRSA), Indian Health Service (IHS), National Institutes of Health (NIH), and the Substance Abuse and Mental Health Services Administration (SAMHSA). The duties of each agency are described in Table 2-4.

Each operating division has numerous bureaus or divisions that operate health programs. For example, the HIV/AIDS Bureau (HAB) is one of five bureaus in HRSA. HAB implements the Ryan White CARE Act,[19] which provides health care to individuals with HIV and AIDS. Similarly, the FDA has eight offices or centers. The one whose job is perhaps most well-known to the general public is the Center for Drug Evaluation and Research, which is responsible for testing and approving new drugs before they can be sold to the public. These are just

two examples of the many subagency units that perform vital functions in our federal health care bureaucracy. Although not shown in Figure 2-3, the 11 operating divisions are divided into two program areas, the Public Health Service Operating Division and the Human Services Operating Division. Three agencies—ACF, AoA, and CMS—are part of the Human Services Operating Division. The remaining eight agencies fall under the Public Health Services Operating Division.

CMS is by far the largest of the HHS agencies; its budget consumed 83% of HHS spending in 2005.[20(p2)] CMS administers the country's major public health insurance programs—Medicaid, Medicare, and State Children's Health Insurance Program (SCHIP)—meaning that most of HHS's funds are spent on individual health care needs. By contrast, just 9% of the HHS budget went to the eight agencies in the Public Health Service Operating Division, and NIH received over half of that funding.[20(p2)]

HHS also includes numerous offices that assist the Secretary of HHS in running the department. The Assistant Secretary of Health is the principal advisor to the HHS secretary on public health matters. This individual oversees the U.S. Public Health Service (PHS), the Commissioned Corps (health professionals used for both emergency responses and as health promoters), and the Office of Public Health and Sciences (OPHS).[n] OPHS consists of 11 offices: Office of the Surgeon General, Office of Women's Health, Office of Population Affairs, Office of Minority Health, Office of HIV/AIDS Policy, Office of Disease Prevention and Health Promotion, National Vaccine Program Office, Office of Human Research Protections, Office of Research Integrity,

FIGURE 2-3 Department of Health and Human Services organizational chart.

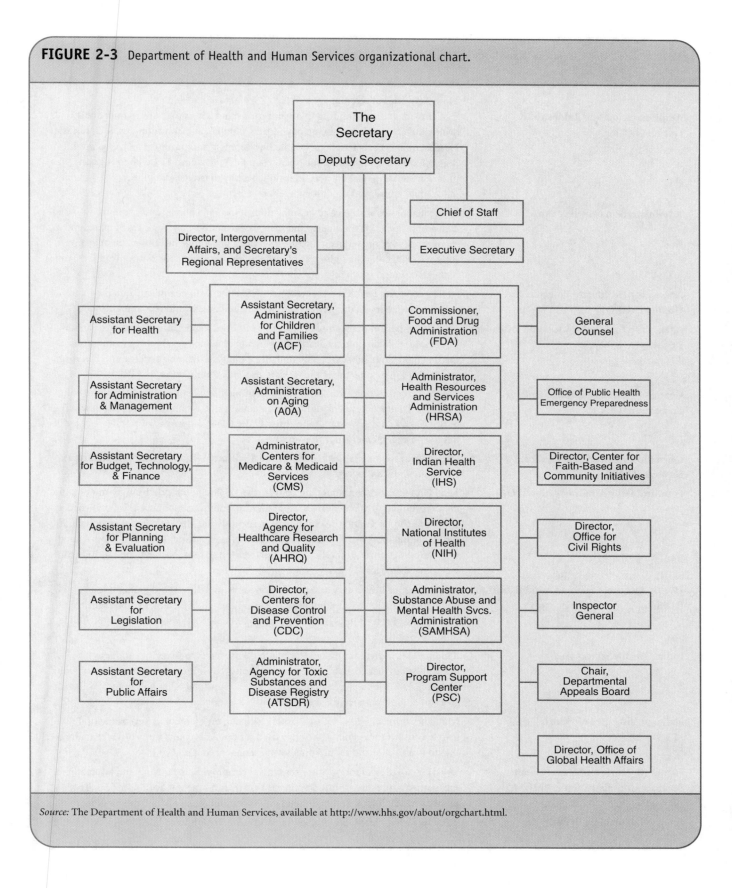

Source: The Department of Health and Human Services, available at http://www.hhs.gov/about/orgchart.html.

TABLE 2-4 Department of Health and Human Services Agency Activities

Agency	Main Activities of Agency
Administration for Children and Families (ACF)	ACF provides federal funding to organizations that have programs to improve the health and economic well-being of children, families, and communities. ACF funds Head Start and Early Head Start (child development programs for low-income children), Temporary Assistance for Needy Families (the country's welfare program), and programs relating to child care, adoption, healthy marriage, disabilities, energy assistance, child abuse, and domestic violence.
Administration on Aging (AoA)	AoA collaborates with service organizations to provide home- and community-based care and support for the elderly and their caregivers. The agency focuses on seven main areas: support services, nutrition services, preventive health services, caregiver support, protecting the rights of vulnerable elderly, services for Native Americans, and connecting elderly with resources in their community.
Agency for Healthcare Research and Quality (AHRQ)	AHRQ conducts health services research with a focus on health care quality, evidence-based medicine, patient safety, increased access, and cost containment.
Agency for Toxic Substances and Disease Registry (ATSDR)	ATSDR focuses on preventing exposure to hazardous substances from waste sites. The agency provides public health assessments of waste sites, health consultations regarding hazardous substances, surveillance, emergency response, research, education, and training. The director of the CDC is also the administrator of ATSDR.
Centers for Disease Control and Prevention (CDC)	The CDC focuses on controlling and preventing disease and injuries and promoting healthy behavior. The agency addresses infectious disease outbreaks, environmental health risks, and behavioral health threats. The CDC also works with states and localities to assist with emergency preparedness.
Center for Medicare and Medicaid Services (CMS)	CMS administers and collects data for the Medicare, Medicaid, and State Children's Health Insurance Programs.
Food and Drug Administration (FDA)	The FDA regulates, conducts, and coordinates research on food, drugs, cosmetics, biological products, medical devices, and radiation-emitting products. It is concerned with both the safety and the efficacy of these products. The FDA shares responsibility for regulating food with the U.S. Department of Agriculture. The FDA's food-related responsibilities cover domestic and imported food, except for meat and poultry (but including shell eggs).
Health Resources Services Administration (HRSA)	HRSA expands health care access to low-income, uninsured, and vulnerable populations. HRSA has five bureaus: Maternal and Child Health, Primary Health Care, Health Professions, HIV/AIDS, and Healthcare Systems, and houses the Office of Rural Health Policy.
Indian Health Service (IHS)	IHS provides individual and public health care services to American Indians and Alaska Natives that are comprehensive and culturally appropriate. About half of IHS's budget is used for the agency's health care system and the other half is given to tribal governments who manage their own health care services.
National Institutes of Health (NIH)	NIH consists of 27 institutes and centers focusing on biomedical and behavioral research. Most of the agency's budget is used for research grants for projects that aim to extend healthy life and reduce disease and illness burdens.
Substance Abuse and Mental Health Services Administration (SAMHSA)	SAMHSA focuses attention and programs on improving the quality and availability of substance abuse prevention, addiction treatment, and mental health services. The agency provides block grants to states and communities to address these needs.

Source: National Health Policy Forum, "The Basics: The Public Health Service," Sultz and Young, *Health Care USA*, 354–355.

President's Council on Physical Fitness and Sports, and Regional Health Administrators.

HHS also has divisions concerned with planning and evaluation, legislation, administration and management, budget and finance, program support, public affairs, and global health affairs. In 2001, President George W. Bush created the Center for Faith-Based and Community Initiatives, which strives to increase participation by faith-based community organizations in providing health and human services.[21] Offices concerned with the legality and efficiency of the department's activities include those of the General Counsel and Inspector General, and the Office of Civil Rights.

As a result of the recent focus on preventing terrorism, HHS recently gained a new office of Public Health Emergency Preparedness. This office is the principle advisor to the Secretary of HHS on matters relating to bioterrorism and other public health emergencies, and helps coordinate efforts in these areas at all levels of government. Other federal departments also have a role in public health emergency preparedness. The new Department of Homeland Security (DHS), which now includes the Federal Emergency Management Agency (FEMA), is tasked with preparing for and coordinating the federal response to emergencies, whether due to natural or man-made disasters.[o] DHS also has an Emergency Preparedness and Response Directorate with duties related to public health, and houses the Strategic National Stockpile of emergency pharmaceutical supplies.[22(pp326–329)] Other agencies, such as the Environmental Protection Agency (EPA), DOD, and VA, play significant roles in emergency preparedness and response.

Department of Veterans Affairs and Department of Defense

Any veteran who does not receive a dishonorable discharge is potentially eligible for health care services through the Veterans Health Administration (VHA). The VHA is the largest health care delivery system in the country, with hundreds of medical centers, nursing homes, and outpatient clinics that serve over 1 million patients each year.[22(p357)]

VHA-sponsored health plans offer a wide array of preventive, ambulatory, and hospital services as well as medications and medical and surgical supplies. VHA providers are organized into integrated networks aimed at providing cost-effective services based on local need. There are no premiums (monthly payments) for the plan, but veterans have to make co-payments (a charge per visit) unless they are exempt based on disability or income level. Unlike most health care plans, the VHA system is completely portable,

meaning that veterans can access VHA facilities anywhere in the country.

Veterans who wish to receive care through the VHA must enroll in the program. Because the VHA receives an annual appropriation from Congress, it may not have sufficient funds to pay for all of the care demanded by eligible veterans. For that reason, the VHA uses a priority system to ensure that veterans who are low-income or have service-related disabilities can be enrolled into a plan. Other veterans may have to wait to be enrolled if there are insufficient funds. In addition, priority in accessing care is given to enrolled veterans who need care for service-related disabilities or have a sufficiently severe service-related disability and need care for any health concern. Veterans not in a priority group may have to wait to see an appropriate provider once they are enrolled.

Although veterans may receive care through VHA, they are not required to do so. If eligible, they may choose to obtain services through other public or private health care programs or health insurance plans. They may also choose to receive some services through VHA and others from non-VHA programs or plans.

The VHA does not provide coverage to veterans' family members, but the DOD does through its TRICARE program. TRICARE provides health care services to current and retired military personnel and their families. TRICARE offers a variety of plans with various eligibility requirements and costs to the patient.

State and Local Governments

As discussed earlier, the Constitution gives states primary responsibility for protecting the public's health. States have health-related agencies that deal with health financing, aging, behavioral health, environmental health, children and family services, veterans, facility licensing and standards, provider credentialing, and more. Although all states have agencies that generally cover the same functions, their structure, responsibilities, and lines of authority vary greatly.

With the variation among state agencies, it is not surprising that there are significant differences across the states in terms of their approach to public health and health services needs. All states have agencies to run their Medicaid and SCHIP programs, as well as other state-specific health services programs. Although a recent review of enabling statutes and mission statements found that only one-fifth of states address most of the concepts identified by PHS as essential public health functions, most states cover the traditional public health tasks such as surveillance, investigation, and education.[23(p154),p]

Local public health agencies (LPHA) carry out the public health functions of the state. Most commonly, LPHAs are formed, managed by, and report to a local government, such as a county commission or local board of health. This structure provides LPHAs with significant latitude to interpret and implement state statutes. In some states, the state and local governments jointly oversee the LPHA. In about one-third of states, the state directly operates its LPHAs or provides services directly.[23(pp155–156)]

LPHAs may provide services directly or, as is increasingly common, may contract or provide support to others who perform the services. The services provided by LPHAs vary considerably, though there is an emphasis on addressing communicable diseases, environmental health, and children's health issues. LPHAs often provide services such as immunizations, community assessments, epidemiology and surveillance, food safety and inspections, and tuberculosis testing. Some, but not all, also provide diabetes care, glaucoma screening, substance abuse treatment, mental health services, and more.[23(pp160–161)]

INTEREST GROUPS

Before leaving the discussion of policy, the policymaking process, and the health bureaucracy, we must say a few words about interest groups. *Interest group* is a general term used for a wide variety of organizations that are created around a particular issue or population and have the goal of influencing policy and educating others about their views and concerns.[4(p117)] Interest groups are different from most of the other stakeholders that have been discussed because interest groups do not have the power to make policy. Although members of the executive and legislative branches of government have a key role in determining which policies are adopted, interest groups have the limited, but still significant, role of trying to influence the decisions of policymakers.

There are many types of interest groups, including trade associations, think tanks, advocacy groups, and lobbying firms. A few examples include the Pharmaceutical Research and Manufacturers of America, whose mission is to "conduct effective advocacy for public policies that encourage discovery of important new medicines for patients by pharmaceutical/biotechnology research companies"[24]; the National Association of Public Hospitals, which has as its goal "educating federal, state and local decision makers about the unique needs of and challenges faced by member hospitals and the nation's most vulnerable populations"[25]; the Center for Budget and Policy Priorities, which "conducts research and analysis to inform public debates over proposed budget and tax policies and to help ensure that the needs of low-income families and individ-

uals are considered in these debates"[26]; the American Association for Retired Persons, which is "dedicated to enhancing quality of life for all as we age . . . through information, advocacy and service"[27]; and the Heritage Foundation, which has as its goal to "formulate and promote conservative public policies based on the principles of free enterprise, limited government, individual freedom, traditional American values, and a strong national defense."[28]

Just as members of Congress do not have the time or ability to become experts in every issue that comes before them, the same is true for the average citizen. Many people do not have the time and ability to learn about all of the issues that are important to them, develop proposals, rally public support for their positions, monitor current activity, lobby to remove issues from the agenda, and reach out to politicians who make policy decisions. Instead, interest groups take on those duties. "Their job is to make the case for their constituents before government, plying the halls of Congress, the executive branch, the courts, and the offices of other interest groups to provide a linkage between citizens and government."[4(p119)]

Interest Group Powers

Interest groups do not have the power to pass laws. However, they can influence policy in a variety of ways throughout the policymaking process. For example, recall all the steps it takes for a bill to become a law. Anywhere along that continuum is an opportunity for interest groups to make their case. The first step for interest groups is often to commission research that they use to support their position. This can be most important in the early stages of policy development, when politicians might have an open mind about various proposals.[4(p131)] However, it does not matter how much information a group has if it is not able to gain access to the decision makers. Even a few minutes with a politician may be a few more minutes than the opposition has to make its case directly to a decision-maker.[4(p131)] Finally, interest groups need to develop a persuasive argument, a way to frame the issue that convinces politicians to agree with their view of a policy matter.

Interest groups have a variety of tools at their disposal when developing strategies for lobbying. They may initiate a *grassroots* campaign, asking their members to contact their representatives with a particular message. Because interest group members are the voters with the power to re-elect public officials, strong grassroots campaigns can be quite effective. Or, they may try a *grasstops* strategy and harness the influence of community leaders and other prominent individuals.[4(p139)] Or, they may join with other interest groups to create coalitions and strengthen their influence through numbers. Interest groups may start a media campaign to align public sentiment with their goals. Of course, providing candidates with money, often through political action committees, is a time-honored way to try to influence the outcome of policy debates.

Whatever methodology they use, interest groups are an important part of the policymaking process. One researcher has called interest groups an "indispensable" part of making policy decisions.[29(p85)] They provide a way to give a voice to their members, who may not otherwise feel able to participate effectively in the policymaking process.

CONCLUSION

This journey through the policymaking process in the United States was intended to provide you with an understanding of policy and a context for your discussions and analysis of health policy issues. It is vital that you become familiar with both the nature of policy and the institutions that make and influence policy. As you have seen, the definition of policy is subject to much debate, yet it is necessary to define what policy means before attempting to engage in policy analysis. We have also walked through the specific duties and powers of the executive and legislative branches of the federal government and included key points about state-level policymaking as well. Finally, all policy students must be aware of and understand the influence of interest groups. They have and use numerous opportunities to influence the policymaking process, and their strength and concerns must be accounted for when analyzing policy issues. As you move through the remainder of this book, use the information provided in this overview to help you think about and frame your own policy positions.

REFERENCES

1. Longest BB Jr. *Health Policy Making in the United States*, 2nd ed. Chicago: Health Administration Press; 1998.

2. Subcommittee on Health and Environment of the Committee on Interstate Commerce, U.S. House of Representatives. *A Discursive Dictionary of Health Care.* Washington D.C.: GPO; 1976.

3. Hanley BE. Policy development and analysis. In: Leavitt JK, Mason DJ, Chaffee MW, eds. *Policy and Politics in Nursing and Health Care*, 3rd ed. Philadelphia: WB Saunders; 1998:125–138.

4. Weissert CS, Weissert WG. *Governing Health: The Politics of Health Policy*, 2nd ed. Baltimore: Johns Hopkins University Press; 2002.

5. U.S. Const. art. 1, § 1.

6. U.S. Const. art. 1, § 8.

7. U.S. Const. art. 1, § 3.

8. U.S. Const. art. 1, § 2.

9. Schneider J. The committee system in the U.S. Congress. *Congressional Research Service.* Washington, D.C.: Library of Congress; 2003:2–3.

10. Senate Committee on the Budget. *The Congressional Budget Process: An Explanation*, 105th Cong., 2nd sess., Committee Print 67; 1998.

11. House Committee on the Budget Majority Caucus. *Basics of the Budget Process.* 107th Cong. Briefing Paper; 2001.

12. U.S. Const., art. 2, § 1.

13. U.S. Const., amend. XXII, §1.

14. Committee on House Administration. *Our American Government.*

House Concurrent Res. 221, 106th Cong., 2nd sess.; 2000. H. Doc. 216.

15. Davidson RH. The presidency and the Congress. In: Nelson M, ed. *The Presidency and the Political System.* Washington, D.C.: Congressional Quarterly Press; 1984:371.

16. Kernell S. *Going Public: New Strategies of Presidential Leadership*, 3rd ed. Washington, D.C.: CQ Press; 1997.

17. Public Law 106-554, relevant sections codified at 42 U.S.C. § 1396a(a).

18. 5 U.S.C. §500.

19. Ryan White Comprehensive AIDS Resources Emergency Act of 1990, amended in 1996 and 2000, 42 U.S.C 300ff.

20. National Health Policy Forum. The basics: the Public Health Service, p. 2. Available at: http://www.nhpf.org/pdfs_basics/Basics_PHS.pdf. Accessed August 1, 2006.

21. Executive Order No. 13198, *Code of Federal Regulations,* title 3, sec. 750–752 (2002).

22. Sultz HA, Young KM. *Health Care USA: Understanding Its Organization and Delivery,* 3rd ed. Gaithersburg, Md.: Aspen; 2001.

23. Turnock BJ. *Public Health: What It Is and How It Works*, 3rd ed. Sudbury, Mass.: Jones and Bartlett; 2004.

24. Pharmaceutical Research and Manufacturing Association. About pharma. Available at: http://www.phrma.org/about_phrma/. Accessed August 1, 2006.

25. National Association of Public Hospitals. About NAPH. Available at http://www.naph.org/template.cfm?Section=About_NAPH. Accessed August 1, 2006.

26. Center for Budget and Policy Priorities. About us. Available at http://www.cbpp.org/info.html. Accessed August 1, 2006.

27. American Association of Retired Persons. Overview. Available at http://www.aarp.org/about_aarp/aarp_overview/a2002-12-18-aarpmission.html. Accessed August 1, 2006.

28. The Heritage Foundation. About Heritage. Available at http://www.heritage.org/About/. Accessed August 1, 2006.

29. Lindbloom C. *The Policy-Making Process.* Englewood Cliffs, N.J.: Prentice-Hall; 1980.

ENDNOTES

a. U.S. Constitution, 10th amendment.

b. Chapter 3 provides an in-depth discussion of federalism issues.

c. Under Article 1 of the Constitution, Congress has jurisdiction over the District of Columbia. Both the Senate and the House have committees that oversee some governmental functions of the District. The District elects two "shadow senators" who are allowed to lobby Congress on issues but who do not have voting rights. In terms of representation, this places the District in a position similar to other political bodies administered by the United States, such as Puerto Rico, the U.S. Virgin Islands, and American Samoa. The District's shadow senators (and a shadow representative in the House) were created by the citizens of the District in anticipation of the passage of the 1978 District of Columbia Voting Rights amendment to the U.S. Constitution, which would have granted the District the same voting rights as the states. The amendment never passed, but the District government has maintained the shadow positions nonetheless.

d. At the time of writing, Congressional committees are considering legislation that would give the District of Columbia its first full voting representative and Utah one additional at-large representative, permanently increasing the number of representatives to 437.

e. In addition to the 435 representatives, Puerto Rico has a resident commissioner; and the District of Columbia, Guam, the U.S. Virgin Islands, and American Samoa each has a delegate who is allowed to sponsor legislation and vote in committees, but may not vote on the House floor. The citizens of the District of Columbia also elect a nonvoting shadow representative.

f. The latter committees are the Homeland Security and Governmental Affairs Committee in the Senate, and the Governance Reform Committee in the House.

g. By contrast, the Senate Rules and Administration Committee does not have a role in shaping the order of business on the Senate floor.

h. White House and executive offices include: Office of the President, Office of the Vice President, U.S. Trade Representative, Executive Resident, Office of Administration, Office of Management and Budget, Council of Economic Advisors, and six policy development offices: National Security Council; National Economic Council; Domestic Policy Council; Science, Technology and Space Office; Environmental Policy Office; and National Drug Council.

i. The separation of powers doctrine is discussed more fully in the next chapter.

j. In circumstances where the president serves two years or less of the term of another president, an individual may hold office for 10 years.

k. States also have administrative agencies, under the control of the governor and acting on authority granted by state legislatures.

l. Other cabinet-level departments are the Department of Agriculture, Department of the Interior, Department of Commerce, Department of Justice, Department of Labor, Department of Transportation, Department of Energy, and Department of Veterans Affairs.

m. Agencies publish proposed and final rules in the *Federal Register*. After complying with the public notice and comment period required by the Federal Administrative Procedure Act, these rules become final and are codified as regulations in the Code of Federal Regulations.

n. PHS employs both commissioned corps members and civilians to run its public health programs. In addition to the Public Health Operating Division in HHS, PHS employees also work in the Bureau of Prisons, U.S. Coast Guard, National Oceanic and Atmospheric Administration, Environmental Protection Agency, Division of Immigration Health Services, and U.S. Marshal Services.

o. Given the widely condemned performance of the federal government in the aftermath of Hurricane Katrina, there have been recommendations to change FEMA's role. As of the time of this writing, none of these recommendations have been implemented.

p. For a full explanation of essential public health services, see Turnock, *Public Health,* Chapter 5. In general, they include monitoring health status, diagnosing and investigating health problems, empowering citizens and their communities, health planning, health-related law enforcement, ensuring access to care, ensuring a quality workforce, program evaluation, and research.

CHAPTER **3**

Law and the Legal System

> *"It is perfectly proper to regard and study the law simply as a great anthropological document."*
>
> —Former U.S. Supreme Court Justice Oliver Wendell Holmes[1](p 444)

INTRODUCTION

The importance and complexity of law and the legal system in the United States cannot be overstated. Law's importance stems from its primary purpose: to function as the main tool with which we organize ourselves as an advanced, democratic society. The complexity of law and the legal process is a function of the multiple sources of law that may apply to any one of the millions of actions and interactions that occur daily in society, the division of legal authority among the federal and state governments and among the branches within them, the language the law and its players use to express themselves,[a] and more.

For all its complexity, however, there is also an undeniable openness, or candor, when it comes to law. We are not left to wonder where it comes from, or how it is made. Generally speaking, we are privy to lawmakers' rationales for the laws they write and to judges' reasoning for their legal opinions, just as we are generally privy to the process by which law is made. And once made, laws are not hidden from us; to the contrary, they are discussed in the media and catalogued in books and online services available for public consumption. (Indeed, one is *expected* to know what the law is, since its violation can have potentially severe consequences.) If you want to know more about law than the average person, you can study it formally in law and other schools. Or, you can consult with one of the million or so lawyers in practice today. In other words, although law is complicated, it is equally ubiquitous and therefore transparent in a way that may not be clear at first blush.

Furthermore, beyond the law's sheer pervasiveness lies another simplicity: As the quote at the outset of this chapter implies, studying law is in essence the study of human beings, particularly their evolving customs, beliefs, and value systems. Because law is the key tool with which we regulate social behavior, it stands to reason that it also reflects our foremost values and normative standards. Indeed, law "takes an understanding, a norm, an attitude, and hardens it into muscle and bone"[4](p29)—subject to change, for as our society evolves, so too does our law. A relevant example of legal evolution can be seen in the updating of state public health laws, which before the tragic events of September 11, 2001 and the subsequent anthrax scare had not been updated in most states for over a century. Soon after the 2001 attacks, however, many states, concerned about new risks to the public's health, reviewed and overhauled these laws.[b]

This chapter begins by briefly considering the role law plays in everyday life, and then turns to defining law and describing its multiple sources. It then discusses several key features of the legal system, including the separation of government powers, federalism, the role of courts, due process, and more.

For some, reading this chapter may bring to mind a course you have taken or a book you have read on civics or government. In this case, the chapter should serve as a helpful refresher. For those of you new to the study of law, consider the following pages a condensed but important introduction to one of the most critical and influential aspects of the society in which you live. In either event, this chapter is designed to better position you to understand the law's application to the specific fields of health care and public health and to digest the health policy and law concepts discussed in this textbook.

THE ROLE OF LAW

The law reaches into just about every corner of American life. Its impact is inescapable nearly from the moment you wake up to the time you go back to sleep at night (and perhaps beyond, if your community has a curfew or other means of controlling activity and noise after dark). Have you ever stopped to think about the regulations pertaining to the flammability of the mattress you sleep on, or the safety of the water you shower with, cook with, and drink? How about the consumer protection laws regulating the quality of the food you eat throughout the day, and the quality of the establishments that serve it? Then there are the laws pertaining to the safety of the cars, buses, and subways you travel in each day, and the traffic laws that control their movement. You encounter laws daily pertaining to the environment, property ownership, the workplace, civil rights, copyright, energy, banking, and much more. And these are just the laws implicated by the relatively mundane actions of day-to-day life. Steering into activities that are not as common—say, international travel, or adoption, or being admitted to a hospital—you encounter the law swiftly and noticeably. If you need final proof of the ubiquitous nature of law, pick up today's newspaper and count how many stories have some sort of legal angle to them. Then do it tomorrow and the next day. What you will almost certainly find is that a great majority of the stories concern law or legal process.

The law's pervasive nature is no surprise, given the important societal role we assign to it—namely, to serve as the tool with which we govern our relationships with one another, our government, and society at large. A society as sprawling and complex as ours needs formal, enforceable rules of law to provide a measure of control (for example, the need to regulate entities or actions that are potentially dangerous or invidious—a polluting power plant, or acts of discrimination based on race or gender). Furthermore, many people believe that law should be used not just to organize and control the society in which we live, but to achieve a more just society; in other words, the country's key organizing principle should not simply be grounded in law, but rather grounded in a legal system designed to affirmatively produce outcomes based on fairness, justice, and equality.[5]

The main way the law governs the many kinds of relationships in society is to recognize and establish enforceable legal rights and responsibilities that guide those relationships, and to create the institutions necessary to define and enforce them. Take constitutional law, for example. Constitutions are charters establishing governments and delineating certain individual and governmental rights and obligations. However, constitutional provisions are triggered only when one party to a relationship works for or on behalf of the government, whether federal or state. Thus, constitutional law governs the relationship between individuals and their government—not, for example, the relationship between two private parties, even when one party's actions are clearly discriminatory or wrongful. Thus, it takes affirmative action by a governmental actor to trigger constitutional protections. So although it would be a violation of a public school student's First Amendment right to be forced by his principal to pray in class, forced prayer in private schools passes constitutional muster.

A legal right (constitutional or otherwise) denotes a power or privilege that has been guaranteed to an individual under the law, not merely something that is claimed as an interest or something that is a matter of governmental discretion. Conceptually, legal rights derive from the fact that the government sometimes creates what are called individual "property rights"—a generic term referring to an entitlement to personal or real property—for specified groups of persons.[6] Importantly, legal rights also presuppose that their *enforcement* can be achieved through public institutions, including state and federal courts, because a person's ability to secure a remedy when a legal right is infringed (e.g., denied, reduced, or terminated) goes to the very heart of what it means to be "entitled" to something. Indeed, whether particular health care benefits rise to the level of being a legal "right," and whether the health care right can be enforced in court, are two of the most fundamental legal questions in the area of health law. For example, the federal Medicare program for the aged and disabled confers on eligible individuals not only the right to health care services, but also the ability to enforce their right to benefits when program violations occur.

THE DEFINITION AND SOURCES OF LAW

Defining "Law"

Although many legal scholars agree on the general function of law in society, there is far less consensus on how to define "the law." As with many legal terms, there are several plausible interpretations of what is meant by the law, and thus there is no single way to correctly define it. For example, Black's Law Dictionary includes the following definitions in its primary entry:

> That which is laid down, ordained, or established. A rule or method according to which phenomena or actions co-exist or follow each other. Law, in its generic sense, is a body of rules of action or conduct prescribed by controlling authority, and having binding legal force. That which must be obeyed and followed by citizens subject to sanctions or legal consequences is a law.[3(p 884)]

However, even these commonly accepted definitions are not entirely satisfactory, because "a body of rules" that "must be obeyed" in the face of "sanctions or legal consequences" necessarily envisions a process by which the rules are created, disseminated, enforced, violated, disputed, interpreted, applied, revised, and so on. Considered in this way, "the law" essentially amounts to a "legal system"—and a system, by definition, entails regularly interacting or interdependent parts and subparts coming together to form a functional, unified whole. As you read this chapter and those that follow, think of "the law" not just as words on a page or as codified statutes or regulations, but as the many interacting parts that are involved in drafting those words and statutes in the first place, and in bringing them to life once they have been enacted as laws. Note that this broad conceptualization of law as a system squares nicely with the primary purpose of law described above, since there must by necessity be a sizeable system in place if law is going to carry out its role as the primary organizing tool in society. This broad definition of law also encompasses key legal doctrines, like separation of powers and federalism, described later in this chapter.

Sources of Law

Regardless of the breadth of the definition attached to the term *law*, there is an essential truth to the fact that at the core of the nation's expansive legal system lays a body of enforceable written rules meant to maintain order, define the outer limits of our interactions with one another and with our governments, and delineate legal rights and responsibilities. These rules derive from several sources, which collectively are called *primary* sources of law. The sources of primary legal authority include constitutions, statutes, regulations, and common law. There are also *secondary* sources of law, which are not laws in the technical sense but rather are a collection of treatises, law review articles, reports, legal encyclopedias, and more that analyze, interpret, and critique primary laws. This section focuses on primary legal sources, and a discussion of each of the four types follows.

Constitutions

A constitution is a charter that both establishes a government and delineates fundamental rights and obligations of that government and of individuals who fall within the territory covered by the constitution. In this country, there is a federal constitution and separate constitutions in each of the 50 states. The Constitution of the United States, completed in 1787 and subsequently ratified in each of the original 13 states, took effect in 1789. It provided for a federal union of sovereign states, and a federal government divided into three branches (legislative, executive, and judicial) to operate the union. This governmental structure was not easily agreed upon, however. Prior to the creation of the federal Constitution, the colonies of the American War of Independence first adopted, in 1777, the Articles of Confederation, which represented the first formal governing document of the United States and which were ratified in 1781. However, a defining feature of the Articles was a weak national government; fairly quickly, a movement for a stronger central government took hold, the colonies elected to throw out their original plan, and the Constitutional Convention—and with it the Constitution—was born.

The federal Constitution is rather short and, for the most part, quite general. One explanation for this is that the framers of the Constitution viewed it as a "document for the ages" that needed to include enduring principles to serve a growing, evolving society that has certainly proved to be more complex than it was at the time of the Constitution's ratification. In the words of former U.S. Supreme Court Justice Robert Jackson, the Constitution is a compilation of "majestic generalities" that collect meaning over a span of many years.[7] But the fact that some of the most important constitutional provisions are written in broad terms leads to many thorny legal controversies, because there are many competing approaches and theories as to how courts should interpret ambiguous constitutional phrases.[c] The most well-known of these interpretational controversies in the area of health pertains to the due process clause of the Fourteenth Amendment, which prohibits states from depriving "any person of life, liberty, or property, without due process of law."[8] This provision rests at the heart of the Supreme Court's "right to privacy" jurisprudence, including the right to obtain an abortion (a topic discussed in detail in Chapter 8).

One of the general principles underpinning the Constitution is that citizens should not be subjected to arbitrary and oppressive government. Given that the Constitution was drafted on the heels of the Revolutionary War, this is no surprise. But one consequence of the prevailing mood of the framers toward the reach of a national government is that they drafted the Constitution with an eye toward limiting federal government, as opposed to viewing the Constitution as a vehicle for extending benefits to the public.[d] This helps explain why several key constitutional provisions were drafted in "negative" terms—the First Amendment prohibits government from abridging free speech, the Fourth Amendment makes unreasonable searches illegal—rather than as conferring positive rights, like a generalized right to receive health care services.[e] At the same time, the First and Fourth Amendments, along with eight others, make up the Bill of Rights, a series of important, specifically guaranteed rights in the Constitution the framers believed to be inalienable.[f]

In addition to the federal Constitution, each state has its own constitution. All state constitutions are like the federal one in that they provide for the organizational structure of the particular state's government, and all contain some measure of a state bill of rights. Here the similarities can end, however. Although state constitutions cannot limit or take away rights conferred by the U.S. Constitution (or by federal statutes), some state constitutions go further than federal law in conferring rights or extending protections. For example, under current Supreme Court case law, the death penalty does not always violate the federal Constitution, but the Massachusetts Supreme Court has ruled that the death penalty is prohibited under the state's constitution in every instance. Maryland's constitution requires that a jury be unanimous in order to convict a person of a crime, a standard that differs from federal criminal law. Furthermore, state constitutions are amended much more easily and frequently than their federal counterpart. For example, Georgia's constitution has undergone some 650 amendments.[4(p34)] Compare this with the fact that the language of the federal Constitution has not been dramatically altered since its inception—there have been just 27 amendments, and the 10 that make up the Bill of Rights were all added by 1791.

Statutes

Statutes are laws written by legislative bodies at all levels of government (federal, state, county, city) that, generally speaking, command or prohibit something. It is the fact of their being legislatively created that sets them apart from other sources of law, because legislatures are understood as creating laws that are forward-looking and apply to large numbers of people. Indeed, the two hallmarks of statutes are their prospectivity and generality. These hallmarks result mainly from the fact that legislatures are in the "regulation business" across an enormous array of issues, and as a result legislators often lack both the time and the substantive expertise to regulate other than in broad fashion.

Because statutes tend to be written as broad policy statements (and because words on a page can never communicate intent with absolute accuracy), there are few statutes that are utterly unambiguous. This, coupled with the fact that our evolving society continuously presents situations that may not have been foreseeable at the time a statute was written, results in the need for courts to interpret and apply general statutes to millions of specific legal cases or controversies. This practice is called "statutory construction." Although it is a tenet of the separation of powers doctrine (discussed later in the section on key features of the legal system) that legislatures represent the law-making branch of government and the judiciary's role is to interpret law, it is commonly understood that judges and courts "make" law as well through statutory construction, because the continual interpretation and application of broad policy statements (i.e., statutes) can put a "gloss" on the original product, potentially altering its meaning over time.

As discussed more fully later in the section on federalism, state legislatures have greater ability than does Congress to use statutes to regulate across a broad range of issues, pursuant to states' plenary authority under the Constitution. For instance, the number of state statutes regarding population health and safety (e.g., disease control and prevention, the creation of public health agencies, the ability of governors to classify public health emergencies)[10] far exceeds congressional output on the same topic. Notwithstanding states' broader regulatory power, however, federal statutes have primacy over conflicting state statutes.

Administrative Regulations

The fact that statutes are written in broad generalities has another consequence beyond their need to be interpreted and applied in vast numbers of unique instances: Specific regulations must be written to assist with the implementation of statutory directives and to promote statutes' underlying policy goals. This is where administrative agencies of the executive branch of government come in. Because these federal and state agencies—the U.S. Department of Health and Human Services, the U.S. Department of Labor, the California Department of Social Services, the Wisconsin Department of Commerce, and so on—have expertise in particular policy and substantive areas, they are tasked with enforcing statutes and with promulgating specific regulations, rules, and orders necessary to carry out statutory prerogatives. Assuming that the process for creating the regulations was itself legal and that the regulations do not stray beyond the intent of the enacted statute, regulations have the force of law.[g]

Administrative law is critically important in the area of health policy and law.[h] Consider the Medicaid program, for example, which functions primarily as a health insurance program for low-income individuals. The Medicaid statute embodies Congress's intentions in passing the law, including standards pertaining to program eligibility, benefits, and payments to participating health care providers.[i] Yet there are literally thousands of administrative regulations and rules pertaining to Medicaid, which over the past 40 years have become the real battleground over the stability and scope of the program. In a very real sense, the Medicaid regulations passed by the federal Department of Health and Human Services and state-level agencies are what bring the program to life and give it vitality. This "operationalizing" function of administrative law can be seen across a wide spectrum of important health issues, including the reporting of infectious diseases, the development of sanitation standards, and the enforcement of environmental laws.[10]

Common Law

In each of the prior discussions about constitutions, statutes, and administrative regulations, we pointed out the generality and ambiguity of much of law, and the corresponding responsibility of courts to interpret and apply law to specific cases. It is via the common law—essay-like opinions written by appellate courts articulating the bases for their decisions in individual cases—that courts carry out this responsibility. Common law is also referred to as case law, judge-made law, or decisional law.

Common law is central to legal systems in many countries, particularly those that were territories or colonies of England, which is how the United States came to rely on common law as part of its legal system. Both historically and in modern times, case law is premised on the traditions and customs of society, the idea being that courts could continuously (and relatively efficiently, compared to the legislative process) interpret and apply law in such a way as to match the values of a society undergoing constant evolution. At the same time, the common law is heavily influenced by legal precedent and the doctrine of *stare decisis*, which refers to the legal principle that prior case law decisions should be accorded great deference and should not be frequently overturned. The importance and function of stare decisis in American law is discussed later in the section detailing the role courts play in maintaining stability in the law.

Although courts are expected to overturn their own prior decisions only in rare circumstances and lower courts can never overturn decisions by higher courts that have jurisdiction over them, legislatures can modify or even overturn common law decisions interpreting statutes and regulations. Imagine that the Supreme Court interpreted a federal civil rights statute as protecting individuals from intentional acts of race discrimination, but not from conduct that has the unintended effect of

discriminating against racial minorities. If Congress disagreed with the Court's interpretation of the statute, it could effectively overturn the Court's decision by amending the statute to make it clear that the law was intended to prohibit intentional discrimination *and* presumably neutral acts that nonetheless resulted in unintended discrimination. However, because the judicial branch has final authority to determine whether statutes violate the Constitution, Congress would be powerless to overturn a federal court decision that ruled the same civil rights statute unconstitutional.[j]

Notice the "checks and balances" at play in this example, with one branch of government acting as a restraint on another. In the next section, we discuss the separation of powers doctrine—including checks and balances—and other key features of the legal system. But first, see Table 3-1, which provides a summary of the sources of law.

KEY FEATURES OF THE LEGAL SYSTEM

Recall the earlier description of the law as something more than just words on a page, something more than statutes and constitutional provisions. Although the laws themselves are obviously critical, they are just one component of a complex, interacting legal system that creates the laws in the first instance and brings them to life after they hit the pages of legal code books, texts, and treatises.

All legal systems rest on unique principles, traditions, and customs. This section describes a handful of the most important features and principles of the U.S. legal system, including the separation of powers doctrine, federalism, the role and structure of federal and state courts, judicial review, due process, and constitutional standards of review.

Separation of Powers

This country's government, both federal and state, has an underpinning structure of three independent and equally powerful branches.[k] The legal doctrine that supports the arrangement of shared governance among multiple branches is the *separation of powers* doctrine. This doctrine is considered one of the most important aspects of both federal and state constitutional design. The framers of the Constitution were well aware that nothing was more likely to foster tyrannical government than the concentration of governing powers in one individual or political party. To guard against a concentration of political power, the framers did two related things: they divided governmental powers and responsibilities among separate, co-equal branches, and they structured the elections of officials for the two political branches of government (legislative and executive) so that they would take place at different intervals and through different mechanisms (e.g., the President

TABLE 3-1 Summary of the Primary Sources of American Law

Source of Law	Key Points
Constitutions	• Establish governments and delineate fundamental rights and obligations of government and individuals. • There is a federal constitution and separate constitutions in each state. • The federal constitution restrains government more than it confers individual rights. • However, the Bill of Rights specifically guarantees several important individual rights. • The Supreme Court has final word on the constitutionality of laws created by the political branches of government.
Statutes	• Created by legislatures at all levels of government. • Two hallmarks: prospectivity and generality. • As broad policy statements, statutes are often ambiguous as applied to specific cases or controversies, requiring courts to interpret them through the practice of statutory construction. • State legislatures can use statutes to regulate across a broader range of issues than can Congress. • However, federal statutes have primacy over conflicting state statutes.
Regulations	• Created by executive branch administrative agencies to implement statutes and clarify their ambiguities. • Play a particularly critical role in health policy and law.
Common law	• Court opinions interpreting and applying law to specific cases. • Also referred to as case law, judge-made law, or decisional law. • Based on the traditions and customs of society, yet heavily influenced by legal precedent and the doctrine of stare decisis.

is elected through the electoral college system, whereas members of Congress are not).

Inherent in the separation of powers doctrine is the important concept of checks and balances. "Checks" refers to the ability and responsibility of one branch of government to closely monitor the actions of the other two, including when one branch grasps at an amount of power not envisioned by the Constitution. The "balance" at work in the separation of powers framework prevents one branch from exerting power in an area of responsibility that is the province of another branch.

The constitutional doctrine of separation of powers represents, in the words of one legal scholar, an "invitation to struggle for the privilege"[11(p171)] of governing the country.[l] For example, at the time of this writing, a debate is taking place in the media and between Congress and President George W. Bush over the meaning of separation of powers and the appropriate role of checks and balances. Since taking office in 2001, President Bush has advocated an expansive view of the powers

of the executive branch vis-à-vis the other two branches, a view that for several years has gone mainly unchecked (in part because the same political party controlled the White House and both chambers of Congress through late in 2006). However, disagreements between members of Congress and the President over topics such as interrogation tactics for foreign enemies and the scope of a White House–supported domestic spying program have touched off a national discussion about whether the executive branch is overreaching.[m]

Throughout this book, there are health policy and law questions that distinctly highlight our government's divided powers. For example, should Congress enact major health reform legislatively, or should reform happen piecemeal through executive branch regulatory channels? And how has the Supreme Court applied its constitutional right to privacy jurisprudence to the matter of abortion in response to federal and state legislative enactments? As you consider these and other health policy and law questions from a separation of powers angle, consider the peculiar roles of each branch of government, taking into account their duties, powers, and limitations. Through this prism, continually reflect on which governmental body is best equipped to effectively respond to health policy problems.[n]

Federalism: Allocation of Federal and State Legal Authority

In the legal system, the powers to govern, make and apply law, and effectuate policy choices are not just apportioned among three governmental branches at both the federal and state levels; they are also divided *between* the federal government and the governments of the various states. This division of authority—which also plays a key role in the development of health policies and laws—is referred to as *federalism*. Like the separation of powers doctrine, federalism derives from the Constitution.

Under the Constitution, the federal government is one of limited powers, while the states more or less retain all powers not expressly left exclusively to the federal government. In essence, this was the deal consented to by the states at the time our federal republic was formed: They agreed to surrender certain enumerated powers (like foreign affairs) to the federal government in exchange for retaining many aspects of sovereignty.

The Constitution's Tenth Amendment states that "the powers not delegated to the United States by the Constitution . . . are reserved to the States respectively. . . ."[13] For example, because the Constitution does not explicitly define the protection and promotion of the public's health as a power of the federal government, public health powers are primarily held by the states.[o] As a result, all states regulate the area of public health through what are known as their "police powers," which allow state and local governments to (among other things) legislate to protect the common good. Examples of the kinds of laws passed under this authority include childhood immunization standards, infectious disease data collection mandates, environmental hazard regulations, and much more. Furthermore, under the Tenth Amendment, states historically have had the power to regulate the practice of medicine and the licensing of hospitals and other health care institutions.

Recall from Chapter 1, however, that the federal government also plays a role in regulating health care and public health. The national government's enumerated powers include the ability to tax, spend, and regulate interstate commerce, all of which have been utilized in ways to improve health care and promote public health. For example, Congress has used its taxing power to increase the cost of cigarettes (in the hopes of driving down the number of smokers) and to generate funds for programs such as Medicare. And congressional spending powers are the legal cornerstone for federal health programs like Medicaid. Furthermore, the sharing of power under the Tenth Amendment notwithstanding, the Constitution's supremacy clause declares that federal laws—the Constitution, statutes, and treaties—are the "supreme" law of the land, and thus preempt state laws that conflict with them.[15,p]

While federalism is built solidly into the nation's political branches through separate federal and state legislatures and executives, it is also on display in the structure of U.S. courts. There are both federal and state court systems, and each has unique authority and jurisdiction. For example, federal courts are limited to ruling only in certain kinds of cases, including those involving federal constitutional or statutory law, those in which the United States is a party to the lawsuit, and those specified by statutory law. State courts, by contrast, have jurisdiction to hear just about any case (unless explicitly precluded from doing so by federal statute), including those over which federal courts also have jurisdiction. This includes cases implicating state statutory and regulatory law, the state constitution, and the U.S. Constitution.[q]

Over the years, defining the boundaries of federalism (i.e., defining the federal government's sphere of authority and determining the scope of state sovereignty) has been a contentious legal and political issue. At the dawn of the country's independence, after the colonies intentionally scrapped the Articles of Confederation in favor of a stronger central government, the Supreme Court decided federalism cases with a nod toward expansive national powers (much to the dislike of some states). Two famous cases make the point. In the 1819 case of *McCulloch v. Maryland*,[16] the Supreme Court enhanced the power of the U.S. government by establishing the principle that federal governmental powers are not strictly limited to those expressly provided for in the Constitution. At issue in the case was whether Congress had the power to charter a national bank to help the federal government shoulder wartime debt. In 1824, the Court for the first time had the opportunity to review the Constitution's commerce clause (which grants Congress the authority to regulate interstate commerce) in the case of *Gibbons v. Ogden*,[17] which resulted from a decision by the state of New York to grant a monopoly to a steamboat operator for a ferry between New York and New Jersey. Again, the Court ruled broadly in favor of the federal government, stating that the commerce clause reserved exclusively to Congress the power to regulate interstate navigation.

By the mid-1800s, however, this approach to defining the relative power of the federal and state governments gave way to one that was more deferential to states and more willing to balance their sovereign interests against the interests of the federal government. This approach, in turn, lost ground during the New Deal and civil rights eras, both of which were marked by an acceptance of federal authority to provide social services and regulate the economy. The arrival of Ronald Reagan's presidency in 1981 marked yet another turning point in the evolution of federalism. For eight years, the Reagan administration acted to restrict national authority over the states, a process that took on even more force after the Republican Party took control of Congress in the mid-90s. Indeed, since the early 1980s and continuing into the new millennium, a defining feature of federalism has been the purposeful devolution of authority and governance over social and economic policy from the federal government to state legislators and regulators.

The Role of Courts

Chapter 2 described the structure and powers of the political branches of government—the legislative and executive branches. The third branch is that of the judiciary, made up of justices, judges, magistrates, and other "adjudicators" in two separate court systems—one federal, one state. Adjudication refers to the legal process of resolving disputes. It is in the context of resolving specific legal disputes that the judiciary interprets and applies the law, and also indirectly "makes" law under its common law authority. The results of adjudication are the common law decisions described earlier. Because U.S. courts are generally not permitted to issue advisory opinions, courts effectively only act in response to a specific "case or controversy" brought before them.[r] This essentially means that in order for a court to rule in a particular case, an individual initiating a lawsuit must assert an enforceable legal right, a measurable violation of that right, actual damage or harm, and a court-fashioned remedy that could appropriately respond to the lawsuit.

Courts play a vital role in the legal system. This role stems in large part from their responsibility to determine what, ultimately, the Constitution means, permits, and prohibits. In discharging this responsibility, courts are asked to protect and enforce individual legal rights, determine whether the political branches of government have acted in a way violative of the Constitution, and maintain stability in the law through the application of legal precedent. The judicial branch is viewed as uniquely able to fulfill these key responsibilities, at least at the federal level, because it is the branch of government most insulated from politics: Federal judges are appointed, not elected, and granted life tenure under the Constitution to shield them from political influences that might otherwise interfere with their impartially.[s] Most state judges, however, are now subject to popular election,[14] either at the time of initial selection or subsequently, when it is determined whether they will be retained as judges.[t]

Enforcing Legal Rights

As described earlier, two main functions of the legal system are to establish legal rights and to create institutions to enforce those rights. The primary enforcers of individual legal rights, and those in the best position to create remedies for their violation, are the courts. For example, the federal courts (and the Supreme Court in particular) were critical to the success of the civil rights movement, during which time federal judges expansively interpreted civil rights laws and maintained close oversight of the implementation of their rulings. At the same time, however, the Supreme Court has not often been at the forefront of advancing individual rights. Certainly there have been times when the Court has played an enormous role in advancing societal expectations with respect to individual equality—*Brown v. Board of Education*[18] being the most obvious example—but this decision, and a few others, are actually quite anomalous, and the Court has been more a follower of evolving attitudes and expectations.

Among the most important rights courts are expected to uphold and enforce is the constitutional right to *due process*, which protects individuals from arbitrary and unfair treatment at the hands of government. Both the Fifth and Fourteenth Amendments to the Constitution make clear that no person can be deprived of "life, liberty, or property, without due process of law," with the Fifth Amendment applying to the federal government and the Fourteenth applying to the states. An important component of due process is the principle that when government establishes a legal right or entitlement for individuals, it may not then decide to deny the right or entitlement unfairly.

When courts consider due process claims, they are often thought of as reviewing *how* laws operate and *why* laws have been established in the first place. This results from the fact that the due process clause has been interpreted by the Supreme Court as including *procedural* due process (the "how") and *substantive* due process (the "why"). Procedural due process requires that laws be enacted and applied fairly and equitably, including procedural fairness when individuals challenge government infringements on their life, liberty, or property. Thus, due process requirements might be triggered if a law is too vague or is applied unevenly, if government threatens to withdraw a previously granted license, or if an individual's public benefits are withheld. For example, before a physician can lose his state-granted license to practice medicine, the state must provide the physician advance notice of the termination and a formal hearing before an impartial examiner with all the usual legal trappings (right to legal representation, right to present evidence in one's defense, right to appeal the examiner's decision, etc.). Similarly, Medicaid beneficiaries must be given notice of, and an opportunity to challenge, benefit coverage denials made by a managed care company participating in the Medicaid program. And the courts' most well-known jurisprudence in the area of health-related due process rights concerns abortion, specifically whether federal and state laws impermissibly infringe on the right to terminate a pregnancy, which is part of the right to "liberty" under the due process clause.

But that clause has been interpreted by courts to require more than just procedural fairness when a law deprives an individual of life, liberty, or property; it also requires that government provide a sound reason for having invaded personal freedoms in the first place. This is termed *substantive due process*. This form of due process serves as a proscription against arbitrary government activity. For instance, when states have been unable to adequately explain the reasoning behind statutes requiring involuntary confinement of mentally ill individuals who were not dangerous to themselves or others, courts ruled the laws unconstitutional on substantive due process grounds. Substantive due process is unquestionably more controversial than its procedural counterpart, because many critics argue that the former gives courts unrestrained power to invalidate on constitutional grounds government actions with which they simply disagree. In other words, some view this form of due process "as a potentially limitless warrant for judges to impose their personal values on the Constitution."[19(p474)]

Reviewing the Actions of the Political Branches

An important piece of the separation of powers puzzle, and one that grants the courts wide authority to enforce individual legal rights in this country, is the doctrine of *judicial review*. Judicial review refers to the power of the courts to declare laws unconstitutional and to determine whether the actions of the legislative and executive branches of government are lawful. The theory behind judicial review is that as the branch of government most independent of the political process, courts can pass judgment on the actions of the political branches free of partisanship.

Judicial review has its roots in the famous 1803 case of *Marbury v. Madison*,[20] in which the Supreme Court ruled that it had the power to review acts of Congress and determine their constitutionality. The facts of the case are fascinating. In 1800, Thomas Jefferson won the presidential election, besting incumbent John Adams. In the final days of President Adams's term, the Federalist-controlled Congress passed, and Adams signed into law, a statute called the Judiciary Act of 1801. Among other things, the law created several new judgeships, and the idea was to fill the new judicial posts with Federalists before Jefferson assumed the presidency. Among the new judicial appointments made by Adams and approved by the Senate before Jefferson took office were 42 justices of the peace, including one for William Marbury. Prior to Jefferson's taking office, Marbury's commission was signed by Adams and by John Marshall—who at the time was Secretary of State under Adams—but not delivered. After his inauguration, Jefferson ruled that Marbury's commission (and those of several other Adams-appointed justices of the peace) were invalid because they had not been delivered during the Adams presidency, and therefore directed his new Secretary of State, James Madison, to withhold delivery. Marbury sued to force delivery of his commission, petitioning the Supreme Court directly to issue a *writ of mandamus*, which is an order by a court compelling a government officer to perform his duties. Marbury was able to ask the Court directly for the writ because the recently enacted Judiciary Act also authorized the Supreme Court to issue writs of mandamus.

The Supreme Court's decision in *Marbury v. Madison*[u] first established the important principle that for every violation of a legal right, there must be a corresponding legal remedy. With this principle in place, the Court ruled that Marbury was in fact entitled to his commission and to a legal remedy for Jefferson's decision to withhold it, "since [Marbury's] commission was signed by the President, and sealed by the secretary of state . . . ; and the law creating the office, gave the officer a right to hold for five years, independent of the executive, the appointment[.] To withhold his commission, therefore, is an act deemed by the court not warranted by law, but violative of a vested legal right."[21]

The *Marbury* Court then did something monumental: It established and justified the power of judicial review. This outcome flowed from the fact that Marbury had filed his legal petition directly with the Supreme Court, and the Court needed to determine whether Congress acted constitutionally in granting the Court power under the Judiciary Act to issue writs of mandamus as a matter of "original jurisdiction."[v] It was not apparent that the mandamus component of the new Judiciary Act was constitutional because Article III of the Constitution—which established the judicial branch of the federal government, including the Supreme Court—says that "In all Cases affecting Ambassadors, other public Ministers and Consuls, and those in which a State shall be a Party, the supreme Court shall have original Jurisdiction. In all the other Cases [subject to Supreme Court jurisdiction], the supreme Court shall have appellate Jurisdiction, both as to Law and Fact, with such Exceptions, and under such Regulations as the Congress shall make."[22] Interpreting this clause, Chief Justice Marshall determined the Court could issue a writ of mandamus under the Constitution only as an exercise of appellate—but not original—jurisdiction, and that Congress had no power to modify the Court's original jurisdiction. As a result, the Court held that the Judiciary Act of 1801 was in conflict with Article III, and thus unconstitutional.

Marbury represented the first time the Supreme Court exercised the power of judicial review and declared unconstitutional a law passed by Congress. Over the years, the Court has exercised this power sparingly, exclaiming in 1867 that although it clearly had the authority to strike down congressional legislation repugnant to the Constitution, this "duty is one of great delicacy, and only to be performed where the repugnancy is clear, and the conflict unreconcilable."[23] For example, the Supreme Court invalidated few congressional acts in the first 50 years after *Marbury*, although the pace picked up somewhat after that, to an average of about one invalidation every two years. During William Rehnquist's term as Chief Justice (1986–2005), however, the Court ruled unconstitutional more than 30 laws or statutory provisions, with most of these decisions occurring between 1995 and 2005. This up-tick in the Court's use of its most powerful judicial review tool has led to a discussion about the Court's proper place in the separation of powers framework. As a recent opinion piece exclaimed, "[d]eclaring an act of Congress unconstitutional is the boldest thing a judge can do. That's because Congress, as an elected legislative body representing the entire nation, makes decisions that can be presumed to possess a high degree of democratic legitimacy."[24(pA19)]

When determining whether a statute violates the Constitution, courts necessarily take into account the subject of the regulation and Congress's purpose in regulating. Certain kinds of laws—say, affirmative action laws, or a law that classifies people on the basis of their gender—require a greater level of governmental justification and thus are held to a higher constitutional *standard of review*. In other words, these laws are scrutinized more closely by the Court and thus stand a greater chance of failing the constitutionality test.

By way of example, the Supreme Court has developed a tiered standard of review framework for equal protection jurisprudence. Under the Constitution's equal protection clause, states are prohibited from denying "to any person within its jurisdiction the equal protection of the laws."[25] The Court employs one of three standards when it reviews whether a particular law satisfies this constitutional mandate. The first, termed *rational basis* or *rational relations* review, is applied to everyday legislation pertaining to things like public safety, tax rates, and consumer protection and thus is the review standard most frequently used. It is nearly impossible for a law to run afoul of this standard, because as long as the challenged statute is *rationally* related to *any* legitimate government purpose in passing the law, it will be upheld as constitutional.

The second standard is that of *intermediate* review. This is the Court's choice when the measure under review classifies individuals or groups on, for example, the basis of gender. The assumption here—and the point of the heightened review standard—is that when politicians legislate with gender (or another potentially baseless characteristic) in mind, there is a greater likelihood they are doing so for nefarious reasons. In order to pass constitutional muster under intermediate review, a statute must serve an *important* government objective and be *substantially* related to that objective. A good deal of legislation reviewed under this standard is found to be unconstitutional.

Finally, the Court has at its disposal in equal protection lawsuits a review standard known as *strict scrutiny*. The Court reserves this standard for laws that tread on fundamental constitutional rights (defined in part as those that are firmly established in American tradition), including an individual's right to be free of governmental discrimination on the basis of race. In theory, otherwise discriminatory laws that are *necessary* to achieve a *compelling* government interest—meaning that the law in question is the least discriminatory way to meet the legislature's compelling objective—can survive this intense form of scrutiny. However, of all the equal protection claims measured against this standard, only one survivor has emerged—when the Supreme Court permitted the federal government to intern individuals of Japanese descent during World War II[26]—and now it is almost universally agreed that this decision was terribly off the mark.[w]

Maintaining Stability in the Law

In addition to enforcing legal rights and passing on the constitutionality of actions of the two political branches of government, courts are expected to maintain a measure of stability, continuity, and predictability in the law. This expectation derives from the idea that those subject to the law should not have to contend with continuous swings in the direction law takes. In theory, the relatively nonpolitical judicial branch of government is in the best position to bring this expectation to fruition.

The way courts implement their responsibility to maintain legal stability is through application of stare decisis, a Latin legal term meaning "let it stand." Stare decisis is a policy of the courts to stand by existing legal precedent; that is, where rules of law have been established in prior judicial decisions, these decisions should be adhered to in subsequent cases where the questions of law and fact are substantially similar to those in the original case. Stability in the law is considered so important that stare decisis is usually applied, and the original judicial decision given deference, *even when the original decision is subsequently determined to be wrongly decided or not legally sound.* This is especially true where the original decision is an old one on which society has come to rest, as opposed to a relatively young decision with few deep roots in terms of societal expectations.[x]

At the same time, legal precedent is not completely sacred, and prior decisions are sometimes reconsidered and, on occasion, overturned. For instance, changes in societal values might outweigh strict application of stare decisis, as was the case with the Supreme Court's 1954 decision in *Brown v. Board of Education*[27] to overturn the invidious idea of "separate but equal" from that Court's 1896 decision in *Plessy v. Ferguson*.[28] Stare decisis is, however, generally understood to trump mere changes in a court's makeup. In other words, courts are expected to remain anchored to precedential rules of law even when current individual members may not be.[y] Indeed, in a well-known Supreme Court case, former Justice John Marshall Harlan II once wrote:

> A basic change in the law upon a ground no firmer than a change in our membership invites the popular misconception that this institution is little different from the two political branches of the Government. No misconception could do more lasting injury to this Court and to the system which it is our abiding mission to serve.[29]

CONCLUSION

This chapter led you on a short journey through the complex world of the legal system. Along the way, you visited several of its essential elements and doctrines: legal rights, the various types of law, separation of powers, federalism, judicial review, and more. To be sure, the trip was abbreviated and in some cases concepts were oversimplified, but above all this is a function of needing to concisely cover a complex and expansive topic.

As you encounter in this textbook myriad health policy and law topics and concepts that are complex in their own right, bearing in mind a few important details about law might help you achieve a greater measure of clarity. First, law's primary purpose is to organize and control an ever-changing, ever-expanding, ever-more-complex society, and it does this in part by regulating a variety of relationships among parties with oftentimes competing interests (e.g., individual citizen and government; patient and physician; beneficiary and public program or private insurance company; physician and managed care organization; individual and her family). This helps explain why in the context of a specific relationship, one party has a legal right and the other party has a legal responsibility to refrain from acting in a way that infringes that legal right. It also helps explain why an individual can justifiably claim a particular legal right in the context of one specific relationship, but not in others (for example, a patient who believes that he has been treated negligently might have a legitimate legal claim against the physician who provided his care, but not against the hospital where the care was provided).

A second detail worth reflecting on periodically is that law is established, enforced, interpreted, and applied by human beings, and thus one must accept that law and the legal process comprise a certain amount of imperfection. This helps explain why statutes and regulations are sometimes difficult to understand; why laws are sometimes enforced sporadically or not at all; why reasonable jurists can disagree about the intended meaning of statutory and constitutional provisions; and why law is too often applied unevenly, or inequitably.

Finally, bear in mind the fact that laws and the broader legal system are reflective of the beliefs and values of the society from which they flow. This *fait accompli*, perhaps more than anything else, provides an object lesson in the role of law across a wide range of subjects, including matters related to health care and public health.

REFERENCES

1. Holmes OW. Law in science and science in law. *Harvard Law Rev.* 1899;12: 443, 444.
2. Friedman LM. Law and its language. *George Wash Univ Law Rev.* 1964;33: 563, 567.
3. Black HC, et al. *Black's Law Dictionary,* 6th ed. St. Paul, Minn.: West; 1990.
4. Friedman LM. *Law in America: A Short History.* New York: The Modern Library; 2002.
5. Smith SD. Reductionism in legal thought. *Columbia Law Rev.* 1991;91:68, 73–75.
6. Reich CA. The new property. *Yale Law J.* 1964;73:733.
7. *Fay v. New York*, 332 U.S. 261, 282 (1947) (Jackson, J., concurring).
8. U.S. Const. amend. XIV, § 1.
9. *Jackson v. City of Joliet*, 715 F.2d 1200, 1203 (7th Cir. 1983).
10. Mensah GA, et al. Law as a tool for preventing chronic diseases: expanding the spectrum of effective public health strategies. *Prev Chronic Dis: Public Health Res Pract Policy.* 2004;1(2):1–6.
11. Corwin ES. *The President: Office and Powers, 1787–1957.* New York: New York University Press; 1957.
12. de Tocqueville A. *Democracy in America.* New York: Vintage Books; 1990.
13. U.S. Const. amend. X.
14. American Bar Association, Governmental Affairs Office. An independent judiciary: report of the ABA Commission on Separation of Powers and Judicial Independence. Available at http://www.abanet.org/govaffairs/judiciary/r5.html. Accessed August 1, 2006.
15. U.S. Const. article VI, paragraph 2.
16. 17 U.S. (4 Wheat.) 316 (1819).
17. 22. U.S. (9 Wheat.) 1 (1824).
18. 347 U.S. 483 (1954).
19. Lazarus E. *Closed Chambers: The Rise, Fall, and Future of the Modern Supreme Court.* New York: Penguin Books; 1999.
20. 1 Cranch (5 U.S.) 137 (1803).
21. *Marbury*, 1 Cranch (5 U.S.) at 162.
22. U.S. Const. art. III, § 2, Clause 2.
23. *Mayor v. Cooper*, 73 U.S. 247, 251 (1867).
24. Gewirtz P, Golder C. So who are the activists? *The New York Times.* July 6, 2005: A19.
25. U.S. Const. amend. XIV, § 1.
26. *Korematsu v. United States*, 323 U.S. 214 (1944).
27. 347 U.S. 483 (1954).
28. 163 U.S. 537 (1896).
29. *Mapp v. Ohio*, 367 U.S. 643, 677 (1961) (Harlan, J., dissenting).

ENDNOTES

a. Although the important role that language plays in law is not a topic we delve into in this chapter, it is, particularly for students new to the study of law, one worth thinking about. Words are the basic and most important tool of the law and of lawyers. Without them, how could one draft a law, legal brief, contract, or judicial opinion? Or engage in oral advocacy on behalf of a client, or conduct a negotiation? Or make one's wishes known with respect to personal matters near the end of life? As one renowned legal scholar puts it, "law is primarily a verbal art, its skills verbal skills."[2]

Of course, one problem with the language of law is that it is full of legal jargon, making it difficult sometimes for lay people to understand and apply to their own particular situation. For example, if government regulation is to be effective, the language used to do the regulating must be understandable to those being regulated. Another problem relates to the interpretation of words and terms used in the law, because both ambiguity (where language is reasonably capable of being understood in two or more ways) and vagueness (where language is not fairly capable of being understood) are common to laws, leaving those subject to them and those responsible for applying them unclear about their true meaning. Furthermore, as the Preface to *Black's Law Dictionary*, under the heading "A Final Word of Caution," states: "The language of the law is ever-changing as the courts, Congress, state legislatures, and administrative agencies continue to define, redefine and expand legal words and terms. Furthermore, many legal terms are subject to variations from state to state and again can differ under federal laws."[3(p iv)]

b. For information on and updates of state legislative activity related to their public health laws, see the Center for Law and the Public's Health, Georgetown and Johns Hopkins Universities, at http://www.publichealthlaw.net/Resources/Modellaws.htm#TP.

c. Broadly speaking, the leading approaches to constitutional interpretation include the "living constitution," the "moral constitution," "originalism," and "strict constructionism." Although a full discussion of these theories is beyond the scope of this chapter, we offer a thumbnail description of each here.

The living constitution model reflects a belief that the broadly written Constitution should be interpreted to reflect current moral, political, and cultural values in society, not the values that were predominant at the time of the Constitution's ratification. Under this view, the meaning of the Constitution is not fixed, but instead evolves along with society. Moral constitutionalists infuse their interpretation of constitutional law with principles of moral philosophy. Originalism technically is an umbrella term referring to a small group of constitutional interpretation theories, all of which share a common belief that constitutional provisions have a fixed and knowable meaning. For example, "original intent," one well-known theory under the originalism umbrella, adheres to the position that constitutional interpretation should be consistent with the intent of the Constitution's original drafters. Finally, strict constructionists limit their interpretation to the Constitution's actual words and phrases, and decline to consider contextual factors such as shifts in societal values or the commentaries or intent of the framers. For in-depth analysis of these and other theories of constitutional interpretation, there is a vast body of literature at one's disposal. See, e.g., Thomas E. Baker, "Constitutional Theory in a Nutshell," *William and Mary Bill of Rights Journal* 13 (2004): 57; Richard H. Fallon, Jr., "How to Choose a Constitutional Theory," *California Law Review* 87 (1999): 535.

d. Federal Judge Richard Posner wrote that "[t]he men who wrote the Bill of Rights were not concerned that government might do too little for the people but that it might do too much to them."[9]

e. This concept of the "negative constitution" is discussed more fully in Chapter 8, which discusses individual rights in the contexts of health care and public health.

f. For an overview of the Bill of Rights in a public health context, see Lawrence O. Gostin, *Public Health Law: Power, Duty, Restraint* (Berkeley: University of California Press, 2000), 62–65.

g. In order to be lawful, regulations must be proposed and established in a way that conforms to the requirements of the federal Administrative Procedure Act of 1946, 5 U.S.C. §500, as described in Chapter 2.

h. For a full description of the intertwined nature of administrative and health law, see Timothy Stoltzfus Jost, "Health Law and Administrative Law: A Marriage Most Convenient," *Saint Louis University Law Journal* 49 (2004): 1.

i. Medicaid is described in detail in Chapter 6.

j. Supreme Court decisions pertaining to the meaning of the Constitution are final, save for two possibilities. First, the Court could issue a subsequent ruling overturning its original decision. Second, Congress and the states could undertake the challenging process of amending the Constitution to alter its meaning. The latter can be achieved in one of two ways. The first is for each chamber of Congress, by at least a two-thirds majority, to pass a bill specifying a constitutional amendment, which then needs to be approved by at least three-fourths of state legislatures; this is how all existing amendments to the Constitution have been passed. The second approach would require that at least two-thirds of state legislatures agree to hold a constitutional convention, use the convention to propose an amendment, and then press for passage of the amendment by at least three-fourths of all state legislatures.

k. The fact that in our system of government the legislature is co-equal to the executive branch sets it apart from parliamentary systems of government—found in Canada, Germany, the United Kingdom, and many other countries—in which the legislature appoints the executive.

l. Alexis de Tocqueville, a French philosopher and political theorist who studied American government in the 1830s, viewed the concept of checks and balances in much starker terms: "The president, who exercises a limited power, may err without causing great mischief in the state. Congress may decide amiss without destroying the union, because the electoral body in which the Congress originates may cause it to retract its decision by changing its members. But if the Supreme Court is ever composed of imprudent or bad men, the union may be plunged into anarchy or civil war."[12(p152)]

m. See, e.g., Linda Greenhouse, "Detainee Case Hits on Limits of Presidency," *The New York Times* (January 10, 2006), page A22 ("When the Supreme Court agreed two months ago to hear an appeal from a Yemeni detainee at Guantánamo Bay, Cuba, named Salim Ahmed Hamdan, it was evident that an important test of the limits of presidential authority to conduct the war on terror was under way."); Dan Eggen and Walter Pincus, "Campaign to Justify Spying Intensifies: NSA Effort Called Legal and Necessary," *The Washington Post* (January 24, 2006), page A04 ("Some experts on intelligence and national security law have said that the president overstepped his authority in ordering the NSA spying, and that the 1978 Foreign Intelligence Surveillance Act (FISA) specifically prohibits such domestic surveillance without a warrant."); Bruce Fein, "Data-Mining Doubts," *The Washington Times*, (January 24, 2006), commentary page ("A president above separation of powers might help to defeat the terrorist enemy. But the nation's constitutional dispensation and bulwarks against tyranny would be destroyed.") Ruth Marcus, "Contempt for Congress," *The Washington Post* (January 25, 2006), page A19 (op-ed) ("[The executive branch] thinks of congressional oversight as if it were a trip to the dentist, to be undertaken reluctantly and gotten over with as quickly as possible. Most astonishingly, it reserves the right simply to ignore congressional dictates that it has decided intrude too much on executive branch power.")

n. For a full discussion of each of the government branches' role in health policy making, see Lawrence Gostin, "The Formulation of Health Policy by the Three Branches of Government," in *Society's Choices: Social and Ethical Decision Making in Biomedicine*, eds. Ruth Ellen Bulger, Elizabeth Meyer Bobby, and Harvey V. Fineberg (Washington, D.C.: National Academy Press, 1995).

o. In fact, compared to the federal government, the states handle the vast majority of all legal matters in this country. Consider just a sampling of typical legal affairs overseen by state government: marriages, divorces, and adoptions; law enforcement and criminal trials; schooling; driving, hunting, medical, and many other licenses; consumer protection; and much more.[4(pp10–11)] Furthermore, 97% of all litigation occurs in state courts.[14]

p. "This Constitution, and the Laws of the United States which shall be made in Pursuance thereof; and all Treaties made, or which shall be made, under the Authority of the United States, shall be supreme Law of the Land; and the Judges in every State shall be bound thereby, any Thing in the Constitution or Laws of any State to the Contrary notwithstanding."

q. Although the federal and state court systems have critically distinctive authority, they do not look very different structurally. The federal court system has three tiers, with cases proceeding from the lowest-level court (a trial court) to two separate, higher-level courts (appellate courts). Federal trial courts are called district courts, and they exist in varying numbers in each state, with the size of the state determining the actual number of "districts," and thus the number of federal trial courts. In total, there are nearly 100 federal district courts. After a district court renders a decision, the losing party to a lawsuit is entitled to appeal the decision to a federal circuit court of appeals. There are 13 U.S. circuit courts of appeals—12 with jurisdiction over designated multi-state geographic regions, or "circuits," and a court of appeals for the federal circuit (residing in Washington, D.C.), which has nationwide appellate jurisdiction over certain kinds of cases, such as patent and international trade disputes. For many individuals, losing a case in a federal circuit court represents the end of the line for their case, since litigants have no entitlement to have their case heard by the U.S. Supreme Court, the highest court in the country. Although parties have a right to *petition* the Supreme Court to hear their case, at least four of the nine justices on the Court must agree to grant the petition. Although the Supreme Court is undeniably the most important court in the country in terms of its authority, it by no means renders the most decisions. The Supreme Court grants approximately 150 petitions annually, whereas the 13 circuit courts collectively decide approximately 62,000 cases annually. This fact is more than trivial; it effectively means that in the huge majority of federal cases, lower appellate courts, and not the Supreme Court, have final say over the scope and meaning of federal law.

As mentioned, each state also has its own court system, most of which are organized like the federal system: one trial court, followed by two separate appellate courts (generally termed "[name of state] court of appeals" and "[name of state] supreme court"). However, some state systems provide for only one appellate court. State systems also tend to include courts that are "inferior" even to their general trial courts; these handle relatively minor disputes (think of the small claims courts frequently shown on daytime television). Furthermore, state trial courts are sometimes divided by specialty, so that certain courts hear cases that involve only family matters, juvenile matters, and the like.

Within the federal and state court system hierarchy, appellate courts have two powers unavailable to trial courts: reviewing lower court decisions to determine whether there were errors of law made during the trial that necessitate a new one, and establishing legal precedents that lower courts are bound to follow. But appellate courts lack trial courts' powers to actually conduct trials, including empanelling juries, hearing testimony from witnesses, reviewing evidence, and the like. Instead, appellate reviews are limited to the written record created at trial by the lower court.

r. Where permitted, advisory opinions are released by courts not in response to a particular legal dispute, but in response to a request from another branch of government regarding the interpretation or permissibility of a particular law. Federal courts are bound from issuing advisory opinions because the Supreme Court has ruled that constitutional provisions establishing the federal courts prevent them from reviewing hypothetical or moot disputes.

Although a couple exceptions exist, state courts are likewise prohibited from issuing advisory opinions.

s. However, since the 1980s the selection (by the president) and approval (by the U.S. Senate) process for federal judges has become highly politicized. There is an extensive body of literature on this topic, as evidenced by a simple Internet search.

t. The potential implications of increasingly injecting politics into the court system are very troubling. See, e.g., Mike France, Lorraine Woellert, and Brian Grow, "The Battle Over the Courts: How Politics, Ideology, and Special Interests are Compromising the U.S. Justice System," *Business Week* (September 27, 2004), page 36; and Ron Sylvester, "Bills Would Alter How Justices Are Picked," *The Wichita Eagle* (February 20, 2006), at http://www.kansas.com/mld/kansas/news/state/13914385.htm ("A vote by the [Kansas] House Judiciary Committee is expected as early as today on one of three constitutional amendments aimed at changing—for the first time in nearly 50 years—the way Kansas selects its Supreme Court justices. But opponents, including organizations that represent most of the attorneys in Kansas, say the proposals are simply intended to give lawmakers control over the court, upsetting the checks and balances built into government.")

u. The decision was written, as it turned out, by Chief Justice John Marshall—the very same person who, as Secretary of State, signed Marbury's commission. Marshall was sworn in as Chief Justice of the United States just before Jefferson took office.

v. A court's "original jurisdiction" refers to cases on which the court rules before any other court does so, contrasted with situations in which the court reviews a decision of a lower court, which is called "appellate jurisdiction."

w. For a fuller discussion of how the equal protection standards of review operate, see Edward Lazarus, *Closed Chambers: The Rise, Fall, and Future of the Modern Supreme Court* (New York: Penguin Books, 1999), 293–294.

x. The role of legal precedent has been described in this way: "Legal doctrines are shaped like family trees. Each generation of decisions is derived from ones that came before as, over time, each branch of the law grows and spreads or, occasionally, withers and dies away. The most recent decisions almost always draw their strength by tracing back through an ancestral line, choosing among parents, uncles, and cousins according to the aptness of their bloodlines. Rarely, a branch of doctrine is disowned, repudiated, and left vestigial until perhaps revived in another legal era."[20]

y. This understanding is often put to the test, however, as seen in the national discussion of the right to abortion that takes place each time a new U.S. Supreme Court nominee is announced whose political stripes seem to clash with the prevailing law that abortion is a constitutionally protected right.

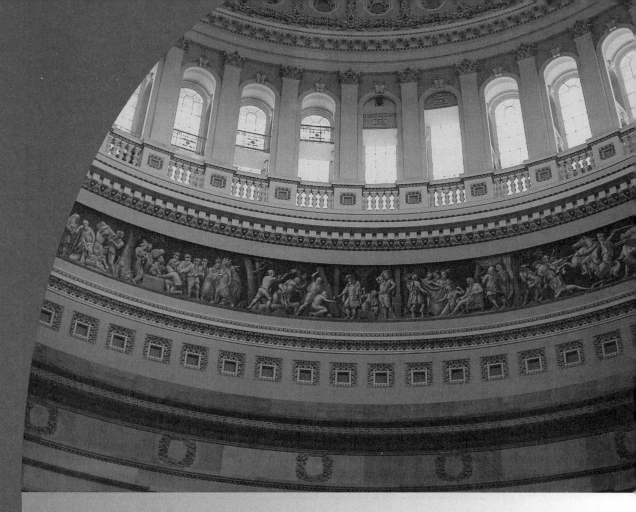

PART II

Essential Issues in Health Policy and Law

Part I of this book introduced frameworks for conceptualizing health policy and law and described basic aspects of policy, the policymaking process, law, and the legal system. Part II covers some of the essential issues in health policy and law. Chapters 4 and 5 address the fundamentals of health insurance and health economics, respectively, and begin a thematic discussion continuing in Chapters 6–8 concerning gaps in health care coverage, coverage reform efforts, and the importance of policy and law to both. After completing Part II, among other things you will understand how health insurance functions, why private employer-based coverage dominates the health insurance market, why enormous gaps in health insurance coverage remain, the consequences of being uninsured, what the federal and state governments have and have not done to fill in insurance coverage gaps, the role of individual legal rights in health care and public health, and various policy and legal dimensions to health care quality.

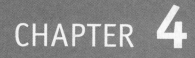

Understanding Health Insurance

By the end of this chapter you will be able to:

- Understand the role of risk and uncertainty in insurance
- Define the basic elements of health insurance
- Differentiate various insurance products
- Discuss incentives created for providers and patients in various types of insurance arrangements
- Discuss health policy issues relating to health insurance

INTRODUCTION

Unlike many other countries, the United States does not have a national health care delivery system; whether individuals have access to health care services—and whether they receive health care of appropriate quantity and quality—often depends on whether they are insured. Even if an individual is insured, the kind of coverage she has can affect her ability to obtain care.

Understanding health insurance, however, requires more than understanding its importance to health care access.

VIGNETTE

Ms. Tevet owns a small business that sells pet food and accessories. She has nine employees and has always made it a priority to offer competitive benefits, including health insurance. Unfortunately, last year one of her employees was diagnosed with cancer, which he continues to fight. Due to the sharp increase in use of health services by her employee group, the insurance company doubled her group premiums for the upcoming year. When Ms. Tevet contacted other carriers, several of them would not consider insuring her group, and most of the others gave her quotes as expensive as her current carrier. One company gave her a lower quote, but it covered only catastrophic care; her employ-

ees would have to pay for the first $5,000 of care out of their own pockets. After reviewing her company's finances, Ms. Tevet is left with several unattractive options: stop offering health insurance; offer comprehensive health insurance but pass on the cost increase to her employees, which would make it unaffordable for most of them; offer the bare-bones catastrophic plan only; or significantly lower wages and other benefits to defray the rising health insurance costs. In addition to wanting to offer competitive benefits, Ms. Tevet is concerned that adopting any of these options will cause her employees to leave and make it hard to attract others, threatening the sustainability of her company.

Policymakers must also know how providers, suppliers, employers, states, and others respond to changes in the health insurance market. For example, if policymakers decide to reduce the number of uninsured by creating a new government-sponsored health insurance program, they must know whether providers will participate in the program and what features will make it more or less attractive to providers. Or, if policymakers want to reduce the number of uninsured by increasing access to employer-sponsored health insurance plans, they must know which policy changes will make it more or less likely that employers will offer (or expand) insurance coverage to their employees. In either case, policymakers might also want to know whether an initiative will affect the financial viability of public hospitals or health centers.

Several themes emerge when considering these types of health insurance–related policy questions. First, insurance is rooted in the concepts of uncertainty and risk; reducing uncertainty and risk by, for example, offering a health insurance product, participating as a provider in a health insurance plan, or purchasing health insurance coverage as a consumer creates various incentives for insurers, the insured, providers, and governments to act or refrain from acting in certain ways. Second, insurance carriers choose the design of their health insurance products, and employers and individuals choose whether to (and what type of) health insurance to purchase. Indeed, insurance carriers have wide latitude to determine the individuals or groups that may join a plan, employers have broad discretion to determine whether to offer coverage and what type to offer, and individuals choose whether to purchase health insurance coverage, although this choice is often illusory due to the high cost of health care. Cutting across these themes is the question of what policy goal (e.g., equity, universal coverage, fiscal restraint, market efficiency) should drive the design and regulation of health insurance.

This chapter begins with a brief discussion of which segments of the population have health insurance[a] and provides a short history of health insurance in this country. It then reviews the health insurance concepts key to understanding the structure and operation of health insurance. It concludes with an overview of managed care, a particular form of health insurance dominant in today's market.

HEALTH INSURANCE COVERAGE

The U.S. does not have a single, national health insurance program that covers the entire population. Instead, as shown in Figure 4-1, people who have health insurance are covered by a patchwork of programs and plans. Overall, 84.1% (247.3 million people) of people living in the United States had health insurance coverage in 2004.[1(p21)] Among the insured, most obtained coverage through their employer; almost 60% had employer-sponsored health insurance in 2005.[1(p21)] Even though employers provide coverage for the majority of insured Americans, the percentage of firms offering health benefits has steadily decreased over the last several years, with an overall decrease of 9% since 2000.[2]

Although the price of insurance varies greatly depending on multiple factors (e.g., number of people covered on a policy, benefit package, geography), it is expensive to purchase private health insurance. The average cost of coverage for a family of four is almost $11,000 annually.[2] Premiums for family coverage increased 9.2% in 2005, which is the first year the cost did not increase by double digits since 2000. Even so, the 2005 increase was much higher than the rate of inflation (3.5%) or the increase in worker earnings (2.7%).[2]

Medicaid and Medicare are the two largest government-sponsored health insurance programs. Both the percentage and number of people covered by public programs was steady from 2004 to 2005. Medicaid covered 38.1 million people (13.9% of the population) in 2005, while Medicare covered 42.3 million people (13.7% of the population) that year.[1(pp16–19),3]

There were 46.6 million people (15.9% of the population) without insurance in 2005.[1(p20)] Among the uninsured, 32.7% were Hispanic, 19.6% were Black, 17.9% were Asian, and 11.3% were non-Hispanic Whites.[1(pp21–22)] In addition, 8.3 million children under 18 (11.2% of the population) were uninsured in 2005, a figure that was slightly higher than the year before. Among uninsured children, 19.9% were at or below the federal poverty line.[1(p21)]

A BRIEF HISTORY OF THE RISE OF HEALTH INSURANCE IN THE UNITED STATES

Although 84% of people in this country are insured today, health insurance was not always an integral part of our society. The initial movement to bring health insurance to the U.S. was modeled after activities in Europe. In the late 1800s and early 1900s, the European social insurance movement resulted in the creation of "sickness" insurance throughout many countries: Germany in 1883, Austria in 1888, Hungary in 1891, Britain in 1911, and Russia in 1912, to name just a few examples. These programs varied in scope and structure, from a compulsory national system in Germany, to industry-based requirements in France and Italy, to extensive state aid in Sweden and Switzerland. Although the Socialist and Progressive parties advocated for the adoption of similar social insurance systems in the U.S. in the early 1900s, their efforts were unsuccessful.[b]

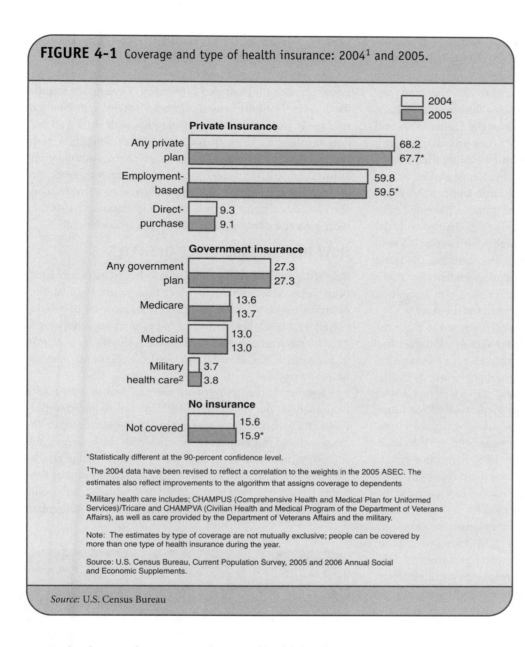

FIGURE 4-1 Coverage and type of health insurance: 2004[1] and 2005.

☐ 2004
■ 2005

Private Insurance

Any private plan: 68.2 / 67.7*

Employment-based: 59.8 / 59.5*

Direct-purchase: 9.3 / 9.1

Government insurance

Any government plan: 27.3 / 27.3

Medicare: 13.6 / 13.7

Medicaid: 13.0 / 13.0

Military health care[2]: 3.7 / 3.8

No insurance

Not covered: 15.6 / 15.9*

*Statistically different at the 90-percent confidence level.

[1]The 2004 data have been revised to reflect a correlation to the weights in the 2005 ASEC. The estimates also reflect improvements to the algorithm that assigns coverage to dependents

[2]Military health care includes; CHAMPUS (Comprehensive Health and Medical Plan for Uniformed Services)/Tricare and CHAMPVA (Civilian Health and Medical Program of the Department of Veterans Affairs), as well as care provided by the Department of Veterans Affairs and the military.

Note: The estimates by type of coverage are not mutually exclusive; people can be covered by more than one type of health insurance during the year.

Source: U.S. Census Bureau, Current Population Survey, 2005 and 2006 Annual Social and Economic Supplements.

Source: U.S. Census Bureau

have reduced the type of physician autonomy described in Chapter 1.[4(p307)]

World War II led to rapid growth in employer-sponsored health insurance. With employees scarce and a general wage freeze in effect, a 1942 War Labor Board ruling that employee fringe benefits of up to 5% of wages did not violate the wage freeze created a strong incentive for employers to provide health benefits to attract new workers and keep their current ones. After the war, labor unions gained the right to bargain collectively, leading to another expansion of employee health plans. In 1954, the Internal Revenue Service declared that employers could pay health insurance premiums for their employees with pre-tax dollars, further increasing the value of the fringe benefit to employers.[c] By 1949, 28 million people had commercial hospital insurance, 22 million had commercial physician insurance, and 4 million had independent hospital plans. At that time, over 31 million had Blue Cross hospital coverage and 12 million had Blue Shield coverage.[4(p327)] Employer-sponsored health insurance, not national health insurance, was well on its way to becoming entrenched as the primary form of health insurance.

The federal government first became a major player in health insurance with the passage of Medicaid and Medicare in 1965. These programs were created, in part, to fill in coverage gaps left by the private insurance market—namely, coverage for the elderly, disabled, and low-income populations who had too little income and too high health risks to be viable candidates for insurance coverage from the insurance carriers' point of view. Like many major policy changes, the passage of these programs was a multi-layered compromise. Before the

In the absence of government-sponsored health insurance plans, the private sector insurance industry flourished with the growth of Blue Cross, Blue Shield, and commercial insurance carriers. Blue Cross established its first hospital insurance plan at Baylor University in 1929 by agreeing to provide 1,500 teachers with 21 days of hospital care per year for the price of $6 per person.[4(p295)] The hospital industry supported the growth of private insurance as a way to secure payment for services during the Depression. Blue Shield, the physician-based insurance plan, began in 1939 as a way to forestall renewed efforts to enact compulsory national health insurance and to avoid growth in consumer-controlled prepaid health plans, both of which would

final design of these programs was established, several proposals were considered. The American Medical Association (AMA) supported a combination federal–state program to subsidize private insurance policies for the elderly to cover hospital care, physician care, and prescription drugs; Representative John Byrnes (R-WI), ranking Republican on the House Ways and Means Committee, endorsed an AMA-like proposal but with federal, instead of federal–state, administration; the Johnson Administration supported hospital insurance for the elderly through Social Security; and Senator Jacob Javitz (R-NY) supported federal payments to state programs to provide health care to poor, elderly individuals.[5(pp46–48)] In the end, the Medicare and Medicaid programs were passed in one bill with features from all of these proposals. For example, Medicare was established as a federally funded program with two parts, one for hospital insurance and one for physician insurance, and Medicaid as a state–federal program for the poor.

By the 1970s a number of factors converged to place rising health care costs on the national agenda: advances had been made in medical technology, hospitals expanded and became more involved in high-tech care, physician specialties became more common, hospitals and physicians had a large new pool of paying patients due to Medicaid and Medicare, wages for medical staff increased, and an aging population required an increasing amount of services.[4(pp383–384)] In addition, the prevailing fee-for-service (FFS) insurance system rewarded health care professionals for providing a high quantity of services. As the name suggests, fee-for-service reimbursement means the providers are paid for each service they provide. The more services (and more expensive services) rendered, the more reimbursement the provider receives. From 1960 to 1970, hospital care expenditures tripled from $9.3 billion to $28 billion and physician service expenditures almost matched that growth rate, increasing from $5.3 billion to $13.6 billion.[6(pp257–258)] Federal and state governments were also feeling the burden of high health care costs. From 1965 to 1970, federal and state governments collectively experienced a 21% annual rate of increase in their health care expenditures.[4(p384)]

As is discussed in more detail later in this chapter, managed care moves away from the FFS system by integrating the payment for services and the delivery of services into one place in an attempt to rein in health care costs and utilization. The federal Health Maintenance Organization Act of 1973 was intended to spur the growth of managed care by providing incentives to increase the use of health maintenance organizations (HMOs). The act relied on federal loans and grants and a mandate that employers with 25 or more employees offer an HMO option if one was available in their area.[6(pp262–263)] Even so, managed care did not flourish due to opposition by patients who did not want their provider and service choices restricted, and by providers who did not want to lose control over their practices.

As health care cost and quality concerns remained a national priority, the managed care industry eventually found a foothold in the health insurance market. Indeed, enrollment in managed care doubled during the 1990s, with almost 80 million enrollees by 1998. In 2005 only 3% of workers were in conventional, nonmanaged care arrangements.[7] Although only about 12% of Medicare enrollees choose managed care arrangements, over 60% of Medicaid beneficiaries are in managed care, though for many of them it is mandatory that they receive services through a managed care arrangement.[8,9]

HOW HEALTH INSURANCE OPERATES

Before delving into the specifics of how health insurance functions, we want to emphasize two critical points: Participation in an insurance plan is a voluntary choice for all parties involved, and many health insurance products are lightly regulated by government. As a result, there is significant variation in the availability, affordability, and comprehensiveness of health insurance.

Insurers and employers are not required to offer health insurance coverage, and individuals are not required to purchase it. Furthermore, insurers have the power to select the employer and individual markets in which they operate, and this power is largely unconstrained by product design regulation. For example, insurers have a significant amount of flexibility to vary coverage by condition or population subgroup. This flexibility stems in part from the Employee Retirement

Box 4-1
Discussion Questions

Most people in this country obtain health insurance through employer-sponsored plans. Although the historical background you just read explains *why* this occurred, it does not discuss whether this is a good or bad thing. Is our reliance on employer-sponsored health insurance ideal for individuals? Providers? Employers? Society? What are the benefits and drawbacks to having employers as the primary source of health insurance? How different are the benefits and drawbacks when considered from various stakeholder perspectives? Would it be better to have more federal government involvement in providing health insurance? What primary policy goal would you use to decide how to answer these questions?

Income Security Act of 1974 (ERISA), a federal law that regulates "welfare benefit programs," including health plans, operated by private employers.[10,d] ERISA broadly (but not completely) preempts state laws that "relate to" employee benefit plans and does not supply federal standards to fill the resulting regulatory vacuum.[11] Because the federal government has largely deregulated private employer-sponsored coverage, and has not built a comprehensive scheme to compensate for the lack of affordable voluntary coverage, individuals often have a limited choice of affordable health insurance plans, no control over the terms of the plan, and little protection from federal or state governments.

This section provides an overview of the purpose and structure of health insurance. It begins with a review of basic health insurance terminology, considers the role of uncertainty and risk in insurance, and concludes with a discussion of how insurance companies set their premium rates.

Basic Terminology

As you read earlier, the health insurance industry first developed when the FFS system was standard. Under this system, not only do providers have incentive to conduct more and more expensive services, but patients are unbridled in their use of the health care system because FFS does not limit the use of services or accessibility to providers. As we will discuss later in this chapter, managed care developed as a response to the incentives created by the FFS system. However, even though there are numerous differences between FFS and managed care, many of the fundamental principles of how insurance operates are applicable to any type of health insurance contract. The following discussion reviews how health insurance works generally, regardless of the type of insurance arrangement.

The health insurance consumer (also known as the *beneficiary*) buys health insurance in advance for an annual fee, usually paid in monthly installments, called a *premium*.[e] In return, the health insurance carrier (or company) pays for all or part of the beneficiary's health care costs if she or he becomes ill or injured and has a covered medical need. (A covered need is a medical good or service that the insurer is obligated to pay for because it is covered based on the terms of the insurance contract or policy.) Insurance contracts cannot identify every conceivable health care need of beneficiaries, so they are generally structured to include categories of care (outpatient, inpatient, vision, maternity, etc.) to be provided if deemed medically necessary. Definitions of the term *medically necessary* vary by contract and are important when determining whether a procedure is covered.

Even if the beneficiary never needs health care services covered by the insurance policy, she still pays for the policy through premiums. The consumer benefits by having financial security in case of illness or injury, and the insurance company benefits by making money selling health insurance.

In addition to premiums, the beneficiary typically pays other costs under most health insurance policies. Many policies have *deductibles*. A deductible is the amount of money the beneficiary must pay on her own for her health care needs each year before the insurance carrier starts to help with the costs. For example, if a policyholder has a $500 deductible, the beneficiary must pay 100% of the first $500 of health care costs each year. The insurance carrier is not liable to cover any costs until the individual's health care bill reaches $501 in a given year. If the individual does not need more than $500 worth of health care in a specific year, the insurance carrier generally will not help that individual pay her health care costs.

Furthermore, a beneficiary generally continues to incur some costs in addition to the premiums even after the deductible has been met. Insurance carriers often impose cost sharing on the beneficiary through *co-payment* or *co-insurance* requirements. A co-payment is a set dollar amount the beneficiary pays when receiving a service from a provider. For example, many HMOs charge their beneficiaries $10 every time a beneficiary sees a primary care provider. Co-insurance refers to a percentage of the health care cost the individual must cover. For example, 20% is a common co-insurance amount. This means the beneficiary pays 20% of all health care costs after the deductible has been met, with the insurance carrier paying the other 80%.

Uncertainty

From a traditional economic perspective, insurance exists because of two basic concepts—risk and uncertainty. The world is full of risks—auto theft, house fires, physical disabilities—and uncertainty about whether any such events might affect a particular individual. As a result, people buy a variety of forms of insurance (e.g., automobile insurance, home insurance, life or disability insurance) to protect themselves and their families against the financial consequences of these unfortunate and unforeseen events.

Although genetic predisposition or behavioral choices such as smoking or working a high-risk job may increase the chances that an individual will suffer from a health-related problem, in general there is a high level of uncertainty as to whether a particular person will become sick or injured and need medical assistance. Health insurance protects the consumer from medical costs associated with both expensive and unforeseen events. Even if the consumer does not experience a negative event, a benefit exists from the peace of mind and reduced uncertainty of financial exposure that insurance provides.

In terms of health status and wise use of resources, when insurance allows consumers to purchase necessary services they would not otherwise be able to afford, it functions in a positive manner. Conversely, when insurance leads consumers to purchase unnecessary health care goods or services of low value because the consumer is not paying full cost, it works in a negative manner. The difficult task is trying to figure out how to set the consumer's share of the burden at just the right point to encourage and make available the proper use of health care, while discouraging improper usage.

Risk

Risk is a central concern in insurance. Consumers buy insurance to protect themselves against the risk of unforeseen and costly events. But health insurers are also concerned about risk—the risk that their beneficiaries will experience a covered medical event.

Individuals purchase health insurance to protect themselves against the risk of financial consequences of health care needs. Because of differences in risk level, individuals who are generally healthy or otherwise do not anticipate having health expenses may place a lower value on insurance than individuals who are unhealthy or those who are healthy but expect to have medical expenses, such as pregnant women. Therefore, healthy individuals tend to seek out lower-cost insurance plans or refrain from obtaining insurance altogether if it is not, in their view, cost effective. Unhealthy individuals or healthy individuals who often use the health care system would obviously prefer a low-cost insurance plan (with comprehensive benefits) but are generally more willing to pay higher premiums because of the value they place on having insurance.

Health insurance carriers are businesses that need to cover their expenditures, including the cost of accessing capital needed to run their company, to stay in the market.[f] They earn money by collecting premiums from their beneficiaries, and they pay out money to cover their beneficiaries health care costs above the deductible amount and to cover the costs of running a business (overhead, marketing, taxes, etc.). One way health insurance companies survive is to make sure the premiums charged to beneficiaries cover these costs. From the insurance carrier's perspective, it would be ideal to be able to charge lower premiums to attract healthy individuals who are less likely to use their benefits, and higher premiums to unhealthy individuals who are more likely to need medical care.

However, insurance companies have difficulty matching healthy people with low-cost plans and unhealthy people with high-cost plans because of the problem of *asymmetric information*. This is the term economists use when one party to a trans-

Box 4-2
Discussion Questions

As a general matter, all types of insurance under traditional economic models cover expensive and unforeseen events, not events that have small financial risk or little uncertainty.[12(p195)] For example, auto insurance does not cover regular maintenance such as an oil change, and home insurance does not protect against normal wear and tear, such as the need to replace an old carpet. Accordingly, many economists argue that health insurance should not cover regular, foreseeable events such as physical exams or low-cost occurrences such as vaccinations. Other economists support a different school of thought. An alternative economic view is that health insurance should insure one's health, not just offer protection against the financial consequences of major adverse health events. Because people without health insurance are less likely to obtain preventive care such as physical exams or vaccinations, these economists believe it is in everyone's best interest, ethically and financially, to promote preventive care. Therefore, it is appropriate for insurance to cover both unpredictable and expensive events as well as predictable and less expensive events.

Which theory do you support? What do you think is the best use of insurance? If insurance does not cover low-cost and predictable events, should another resource be available to assist individuals, or should people pay out of their own pockets for these health care needs?

action has more information than the other party. In the case of insurance, the imbalance often favors the consumer because insurance carriers generally do not know as much as the individual does about the individual's health care needs and personal habits. Although relatively healthy low-cost individuals want to make their status known because insurance carriers might be willing to sell them an insurance product for a lower price, relatively unhealthy individuals do not want their status known because insurance companies might charge them higher premiums. For this reason, when an insurance carrier lacks complete information it is more beneficial to unhealthy beneficiaries than to healthy ones.

Together, uncertainty about risk and the presence of asymmetric information lead to the problem of *adverse selection*. In terms of health insurance, adverse selection is when unhealthy people over-select (that is, select beyond a random distribution) a particular plan. This occurs because people at risk for having high health care costs choose a particular plan because of that plan's attractive coverage rules.[13(pp12–13)] The consumer who knows he is a high risk for needing services will be more likely to choose a more comprehensive plan because it covers more services, even though it is probably a more expensive option. This leaves the insurer that offers the comprehensive plan with a disproportionate number of high-risk beneficiaries. As a result of the relatively high-risk pool, beneficiaries will have high service utilization rates and, in turn, the insurance carrier would need to raise premiums to be able to pay for the increased cost of covering services for beneficiaries. In turn, some of the healthier individuals might choose to leave the plan because of the higher premiums, resulting in an even riskier beneficiary pool and even higher premiums, and the cycle continues. The healthier consumers may find a lower-cost plan or may choose to go without health insurance, while the insurance plan is left with an increasingly higher percentage of relatively unhealthy people. This is the problem of adverse selection.

One instance where adverse selection is a key concern is with an increasingly popular type of health plan, the high deductible health plan (HDHP). As the name suggests, these plans have very high deductibles (usually defined as at least $1,000 for an individual or $2,000 for a family). Annual premiums for the average HDHP plan cost individuals over $3,000 and families over $7,000.[14] As with other insurance plans, consumers pay most of their health care expenses out-of-pocket until they reach the deductible.[g] HDHPs are often used in conjunction with health reimbursement arrangements (HRAs) or health savings accounts (HSAs), which allow individuals to set aside money for future health care needs. HRAs are funded solely by employers, who usually commit to making a specified amount of money available for health care expenses incurred by employees or their dependents. HSAs are created by individuals, but employers may also contribute to HSAs if the employers offer a qualified HDHP. Individual contributions to HSAs are made with pre-income tax dollars, and withdrawals to pay for qualified health care expenses are also not taxed. High-deductible plans are increasingly popular with employers, with 20% of them offering one in 2005 and another 26% indicating they might offer one in 2006.[14] However, only 2.4 million workers were enrolled in an HDHP in 2005.[14]

Those who support HDHPs assert that high deductible plans promote personal responsibility because enrollees have a financial incentive to avoid overutilizing the health care system and to choose cost-effective treatment options. As a result, HDHPs are favored by employers and others as a cost-cutting strategy. Others are concerned that HDHPs will result in adverse selection, harming low-income and unhealthy individuals. Critics argue that enrollees of high deductible plans are more likely to be wealthier and healthier individuals who can afford high out-of-pocket expenses and are less likely to use the health care system.[15] As a result, relatively poorer and sicker individuals will choose a comprehensive group health insurance plan (assuming one is available and affordable), resulting in plans facing the possibility of adverse selection due to having a relatively high-risk insurance pool. In addition, there are concerns that employers will replace their more expensive comprehensive plan options with HDHPs, potentially resulting in less affordable health care for poorer and sicker individuals. Finally, critics also contend that the lower service utilization associated with HDHP enrollees is due to their better health status, not price sensitivity, undermining one of the main arguments in support of these plans.[15]

Setting Premiums

Assuming that insurance companies make their decisions in the context of asymmetric information, they cannot determine with certainty the appropriate amount of premium to charge each individual. Instead, insurance companies rely on making educated guesses about the risk each individual or group of individuals has of needing health care services. The two main methods of setting premiums are *experience rating* and *community rating*.

Box 4-3
Discussion Questions

In general, people with low incomes or no health insurance (or both) tend to be less healthy than those who are financially better off or insured (or both). As a result, policy proposals that suggest including poor, uninsured individuals in already-existing insurance plans are met with resistance by individuals in those plans and by carriers or employers who operate them. Yet, if an insurance plan is created that only subscribes a less healthy poor or uninsured population, it is likely to be an unattractive business opportunity because beneficiaries are likely to need a high quantity of health care that will be costly to provide.

Given what you know about adverse selection and risk, what, in your opinion, is the best way to provide insurance coverage to the poor and uninsured? Should they be included in current plans? Should the government provide financial incentives for private carriers to insure them? Should a separate plan or program be created to serve them? In these various scenarios, what incentives are created for plans, current plan members, government, and so on? Can HDHPs work for a low-income population?

When insurance companies use experience rating to make an educated guess about the risk of someone's needing health care services, they are relying on how much a beneficiary or group of beneficiaries spent on medical services previously to determine the amount of the premium for each member or group. Thus, if an individual or group had very high medical costs in a given year, premiums are likely to rise the following year. Conversely, community rating does not take into account health status or claims history when setting premiums. In "pure" community rating insurers use only geography and family composition to set rates. In "modified" community rating, insurers may be allowed to consider other characteristics such as age and gender. Regardless of how community rating premiums are set, each person in the group is charged the same rate.

Which rating system makes more sense from a policy perspective as a basis for setting premiums may depend on whether you evaluate the insurance market based on efficiency or equity (think back to the first chapter and the discussion of competing conceptual frameworks). If the market is judged based on efficiency, then the key issue is whether the optimal amount of risk has shifted from consumers to insurers. If there are individuals willing to pay a higher amount for greater coverage and insurers willing to provide greater coverage for the higher amount, but something in the market prevents this transaction from occurring, then the optimal amount of risk shifting has not occurred. Or, if individuals value a certain level of insurance coverage at a price that is less than the price at which insurers are willing to provide that coverage, but individuals buy coverage anyway at the higher price, the market is not optimally efficient (due to excess coverage).

Conversely, the market may be judged based on equity or fairness. Even the most efficient market may result in some inequities. Some individuals may be uninsured, some may have

to pay more than other individuals for the same level of insurance, some may not be able to purchase the level of coverage they desire, and some individuals may not be able to join a particular plan. These inequities are often a concern in the context of the uninsured, especially as uninsurance relates to low-income individuals or those with high health needs due to random events, such as an accident or genetic condition.

Regardless of the underwriting methodology used, premiums are cheaper for people purchasing insurance as part of a large group rather than buying health insurance individually or as part of a small group. Due to the law of averages,[h] larger groups of people are more likely to have an average risk rate. When people join a group for reasons unrelated to health status, such as working for the same company, it is also more likely that the group will have an average risk rate. Groups with average risk rates are attractive to insurers because the cost of insuring a few unhealthy people will probably be offset by savings from insuring many healthy ones. Conversely, in smaller groups it is more likely that the group will have a relatively high risk rate and less likely that the cost of insuring an unhealthy person can be offset by the savings of insuring a few other healthy people.[i] This is the problem faced by Ms. Tevet, the small business owner described at the outset of the chapter who has one high-cost employee. Even though she would like to offer health insurance coverage to her employees, Ms. Tevet and other small business owners like her often are able to offer only expensive or limited coverage, if they can offer any health insurance benefit at all. In order to help individuals and small business owners like Ms. Tevet, some states require insurers to use a community rating system to set premiums for these groups.

Carriers also prefer to insure large groups because most of the administrative costs associated with insurance are the same whether the carrier is covering a few people or a few thousand.[16(pp342–344)] In fact, group coverage has traditionally required fewer marketing resources than individual coverage, which targets customers one at a time. However, the proliferation of information on the Internet may change this equation.

Medical Underwriting

The prior discussion about rate setting assumed asymmetric information (i.e., where the insurer has little information about the consumer's health status and the consumer has substantial information about his or her own health care needs.) Of course, there are ways for insurers to gain information about the medical needs of a consumer looking to join a health plan: Physical exams, questionnaires, medical records, occupation, and demographics all provide clues about the health status of the consumer. Although it is much more difficult to accomplish, insurers may also try to predict an individual's future

Box 4-4
Discussion Questions

What populations or types of people pay more under experience rating? Does experience rating create any incentives for individuals to act in a certain way? What populations or types of people pay more under community rating? Does community rating create any incentives for individuals to act in a certain way? Which rating system seems preferable to you? What trade-offs are most important to you? Should the focus be on the good of the individual or the good of the community? Are these mutually exclusive concerns?

costs through questionnaires that ask, for example, whether an individual engages in risky activities (e.g., riding a motorcycle) or through genetic testing (which is itself an emerging health policy and law issue).

Whether companies are allowed to consider an applicant's medical history or other personal information to help assess risk of health care needs in the future—a practice referred to as medical underwriting—is a somewhat complicated legal question that involves both federal and state law. In terms of federal law, the Health Insurance Portability and Accountability Act of 1996 (HIPAA)[17] includes an important protection for consumers by prohibiting group health plans from excluding or limiting otherwise qualified individuals due to pre-existing conditions. A pre-existing condition is a medical condition, such as cancer or diabetes, that is present at the time an individual applies to enroll in an insurance plan. Prior to HIPAA, many individuals with pre-existing conditions were denied insurance altogether, denied coverage for particular medical care, or charged very high premiums if they sought to purchase a policy. These practices led to a problem referred to as "job lock." Because most Americans receive insurance coverage through their employers, many employees with pre-existing conditions could not switch jobs for fear that their new company's insurance policy would be denied to them on account of their pre-existing condition. One study estimated that job lock resulted in a 4% reduction in voluntary turnover.[16(p341)]

Under HIPAA, however, group policies are no longer allowed to deny coverage to an applicant due to a particular condition, or charge varying premiums based on medical conditions. Furthermore, although HIPAA does not regulate the amount of premiums that may be charged, all members of a group generally pay the same premium due to HIPAA's nondiscrimination provisions. These provisions prohibit plans or insurance carriers from requiring any individual to pay a higher premium or contribution than another "similarly situated" individual[18,j] in the plan based on eight health factors: health status, physical or mental medical conditions, claims experience (i.e., the individual has a history of high health claims), receipt of health care, medical history, genetic information, evidence of insurability, and disability.[19,k] However, recall that those who purchase individual health insurance plans are not covered by HIPAA's protections.

As noted in the beginning of this section, states play the primary role in insurance regulation. Whether insurers are allowed to use any or all of the medical underwriting techniques described above on purchasers of individual policies is generally a matter of state law. Consumers who purchase individual insurance policies are generally provided fewer protections than those in group plans. In most states, insurance companies

Box 4-5
Discussion Questions

As discussed earlier, risk and uncertainty are important concepts in health insurance. Individuals purchase health insurance policies to protect themselves financially against health care costs, and insurance carriers try to set premiums that will cover the cost of the services used by their beneficiaries. Currently (when allowed by law), insurance carriers may consider factors such as medical history, demographics, type of occupation, size of the beneficiary pool, and similar criteria when setting the terms of an insurance policy. Should health insurance carriers also have access to and be able to use genetic testing results when carriers decide whether to insure an individual, what premiums to charge, or which services to cover?

If you think the answer to that question should be "no," why is genetic information different from all of the other kinds of information insurance carriers may take into account when making those decisions? Conversely, what is the strongest argument you can make in favor of allowing insurance carriers to consider an applicant's genetic information? How would allowing genetic testing alter an individual's or a provider's diagnosis and treatment decisions? What is the primary policy goal that affects your view?

are allowed to use medical underwriting for individual plan purchasers and reject an applicant as too high a risk, impose limitations on coverage, or charge relatively high premiums based on medical conditions.[20] However, many states have passed laws restricting the use of genetic testing by insurers. The type of restrictions in place and type of insurance policy regulated (i.e., group and/or individual policy) varies by state.[21]

MANAGED CARE

The prior sections reviewed the history, basic structure, and purpose of health insurance generally. In this section, we discuss a specific kind of health insurance structure that has come to dominate the American market—managed care. We will describe why managed care emerged, some of the frequent cost-containment strategies used by managed care organizations, and the most common managed care structures in the market today.

Managed care became the predominant health care financing and delivery arrangement in the United States because health care costs had risen to alarming levels and there were few mechanisms for containing costs under the FFS system. As mentioned earlier, FFS does not create incentives for providers or patients to utilize health care services sparingly. Providers have an incentive under FFS to provide more services and more expensive services (but not necessarily higher quality services), because their income rises with each procedure or office visit and fees are higher for more expensive services. As long as providers are accessible, insured patients can request services and assume their insurance company will pay most or all of the costs to the extent that the services are covered by the health plan and medically necessary.

In addition, the FFS system does not create incentives for providers or patients to use the lowest-cost quality care available. Many people believe specialists provide higher quality care and turn to them even for minor needs that do not truly require expensive specialty services, and the FFS system does not discourage this behavior. Furthermore, because traditional insurance coverage requires a specific diagnosis for reimbursement, patients are discouraged from seeking preventative services when they are symptom-free under FFS.[22(p332)] At the same time, traditional insurance companies do not have the ability to control costs or quality of care under FFS. Their job is limited to determining whether a service is covered and medically necessary and providing the agreed-upon reimbursement. They have little ability to measure or improve the quality of care provided by health care professionals and cannot control costs by limiting the amount or type of services received; instead they can only raise premiums and other rates in the future to cover increasing costs.

To alter the inherent incentives under FFS and to grant insurers some ability to control the quality and utilization of services, managed care integrates the provision of and payment for health care services. Through various strategies discussed in the following sections, managed care organizations (MCOs) and managed care plans create incentives to provide fewer services and less expensive care, while still maintaining the appropriate level of health care quality. MCOs also attempt to alter patients' decision making through cost-sharing requirements, cost containment tools, utilization restrictions, and free or low-cost coverage for preventive care.

MCOs take various forms, but certain general features apply to all of them to varying degrees. All MCOs provide a comprehensive, defined package of benefits to the purchaser/member for a pre-set fee (including both monthly premium and cost-sharing requirements). Services are offered to members through a network of providers, all of whom have a contractual relationship with the MCO. MCOs choose which providers to include in their networks and what services are rendered by network providers. Most notably, they also use fi-

nancial incentives and other mechanisms to control the delivery, use, quality, and cost of services in ways that are not present in FFS insurance systems.[6(p260)]

Cost Containment and Utilization Tools

Managed care introduced a variety of tools in its attempt to contain costs and control health care service utilization. The cost containment strategies of *performance-based salary bonuses or withholdings*, *discounted fee schedules*, and *capitated payments* shift financial risk or limit payments to providers who, in turn, have an incentive to choose the least costly but still effective treatment option. The utilization control strategies of *gatekeeping* and *utilization review* focus on making sure that only appropriate and necessary care is provided to patients. Another type of strategy, *case management*, is designed to make sure that necessary care is provided in the most coordinated and cost-effective way possible.

Provider Payment Tools

Depending on the structure of the MCO, providers are paid by salary, discounted fee schedule, or capitation rate. Providers in what are called staff-model MCOs are employees of the MCO and are paid an annual salary. The salary structure often includes bonuses or salary withholdings that are paid (or withheld) upon meeting (or not meeting) utilization or performance goals, thus shifting some financial risk from the MCO to the provider. A discounted fee schedule is a service-specific fee system as is used in FFS. However, an MCO-style fee schedule pays lower reimbursement rates than is true in FFS systems; providers agree to accept less than their usual fee in return for the large volume of patients available to them by being a part of the MCO provider network. The MCO retains the financial risk in a discounted fee system, but the costs are lower for the company due to the discounted rate paid to providers. Finally, a capitated payment rate is a fixed monthly sum per member that the provider receives regardless of the number or type of services provided to patients. The physician receiving the capitated rate is responsible for providing all of the care needed by his or her MCO patients, within the provider's scope of practice. As a result, the financial risk in the case of capitated arrangements is shifted entirely from the MCO to the provider. Depending on the contract between the provider and MCO, the insurance company may or may not guarantee the provider a minimum number of patients in exchange for accepting a capitated rate. These provider-focused cost containment strategies are summarized in Table 4-1.

Both the salaried and capitation payment methods have very different incentives for providers than is the case under the FFS system. Instead of being paid more for doing more, MCO

TABLE 4-1 Provider Payment Cost Containment Strategies

Strategy	Provider Payment Method	How Costs Are Controlled	Who Assumes Financial Risk
Salary and bonuses/withholds	Provider receives a salary as an employee of an MCO	Incentive for provider to perform fewer and/or less costly services	MCO and provider
Discounted fee schedule	Provider receives a lower fee than under FFS for each service to members.	Pays provider less per service rendered than under FFS	MCO (but also has lower costs)
Capitation	Provider receives a set payment per month for each member regardless of services provided	Incentive for provider to perform fewer and/or less costly services	Provider

providers are paid the same amount regardless of the number or type of services they provide. Given the use of bonuses and withholdings, salaried providers may be paid more if they make treatment decisions deemed favorable by an MCO. By using these incentives, MCOs encourage providers to render the fewest and most cost-effective services necessary.

Critics of managed care payment methodologies argue that MCO plan members will not receive all necessary care if providers are incentivized to provide fewer services and less costly care. Instead of treating patients using both the most cost-efficient and medically necessary services, critics claim MCOs encourage providers to save money by providing fewer services and less specialized care than necessary. MCOs counter that their own incentive is to keep their members healthy so they do not need expensive services in the future. In addition, MCOs point to their ability to impose quality control measures on providers as a way to ensure that patients are properly treated. In response, critics argue that because members switch health plans relatively frequently, MCOs do not have an incentive to keep their members healthy because the MCOs will not realize the long-term savings as members come and go.

Which side has the better argument? There is no definitive answer. On the one hand, studies have found that treatment decisions under MCO arrangements are mostly influenced by clinical factors (not economic ones), that there is little or no measurable difference in the health outcomes of patients in FFS versus managed care plans, that the quality of care provided under FFS and managed care plans is basically equal, and that most Americans are satisfied with their health plan, whether it is FFS or through an MCO.[22(pp351–352)] On the other hand, studies have also shown that mental health patients do not fare as well in MCOs as in FFS plans; that nonprofit HMOs

(a type of MCO) score better on quality measures than for-profit ones; and that managed care enrollees are less likely than FFS patients to give excellent ratings to their plan overall, the quality of services they receive, access to specialty care, and time spent with physicians.[22(pp351–352)]

Utilization Control Tools

MCOs also employ other techniques, not related to provider payment methods, to control use of health care services. Once again, the goal in using these tools is to reduce the use of unnecessary and costly services. We review three common utilization control tools: gatekeeping, utilization review, and case management.

Gatekeepers monitor and control the services a patient receives. Members of managed care plans are often required to select a primary care provider from the MCO network upon enrollment. This provider acts as the member's "gatekeeper" and is responsible for providing primary care, referring patients for additional care, and generally coordinating the patient's care. Having a gatekeeper allows the MCO, not the patient or specialty provider, to determine when a patient needs additional or specialty services, diagnostic tests, hospital admissions, and the like. As with the cost containment strategies discussed earlier, there are critics who contend that utilization-based bonuses or salary withholdings give gatekeepers financial incentive not to provide specialty referrals even when it is in the best interest of the patient.

Utilization review (UR) allows an MCO to evaluate the appropriateness of the services provided and to deny payment for unnecessary services. MCO personnel review and approve or deny the services performed or recommended by network providers. UR specialists are often health care professionals, and MCOs generally use existing clinical care guidelines to determine whether services are appropriate.

UR may occur prospectively, concurrently, or retrospectively. Prospective UR means that an MCO reviews the appropriateness of treatment before a service is rendered. A request for a recommended service is sent to a UR panel for approval or denial. A denial does not mean a patient cannot move forward with his preferred treatment plan; however, it does mean that the patient will have to pay for the treatment out of his own pocket. Prospective UR is distinguished from concurrent UR, which is when the MCO review of the appropriateness of treatment occurs while treatment is being rendered. For example, a patient may need a procedure that requires hospitalization. Even though the procedure is performed and covered, a UR specialist might still determine the number of days the patient may remain in the hospital or whether certain services, such as home care or physical therapy, will be covered upon discharge from the hospital. Finally, retrospective review means the MCO reviews the appropriateness of treatment (and therefore its coverage) after a service is rendered. In this case, a patient's medical records are reviewed to determine whether the care provided was appropriate and billed accurately; MCOs will not provide reimbursement for services deemed inappropriate or unnecessary. This latter type of review may also be used to uncover provider practice patterns and determine incentive compensation.[22(p339)] Regardless of when the review occurs, the use of UR is controversial because it may interfere with the patient–provider relationship and allow for second-guessing of provider treatment decisions by a third party who is not part of the diagnosis and treatment discussions.

Case management is a service utilization approach that uses trained personnel to manage and coordinate patient care. Although gatekeeping serves as a basic form of case management for all members, many patients with complex or chronic conditions, such as HIV/AIDS or spinal cord injuries, may benefit from more intensive case management. These patients may have frequent need for care from various specialists and thus benefit from assistance by personnel who are familiar with the many resources available to care for the patient and who are able to provide information and assistance to patients and their families. A case manager works with providers to determine what care is necessary and to help arrange for patients to receive that care in the most appropriate and cost-effective settings.[22(pp336–337)] Although the general idea of case management is not controversial, some people believe it can be implemented in a manner that acts more as a barrier than an asset to care because additional approval is needed before a patient receives care and because another layer of bureaucracy is placed between the patient and the provider. Table 4-2 summarizes the three service utilization control strategies just discussed.

As you might imagine, managed care's use of service utilization control mechanisms frequently leads to disputes between patients and their managed care company over whether the company is improperly affecting the provider–patient relationship (and negatively impacting the quality of care provided) by making decisions as to the type or quantity of care a patient should receive. This is both a highly charged health policy issue and a complicated legal issue, and one we discuss in more detail in Chapter 8. For purposes of this chapter, it is enough to note that MCOs must have a grievance and appeal process to at least initially handle these sorts of disputes. Although companies' processes differ in their specifics, they generally allow members to appeal a coverage decision, provide evidence to support the appeal, and receive an expedited resolution when medically necessary. The need for adequate grievance and appeal procedures can be particularly acute for patients with special health care needs, such as those with physical or mental disabilities, and patients who otherwise use the health care system more frequently than most.

TABLE 4-2 Service Utilization Control Strategies

Strategy	Description	Potential Concerns
Gatekeeper	Uses a primary care provider to make sure only necessary and appropriate care is provided.	Gatekeepers may have financial incentive to approve fewer services or less costly care.
Utilization review	Uses MCO personnel to review and approve or deny services requested by a provider to make sure only necessary and appropriate care is provided.	Interferes with patient–provider relationship; someone other than the patient's provider decides whether treatment is appropriate.
Case management	Uses MCO personnel to manage and coordinate patient care to make sure care is provided in the most cost-effective manner.	May act as a barrier to receiving care if the case manager does not approve a desired service or service provider.

Common Managed Care Structures

There are three managed care structures common in the market today: health maintenance organizations (HMOs), preferred provider organizations (PPOs), and point-of-service
plans (POS). All three provide preventive and specialty care,
but the rules relating to accessing care differ for each. In general, HMOs have the most restrictive rules pertaining to patients and providers, PPOs have the least restrictive rules, and
POSs fall in the middle.

Initially, HMOs were the most common MCO structure,
but PPOs have gained popularity in recent years; in 2005, PPOs
insured 61% of employees with health insurance, followed by
HMOs at 21% and POSs at 15%.[23] Only 3% of workers are in
conventional FFS plans today, a striking decrease from the 46%
covered by such plans in 1993.[22(pp336–337),7] In general, the
more control an HMO has over its providers and members, the
easier it is to control utilization of services and, therefore,
health care costs and quality. Conversely, providers and patients prefer to have as much autonomy as possible, so the
more restrictive HMO structures may be less desirable in that
respect. However, the distinctions among managed care structures have become blurred recently because of the consumer
and provider backlash against MCO restrictions.

Health Maintenance Organizations

When managed care first became prominent in the 1970s,
HMOs were the most common type of MCO. There are several characteristics shared by all HMOs:

- They pay providers a salary or a monthly capitated rate
  per member to cover the cost of any and all services that
  beneficiaries need within a provider's scope of practice.

- They coordinate and control receipt of services.
- They arrange for care using only their network providers.
- They are responsible for providing care according to es-
  tablished quality standards.

Despite these commonalities, HMOs may be structured
through a variety of models, including staff-model/closed panel,
group model, network model, individual practice associations
(IPAs), and direct contract model.[22(pp340–344)] Each model has
advantages and disadvantages from the perspective of the
HMO, its providers, and its members, as shown in Table 4-3.

Preferred Provider Organizations

As is evident from Table 4-3, every form of HMO is fairly restrictive. In all models, the HMO provides coverage only if
members seek care from network providers and providers may
or may not be limited to serving only HMO members. As both
patients and providers began rebelling over these restrictions,
new forms of MCOs emerged, often formed by providers and
hospitals themselves.

Like HMOs, PPOs have a provider network, referred to
as preferred providers. Unlike HMOs, however, PPOs provide
coverage to patients seeking care from any provider, regardless
of whether the provider is part of the member's PPO preferred
provider network. However, the amount of the service price
that the PPO will cover is greater for an in-network provider
than an out-of-network provider. For example, a PPO may
agree to cover 80% of the cost for an in-network physician
visit but only 70% of the cost for a similar, but out-of-network
physician visit. PPO patients thus have the option of paying
more but choosing among a greater number of providers or
paying less but choosing among a more limited number of
(in-network) providers. In addition, a PPO member's cost-
sharing responsibilities are often higher than is the case for
HMO members.

In exchange for being in the network, providers agree to
accept a discounted rate for their services, often 25–35% below
their usual rates.[21(p345)] Because PPO members have a financial incentive to seek providers who are in-network, these
health care professionals find it worthwhile to accept a reduced
rate from the PPO in exchange for the higher likelihood that
PPO members will select them over non-network providers.
Furthermore, unlike the capitation system found in HMOs,
PPO providers do not assume financial risk for providing services. Depending on the terms of their contract with the PPO,
preferred providers may or may not agree to limit their practice to PPO members. Although it is rare, PPOs may choose to
guarantee preferred providers a minimum number of patients.

Even though an MCO has much less control over service
utilization in the PPO model than the HMO model, PPOs still

TABLE 4-3 Key Characteristics of Common HMO Models

HMO Model	HMO–Provider Relationship and Payment Type	Provider Employment Arrangement	Must Members Seek Care from Network?	May Providers Care for Nonmembers?	General Comments
Staff-model/ closed panel	HMO employs providers, pays a salary, often includes bonuses or withholds.	Employed by HMO.	Yes	No	Provides services only in HMO's office and affiliated hospitals. Relatively speaking, HMO has the most control over providers and service utilization, but has fixed costs of building and staff. HMO may contract with outside providers if necessary. Providers and consumers often do not like restrictions imposed by HMO. Providers do not need to solicit patients. Consumers may find it most cost-effective option.
Group	HMO contracts with one multi-specialty group for a capitated rate.	Employed by own provider group.	Yes	Depends on terms of contract	HMO has less control over utilization. HMO contracts for hospital care on a prepaid or FFS basis. Providers may prefer this model because they remain independent as opposed to becoming an employee of the HMO and because they may serve nonmembers if their contract permits.
Network	HMO contracts with several group practices (often primary care practices) for a capitated rate.	Employed by own provider group.	Yes	Depends on terms of contract	The group practices may make referrals, but are financially responsible for reimbursing outside providers. HMO has less control over utilization due to greater number of contracts and ability of providers to subcontract. Providers may prefer additional autonomy, but also take on financial risk of providing primary and specialty care. Members may have a relatively greater choice of providers.
IPA	HMO contracts with IPA for a capitated rate.	IPA is intermediary between HMO and solo practitioners and groups. IPA pays providers a capitated rate.	Yes	Depends on terms of contract	HMO has reduced control over providers but may have less malpractice liability because IPA is an intermediary.[1] HMO may contract with specialty physicians as needed and for hospital care on a prepaid or FFS basis. Providers may prefer contracting with IPA instead of HMO to retain more autonomy. Members may have greater choice of providers.
Direct contract	HMO contracts directly with individual providers for a capitated rate.	Self-employed.	Yes	Depends on terms of contract	HMO has more leverage over providers because it contracts with them as individuals, but its administrative costs are much higher than having one contract or a few contracts with groups. Providers have less leverage regarding practice restrictions when contracting on an individual basis.

Box 4-7
Discussion Questions

In terms of containing health care costs and improving health care quality, do you think health care consumers and professionals need even more restrictions than are currently used in managed care? Are there any reasons to revert back to the FFS system, even knowing its inflationary qualities? If you think that managed care is not the answer to our still-rising health care costs and quality concerns, what other tools might help lower costs and improve the quality of care? Should any tools be imposed by government regulation or agreed to voluntarily by insurers and the insured?

provide more incentives to use care judiciously than is the case in an FFS system. For example, in-network PPO providers are paid less than their customary rate by the company when they provide care to PPO members and often agree to abide by any utilization review strategies used by the PPO. In addition, PPO patients have an incentive to use certain lower-cost providers who will cost them less and have cost-sharing requirements unlike anything found under FFS. The PPO model attempts to locate a middle ground between the very restrictive HMO models and the FFS structure that resulted in very high health care utilization and costs.

Point of Service Plans

In another effort to contain costs while still providing patients the freedom to choose their provider, POS plans combine features of HMOs and PPOs. Like an HMO, POS plans have a provider network, use a capitated or other payment system that shares financial risk with providers, and requires members to use a gatekeeper to help control service utilization. However, designated services may be obtained from out-of-network providers who are paid on an FFS basis, but use of these providers costs the member more money, as with the PPO model. A POS gatekeeper must approve all in-network care and may also have some control over out-of-network care, depending on the terms of the plan. The call by many consumers for increased choice in providers has become forceful enough that some HMOs are now offering POS plans, which they may refer to as open-ended (as opposed to closed panel) models.

The Future of Managed Care

Managed care is likely to remain an integral part of the health system despite its drawbacks. Patients chafe at utilization restrictions, as is evident by the increase in PPO popularity and the emergence of the hybrid HMO/POS. Accurate or not, there is a widespread perception that managed care plans deny necessary care and provide lower quality care.[22(p352)] Providers also complain that managed care interferes with their ability to practice medicine in a manner of their choosing, placing them in ethical dilemmas due to the use of financial incentives and possibly lowering the quality of care they provide due to limits on tests and procedures they order. Yet, the key circumstance that led to the creation of managed care—high health care expenditures—has not abated. While the country struggles with ever-growing health care costs, even under managed care, the willingness to experiment with various cost and utilization containment strategies is likely to remain in place.

CONCLUSION

This introduction to health insurance serves as a building block for subsequent chapters, which expand upon many of the key health policy and law themes mentioned here. Even at this early stage, it should be clear to you that health policy analysts and decision makers must be particularly attuned to health insurance issues; without knowing both the basic structure of health insurance and how various incentives impact the actions of health care consumers, professionals, and insurance carriers, they cannot make informed recommendations and policies addressing the key health issues of the day.

REFERENCES

1. U.S. Bureau of the Census. *Income, Poverty, and Health Insurance Coverage in the United States: 2005.* Washington, D.C.: Economics and Statistics Administration, Bureau of the U.S. Census; 2006.

2. Kaiser Family Foundation and Health Research and Educational Trust. *Employer Health Benefits Survey 2005.* Menlo Park, Calif.: Kaiser Family Foundation; 2005: Section 2. Available at: http://www.kff.org/insurance/7315/sections/ehbs05-sec2-1.cfm. Accessed August 1, 2006.

3. Kaiser Family Foundation. State health facts—total Medicare beneficiaries. Available at: www.statehealthfacts.org/cgi-bin/healthfacts.cgi?action=compare&category=Medicare&subcategory=Medicare+Enrollment&topic=Total+Medicare+Beneficiaries. Accessed August 1, 2006.

4. Starr P. *The Social Transformation of American Medicine: The Rise of a Sovereign Profession and the Making of a Vast Industry.* New York: Basic Books; 1982.

5. Stevens R, Stevens R. *Welfare Medicine in America: A Case Study of Medicaid.* New Brunswick, N.J.: Transaction Publishers; 2003.

6. Sultz HA, Young KM. *Health Care USA: Understanding Its Organization and Delivery,* 3rd ed. Gaithersburg, Md.: Aspen Publishers; 2001.

7. Kaiser Family Foundation and Health Research and Educational Trust. *Employer Health Benefits Survey 2005.* Menlo Park, Calif.: Kaiser Family Foundation; 2005: Exhibit 5.1. Available at: http://www.kff.org/insurance/7315/sections/ehbs05-5-1.cfm. Accessed August 1, 2006.

8. Kaiser Family Foundation. *Medicare at a Glance.* Menlo Park, Calif.: Kaiser Family Foundation; 2005. Available at: http://www.kff.org/medicare/1066-08.cfm. Accessed August 1, 2006.

9. Center for Medicare and Medicaid Services. 2004 Medicaid managed care enrollment report, managed care trends. Available at http://www.cms.hhs.gov/medicaid/managedcare/trends04.pdf. Accessed August 1, 2006.

10. 88 Stat. 832.

11. ERISA § 514, 29 U.S.C. § 1144.

12. Council of Economic Advisors. Health care and insurance. In: *Economic Report of the President.* Washington, D.C.: GPO; 2004:195.

13. Penner S. *Introduction to Health Care Economics and Financial Management: Fundamental Concepts with Practical Application.* Philadelphia: Lippincott Williams and Wilkins; 2004.

14. Kaiser Family Foundation and Health Research and Educational Trust. *Employer Health Benefits Survey 2005.* Menlo Park, Calif.: Kaiser Family Foundation; 2005: Section 8. Available at: http://www.kff.org/insurance/7315/sections/upload/7315Section8.pdf. Accessed August 1, 2006.

15. Davis K. Consumer-directed health care: will it improve system performance? *Health Serv Res.* 2004;39:1219–1233.

16. Phelps CE. *Health Economics,* 3rd ed. Boston: Addison-Wesley; 2003.

17. Pub. L. No. 104-191, 110 Stat. 1936 *codified* in sections 18, 26, 29, and 42 U.S.C.

18. Nondiscrimination in Health Coverage in the Group Market; Interim Final Rules and Proposed Rules, 66 Fed. Reg. 1378, 1382 (January 2001) *codified* in 29 CFR 2590.702.

19. 42 U.S.C. § 300gg-1; Nondiscrimination in Health Coverage in the Group Market; Interim Final Rules and Proposed Rules, 1378–1384, 1396–1403.

20. Pollitz K, Sorian R. Ensuring health security: is the individual market ready for prime time? *Health Affairs.* Oct. 23, 2001; Web Exclusive:W372–W376. http://content.healthaffairs.org/cgi/reprint/hlthaff.w2.372v1?maxtoshow=&HITS=10&hits=10&RESULTFORMAT=&author1=pollitz&andorexactfulltext=and&searchid=1&FIRSTINDEX=0&resourcetype=HWCIT. Accessed October 11, 2006.

21. National Conference of State Legislatures. Genetics and health insurance—state anti-discrimination laws. Available at: http://www.ncsl.org/programs/health/genetics/ndishlth.htm. Accessed August 1, 2006.

22. Shi L, Singh DA. *Delivering Health Care in America: A Systems Approach,* 3rd ed. Gaithersburg, Md.: Aspen Publishers; 2004.

23. Kaiser Family Foundation and Health Research and Educational Trust. *Employer Health Benefits Survey 2005.* Menlo Park, Calif.: Kaiser Family Foundation; 2005: Section 5. Available at: http://www.kff.org/insurance/7315/sections/upload/7315Section5.pdf. Accessed August 1, 2006.

ENDNOTES

a. A lengthier discussion about the uninsured can be found in Chapter 7, which discusses the uninsured and health reform.

b. Chapter 7 provides a more in-depth discussion of attempts to create a national health insurance system. For a thorough discussion of the social insurance movement in the United States, see Paul Starr, *The Social Transformation of American Medicine: The Rise of a Sovereign Profession and the Making of a Vast Industry* (New York: Basic Books, Inc., 1982).

c. Section 106 of the IRS Code of 1954 states that employers who pay a share of premiums for employees' hospital and medical insurance may exclude that amount from the gross income of employees.

d. ERISA is discussed in more detail in Chapter 9.

e. As is discussed in Chapter 6, low-income individuals may have different financial obligations under federal and state programs designed to provide health insurance to the indigent.

f. There are both for-profit and not-for-profit insurance companies. Both types of companies seek to earn enough revenues to cover expenses and the cost of accessing capital. However, for-profit companies return excess revenue to their investors whereas not-for-profit companies put excess revenue back into the company.

g. In some plans, select preventive services are covered by the plan before the employee meets the deductible.

h. The "law of averages" is a lay term used to convey the notion that eventually everything evens out. For example, if you flip a coin 1,000 times, you will average around 500 heads and 500 tails, within some variation (e.g., you could end up with 540 heads and 460 tails or 595 heads and 405 tails).

i. Insurers may purchase reinsurance (when the insurer purchases insurance from another insurer) to cover the cost of individuals who have very high expenditures.

j. Individuals are similarly situated based on usual employment classifications (e.g., full-time, part-time, length of employment, member of collective bargaining unit, geographic location).

k. Evidence of insurability includes things like participation in high-risk activities such as riding a motorcycle or a snowmobile. HIPAA includes an exception to the nondiscrimination provisions that allows plans to provide discounts or reduce contributions if beneficiaries adhere to qualified health promotion/wellness programs.

l. Because the IPA is an intermediary, the HMO has a buffer between itself and provider treatment decisions. If a patient sues a provider for medical malpractice, the HMO can point to the IPA as the entity with more direct control over provider decisions. This and related concepts are discussed in Chapter 8.

CHAPTER 5

Health Economics in a Health Policy Context

LEARNING OBJECTIVES

By the end of this chapter you will be able to:

- Understand why it is important for health policymakers to be familiar with basic economic concepts
- Understand how economists view decision making and options analysis
- Describe the basic tenets of supply, demand, and markets
- Understand how health insurance affects economic conditions
- Apply economic concepts to health policy problems

INTRODUCTION

The prior chapters introduced you to several disciplines that may be used to assist you in analyzing health policy problems. In addition to the three frameworks described in the Introduction, Chapters 1 and 2 illustrated how and why you may consider policy problems using political and legal analysis. Furthermore, throughout the text issues are viewed through a social framework by asking you to consider what policies guide your decision making. In other words, what do you think should happen? This chapter informs you about yet another discipline—economics—that is useful when conducting health policy analysis.

VIGNETTE

You are Governor Galway's chief health policy analyst. The governor is interested in reducing the number of uninsured residents in the state, but is also concerned about the impact any new initiative will have on the state's economy. She asks you to compare the economic consequences of three options: tax incentives for individuals to purchase insurance, tax incentives for employers to offer more affordable and more comprehensive insurance options, and a mandate requiring residents to purchase health insurance. Fortunately, you have a background in economics and know that you need to be concerned with basic principles of supply, demand, and market functions to help your governor make the best choice. This knowledge will lead you to ask questions such as: How big a tax incentive is necessary to compel individuals or employers to act? Will tax incentives encourage people to join a plan or employers to offer benefits that they would not otherwise, or will the government simply be subsidizing transactions that would take place anyway? Is the problem that health insurance is not available and affordable, or are individuals simply making the choice not to purchase insurance because they prefer to spend their money on other goods and services? Will a mandate lead to the proliferation of bare-bones insurance policies that do not provide adequate coverage? The answers to these questions will help you supply the governor with informed policy recommendations.

Students just beginning their health policy studies often question why it is necessary to study economics. Most would rather think about and discuss what policies they support and what values should govern decision making, not about competitive markets, equilibriums, and externalities. What may not be clear initially to students is that economic theory provides one of the fundamental building blocks for making policy choices, both generally and in the context of health care and public health. For instance, economic tools help policymakers predict how consumers and producers will react if they implement certain policies. Knowing this may help policymakers choose the most effective and efficient policy to achieve their goals. Governor Galway's request provided one example of how economic knowledge would prove helpful in health policy decision making. Other examples include:

- When federal officials decide which communities should receive grants to support primary care clinics, they need to know if appropriate providers are available to staff clinics. Economic theory can help explain why some providers prefer to locate in urban or suburban Maryland instead of rural West Virginia, why there is a shortage of qualified nurses but an abundance of cardiologists, and how to change this situation and help a rural primary care clinic remain viable.
- In the face of a flu vaccine shortage, the president considers launching an initiative to ensure that every American can be vaccinated against the flu in the case of an epidemic. Economic theory sheds light on why there are so few vaccine producers supplying the U.S. currently and what could be done to entice manufacturers to participate in the flu vaccine market.

Entire books and courses are devoted to the concept of health economics, and this chapter is not an attempt to distill all the theories and lessons of those texts and courses. Instead, our goal is to introduce you to the basic concepts of health economics, because understanding how economists view health-related problems is one essential component of being a good health policy analyst and decision maker. This chapter begins with an overview of what health economics is, how economists view health care, and how individuals determine whether obtaining health insurance is a priority in their lives. It then moves to a review of the basic economic principles of supply, demand, and market structure. As part of this discussion, you will learn what factors make supply and demand increase or decrease, how the presence of health insurance affects supply and demand, how different market structures function, and what interventions are available when the market fails to achieve desired policy goals.

HEALTH ECONOMICS DEFINED

Economics is concerned with the allocation of scarce resources as well as the production, distribution, and consumption of goods and services. Macroeconomics studies these areas on a broad level, such as how they relate to national production or national unemployment levels. Microeconomics studies the distribution and production of resources on a smaller level, including individual decisions to purchase a good or a firm's decision to hire an employee. Microeconomics also considers how smaller economic units, such as firms, combine to form larger units, such as industries or markets.[1(p3)] "Health economics," then, is the study of economics as it relates to the health field.

How Economists View Decision Making

Economists assume that people, given adequate information, are rational decision makers. Rational decision making requires that people have the ability to rank their preferences (whichever preferences are relevant when any sort of decision is being made) and assumes that people will never purposely choose to make themselves worse off. Instead, individuals will make the decision that gives them the most satisfaction, by whatever criteria the individual uses to rate his level of satisfaction. This satisfaction, referred to as *utility* by economists, may be achieved in many ways, including volunteering time or giving money to charities. Utility in a health context takes into account that individuals have different needs for and find different value in obtaining health care goods and services, and that whether and which health resources are purchased will depend on the individual's preferences and resources.

Utility Analysis

What does utility mean in terms of health care? Most people do not enjoy going to the doctor or taking medicine. It seems strange to think that individuals are happy as a result of or maximize their utility by, for example, receiving weekly allergy shots or getting chemotherapy treatments. However, health care can be discussed in terms of utility because most people enjoy being healthy.

Everyone has a different level of health, some due to their status at birth (e.g., infants born prematurely may have problems with their lungs or mental development) and others due to incidents that occur during their lives (e.g., an individual who is in a serious car accident may suffer from back pain in the future). In addition, people have various tolerance levels for being unhealthy. In other words, the willingness to pay for a particular health care good or service will vary among individuals based on their circumstances and preferences.

Furthermore, at some point, obtaining additional "units" of a particular good will bring less satisfaction than the previous units did. For example, although icing a sore knee for 20 minutes may reduce swelling, icing the same knee for 40 minutes will not reduce swelling twice as much. Or, although buying one pair of glasses may bring high satisfaction, buying two pairs of glasses will not double the consumer's satisfaction because the second pair of glasses can't do more than the first. This is called *diminishing marginal utility*, and it also affects what goods and services a consumer purchases.

In addition, consumers must consider the *opportunity costs* of their decisions. Opportunity costs refer to the cost associated with the options that are not chosen. For example, if a consumer decides not to purchase any medication to ease her back pain, there is zero accounting or monetary cost; that is, it did not cost the consumer any money because she did not purchase the medication. However, there may be opportunity costs, monetary or otherwise, because she is not pain-free. She may endure a monetary loss if she has to take time off from work due to her injury. Or, she may endure a nonmonetary loss because she cannot enjoy walking or exercising due to her back pain. Opportunity costs are the hidden costs associated with every decision, and in order to fully assess the cost and benefits of any decision, these hidden costs must be included in the calculation.

In terms of health care goods only, an individual's utility can be thought of as a function of their health and the health care goods and services they desire. Utility maximization in health care is the ideal set of health-related goods and services that an individual purchases. However, people need to purchase a variety of goods and services, not just those relating to health care. Overall, consumers maximize their utility by purchasing what they consider to be an ideal bundle of health care goods and services as well as other goods and services, based on their desire for each good and service and subject to the income they have available to make these purchases.

Scarce Resources

In the health care arena, consumers have to make choices about the production, distribution, and consumption of health care resources. There are many types of health care resources. Health care goods include items such as eyeglasses, prescription drugs, and hospital beds. Health care personnel include providers such as physicians, nurses, and midwives, as well as lab technicians, home health care workers, and countless others. Health care capital inputs (resources used in a production process) include items such as nursing homes, hospitals, and diagnostic equipment (such as an X-ray machine). All of these things (and others) are considered health care resources.

If there were unlimited health care resources and an unlimited ability to pay for goods and services, the questions confronted by health policy analysts about what health care items should be produced and who should have access to them would still exist, but the answers would be less dire because there would be enough health care available for everyone. In reality, however, there is a finite amount of health care goods, personnel, and capital inputs. The financial resources are not available to provide all of the health care demanded by the entire population and still provide other goods and services that are demanded. As a result of this scarcity of resources, choices and very apparent trade-offs must be made.

In general, consumer choices are based on individual preference, as discussed earlier, and the concept of efficiency. In economic terms, an efficient distribution of resources occurs when the resource distribution cannot be changed to make someone better off without making someone else worse off.[a] There are several types of efficiency, such as *allocative efficiency*, *production efficiency*, and *technical efficiency*.[2(pp9–10),3(p5)] Allocative efficiency focuses on providing the most value or benefit with goods and services. Production efficiency focuses on reducing the cost of the inputs used to produce goods and services. Technical efficiency focuses on using the least amount of inputs to create goods or services.

The notion of efficiency raises many questions because there are always trade-offs to be made when producing goods and services. For example, should the production be more automated or more labor-intensive? Should the production sites be located in the U.S. or overseas? Can a service be provided in a less costly setting? Is there any additional or different service or product that will enhance the benefits of the goods or services consumers receive?

Although they may not use this technical economic jargon, public and private policymakers often consider concepts of efficiency when they answer these types of questions. The answers, in turn, help identify which goods and services should be produced overall in society and which of those goods and services should be related to health care. Because there is a finite amount of resources available, the choice to produce more health care goods and services would result in the production of fewer non-health care goods and services, and vice versa. Similarly, the choice to produce more of one kind of health care good or service will lead to the production of fewer health care goods and services of other types.

Finally, policymakers must also decide whether equity or fairness concerns should be taken into account, and in response alter their production and distribution decisions in ways that may make some people better off at the expense of others. For example, when a U.S. flu vaccine shortage occurred in 2004, some states required that vaccines be given only to individuals in high-risk groups. Individuals who had access to the vaccine but were not in those high-risk groups were made worse off by this decision because they were no longer allowed to receive the inoculation. On the other hand, some individuals in the high-risk group who otherwise would not have been able to obtain the vaccine were made better off under the new policy. The point is not that efficiency is more important than equity or vice versa. However, it is important to understand that these are distinct and not always complementary concerns, and whether and how one decides to influence the market will depend, in part, on how much the decision maker values efficiency and equity. In a world of limited resources, balancing consumer preferences, efficiency, and equity concerns can be a very difficult task for policymakers.

How Economists View Health Care

Health economics helps explain how health-related choices are made, what choices should be made, and the ramifications of those choices. Evaluating the consequences of these choices is referred to as *positive* economics. Positive economics identifies, predicts, and evaluates who receives a benefit and who pays for a public policy choice. Positive economics answers the questions, "What is the current situation?" and "What already happened?" *Normative* economics discusses what public policy should be implemented based on the de-

cision maker's values. It answers the question, "What should be?"[3(p14),4(p5)] For example:

> *A positive statement:* In 2003, approximately 45 million people in the U.S. did not have health insurance.
>
> *A normative statement:* All people living in the U.S. should have health insurance.

As shown by the concepts of positive and normative economics, health economists, like other analysts, cannot avoid discussing how health care *should* be perceived. Is health care a good or service like any other good or service such as food, shelter, or clothing that consumers obtain or refrain from obtaining based on availability, price, resources, and preference? Or is health care a special and unique commodity for reasons such as its importance to individuals' quality of life or how the health care market is structured? Bear in mind that health policymakers take their own view of health care's place in the market into account when they argue for or against a policy.

Box 5-1 identifies two theories of how to view health care. Many economists' views fall somewhere in the middle of these two theories or combine aspects of the two theories to create a hybrid theory. These theories were not presented to be an either/or choice, but to illustrate that even within the field of economics there is a fundamental debate about how to view health care.

Box 5-1
Discussion Questions

Consider each issue below and discuss whether you support Theory X, Theory Y, neither theory, or some combination of them.

Issue	Theory X	Theory Y
Your view about how an individual's health is determined	Whether a person is healthy or sick is determined randomly.	Whether a person is healthy or sick depends on lifestyle choices such as whether a person smokes, drinks, or wears a seatbelt.
Your view of medical practice	Medicine is a science, and experts will ultimately discover the best means for treating every illness.	Medicine is an art and there will never be one best way to treat every illness because illnesses are often patient-specific and because there will always be demand for lower-cost and less painful treatments.
Your view of medical care	Medical care is a unique commodity.	Medical care is similar to any other good or service.
Your view of the government's role in health care	Government regulations are necessary to protect this unique commodity, to cou profiteering at the cost of patient care, to control the resources spent on health care, and to improve information sharing.	Government regulations are not necessary, technological advances and more services are desirable, and competition, not regulation, should drive the market.

Source: Gerald L. Musgrave. Health Economics Outlook: Two Theories of Health Economics. *Bus Econ.* 1995;30:7–13.

Health Care Spending in the United States

In 2004, the United States spent approximately $1.9 trillion in aggregate health spending, representing about 16% of the Gross Domestic Product (GDP), as shown in Figure 5-1.[5] The rate of spending on health care services was relatively stable in the 1990s, fluctuating between 12% and 13% of the GDP. Although there has been a slowdown in health spending growth in recent years, national health spending is expected to grow faster than the GDP from 2003 until 2014, and is projected to reach 18.7% of GDP by 2014.[6]

As you can see from Figure 5-2, the largest portion of national health care spending in 2004 resulted from providing hospital care services, followed by the amount spent on physician and clinical services. The greatest increase in national health care spending from 1994 to 2004, however, is represented by expenditures on prescription drugs.

From 1994 to 2004, spending by private insurance plans and Medicaid increased, while consumer out-of-pocket spending decreased (see Figure 5-3). In 2004, slightly over half (55%) of the nation's health care expenditures were by private sources, including 15% from consumer out-of-pocket spending. Public sources accounted for the remaining 44% of expenditures, due in large part to Medicaid and Medicare spending.[5]

ECONOMIC BASICS: DEMAND

Consumers, whether an individual, firm, or country, purchase goods and services. *Demand* is the quantity of goods and services that a consumer is willing and able to purchase over a specified time. In the case of health care, for example, demand equals the total demand for health care goods and services by all the consumers in a given market.

Demand Shifters

In general, as the price of a good or service increases, demand for that good or service will fall. Conversely, as the price of goods or services decreases, demand for those goods or services will rise.

Various factors in addition to price also increase or decrease the demand for a product. Insurance is an important demand

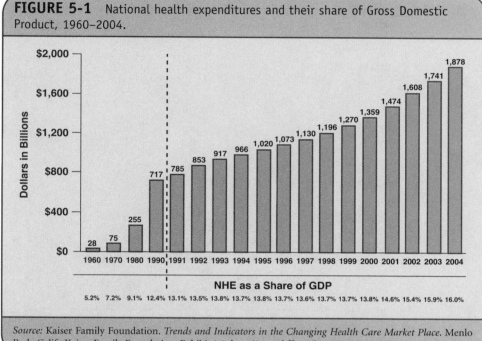

FIGURE 5-1 National health expenditures and their share of Gross Domestic Product, 1960–2004.

Source: Kaiser Family Foundation. *Trends and Indicators in the Changing Health Care Market Place.* Menlo Park, Calif.: Kaiser Family Foundation, Exhibit 1.1, http://www.kff.org/insurance/7031/ti2004-1-1.cfm.

shifter that is discussed separately later in this chapter. A few of the other factors that may shift the demand for a product include:

- *Consumer's income:* As a consumer's income increases, demand for a product may increase. For example, a consumer may desire a new pair of eyeglasses but cannot afford it. Once the consumer's income increases, the consumer can purchase the eyeglasses.
- *Quality:* Consumers have preferences based on quality, both actual and perceived. In addition, a change in quality will likely result in a change in demand. A decrease in the quality of a product may result in a decrease in demand because consumers decide the product is no longer worth the price charged. For example, a consumer may discover that the eyeglasses he wants fall apart easily, thus he may decide not to buy the product.
- *Price of substitutes:* A substitute is a different product that satisfies the same demand. For example, contact lenses may be a substitute for eyeglasses. As the price of contact lenses drops, a consumer may decide he prefers contact lenses to eyeglasses.
- *Price of complements:* A complement is a product associated with another product. For example, cleaning solution is a complement to contact lenses. The price and quality of cleaning solution (the complement) may be an important factor when a consumer is debating whether

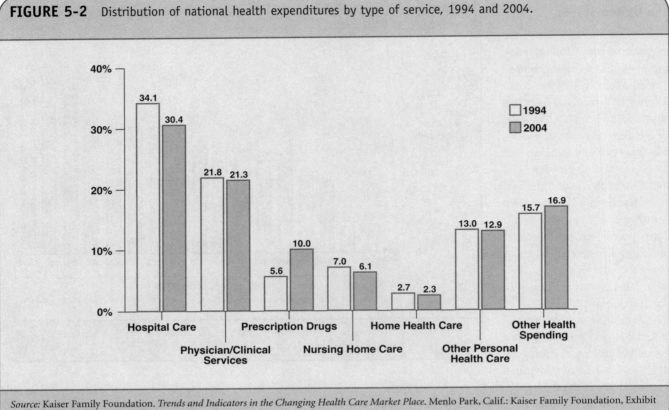

FIGURE 5-2 Distribution of national health expenditures by type of service, 1994 and 2004.

Source: Kaiser Family Foundation. *Trends and Indicators in the Changing Health Care Market Place.* Menlo Park, Calif.: Kaiser Family Foundation, Exhibit 1.5, http://www.kff.org/insurance/7031/ti2004-1-5.cfm.

to keep wearing glasses (the original product) or switch to contact lenses (the alternative product). If the price of cleaning solution increases, even though the price of contact lenses stays the same, the consumer may decide to purchase eyeglasses instead of contact lenses. In other words, demand for complements and alternative products shifts in opposite ways, so an increase in the price of a complement will decrease the demand for the alternative product, and vice versa.

The physical profile of a consumer has an impact on demand for health care services in some predictable ways. Women generally demand more health care services than men before reaching age 65, primarily due to health needs related to childbearing, whereas men over age 65 use more care than do women in the same age group. In addition, many diseases are more prevalent in women than in men, resulting in an expected increase in demand for health services by women. Some of these diseases include cardiovascular disease, osteoporosis, and immunologic diseases.[3(p111),7(pp149–150)] Regardless of gender, an individual who is born with a med-

ical problem, or who develops one at a relatively young age, can be expected to have a higher than average demand for health care services. Aging consumers are more likely to have higher health care needs than younger consumers. Of course, any factor that usually leads to increases in demand for health care services may be offset by lack of financial resources or lack of access to providers.

In addition to the physical profile of a consumer, interesting research is being conducted in relation to consumers' level of education and their demand for services. Although there is no consensus on the direct impact of general education on demand for health services, some studies show a positive relationship between medical knowledge and demand for health care services. That is, the more the consumer knows about medicine, the higher the level of consumption of health care services. This association may indicate that consumers without as much medical knowledge underestimate the appropriate amount of health services they need. Or, it may mean that consumers with more medical education have a greater ability to purchase medical care. Other explanations are possible as well.[3(p127)]

Elasticity

Two of the demand shifters discussed previously are changes in price and changes in income. *Elasticity* is the term used to describe how responsive the change in demand or supply is when there is either a change in price or a change in income. The concept of elasticity is important to understand as a policy analyst because it is essential to know whether changes in consumers' incomes (say, through a tax credit) or changes in the price of a product (perhaps through incentives given to producers) will result in the desired outcome. The desired outcome may be increased consumption, which might be the case if the service is well-child checkups. Conversely, the desired outcome may be decreased consumption, which might be the case if cigarettes are the product being consumed.

Demand Elasticity

Demand elasticity is based on the percentage change in the quantity demanded resulting from a 1% change in price or income. In other words, does consumer demand for a product, such as a vaccination, increase as the price of a product decreases by 1%? Or, how much does consumer demand for the vaccine decrease as the consumer's income drops 1%? The calculation to determine elasticity is:

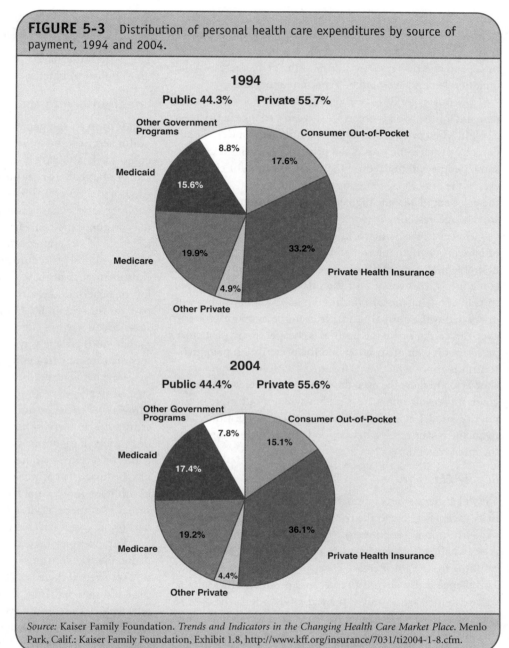

FIGURE 5-3 Distribution of personal health care expenditures by source of payment, 1994 and 2004.

Source: Kaiser Family Foundation. *Trends and Indicators in the Changing Health Care Market Place.* Menlo Park, Calif.: Kaiser Family Foundation, Exhibit 1.8, http://www.kff.org/insurance/7031/ti2004-1-8.cfm.

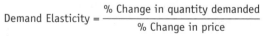

$$\text{Demand Elasticity} = \frac{\%\text{ Change in quantity demanded}}{\%\text{ Change in price}}$$

Demand for a product is considered elastic if the sum is greater than 1 or greater than −1; it is inelastic if the calculation results in a sum that is between 0 and 1 or 0 and −1.

For example, suppose a vaccine costs $20 per dose and at that price a family buys four doses for a total of $80. The next year the price increases 20% to $24 per dose and the family only buys three doses for a total of $72.

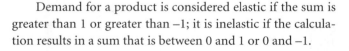

$$\text{Elasticity} = \frac{-25\%\text{ change in demand}}{20\%\text{ change in price}}$$

$$\text{Elasticity} = -1.25$$

Because elasticity equals –1.25, the product is considered elastic (because the result of the elasticity calculation is greater than –1). In this example, for every 1% increase in vaccine price, demand decreases by 1.25%. If the price decreases, the quantity demanded would be expected to increase.

Of course, goods may also be inelastic, which means the demand for the good is not as sensitive to a change in price. As a result, when price increases the quantity demanded will not decrease at the same rate as the price increases. For example, some people will not reduce their consumption of cigarettes even if the price of cigarettes increases. However, at some point the price could become high enough that consumer behavior will change, resulting in a decrease in demand.

However, elasticity works in the opposite way in the case of *inferior goods*. An inferior good, as the name suggests, is less desirable than a *normal good*. As a result, as a consumer's income increases, demand for the inferior good will decrease. Instead of buying more of the inferior good, the consumer will prefer to buy the normal good. For example, suppose a generic over-the-counter pain medication is cheaper than a particular prescription pain medication, but the prescription pain medication is more effective. Consumers with low income may choose to purchase the over-the-counter medicine, the inferior good. If their income increases, they will not buy more of the inferior good, but instead will switch to the prescription pain medicine because it is a better good, for their purposes, than the inferior good.

Supply Elasticity

Supply elasticity works in much the same way as demand elasticity except it refers to the relationship between the quantity of goods supplied and the price of the goods. Supply elasticity is often defined as the percentage change in quantity supplied resulting from a 1% increase in the price of buying the good. The change is usually positive because producers have an incentive to increase output as the price they will receive for the good rises. However, if supply elasticity refers to variables other than the price of the good, such as the cost of raw materials or wages, then the supply elasticity will be negative; that is, as prices of labor or other inputs rise, the quantity supplied will fall (all other things being equal).

$$\text{Supply Elasticity} = \frac{\% \text{ Change in quantity supplied}}{\% \text{ Change in price}}$$

Supply elasticity (with respect to price) is calculated as the quantity of the good supplied divided by the percentage change in its price. For example, assume a medical device supplier is selling 25 needles for $20. Based on the above formula, the needles have a supply elasticity of 1.25.

$$\text{Elasticity} = 25/20$$

$$\text{Elasticity} = 1.25\%$$

Therefore, if the market price increases 10% to $22, the quantity supplied will increase 12.5% to 28 needles.

Health Insurance and Demand

In addition to the general economic rules of demand for health services, the presence of health insurance affects demand for health care goods and services. Health insurance acts as a buffer between consumers and the cost of health care goods and services. In an insured consumer's view, health care goods or services cost less because instead of paying full price, the consumer may only have to pay, for example, a co-insurance rate of 20% (after satisfying the deductible). For example, if a surgical procedure normally costs $10,000, the insured consumer may only have to consider the cost of paying $2,000 for the benefit of the surgery because his insurance company pays for the remainder. In this way, the presence of health insurance can have an effect on the consumer—to increase demand—in the same way that an increase in the consumer's income can increase demand.

In general, insured consumers are not as sensitive to the cost of health care goods and services as uninsured consumers.[2(p38)] Because of this, the presence of health insurance creates the problem of *moral hazard*. Moral hazard can occur in a variety of economic situations when consumers buy more goods or services than necessary because they do not have to pay the full cost of acquiring the good or service. In relation to health insurance, moral hazard results when an insured consumer uses more services than she would otherwise because part of the cost is covered by insurance.

For example, if a consumer has a $500 health insurance deductible, the consumer pays 100% of the first $500 of health care received. If there is a 20% co-insurance charge after that, the consumer pays only $.20 per dollar for every dollar spent after $500. If the consumer values a particular health care service, such as a preventive dental exam, at $50 but the service costs $100, the consumer will not purchase the service before meeting the deductible. However, after the deductible has been met, the dental exam (assuming it is a covered benefit) will cost the consumer $20 (20% of $100), so the consumer will purchase the service because it is under the consumer's $50 value threshold.

As the portion of the health care cost that a consumer pays based on co-payments or co-insurance decreases, the consumer becomes less sensitive to changes in the price of the product. Say a consumer decides he is unwilling to pay more than $2,500 for surgery. If the consumer owes a 10% co-insurance charge, the consumer will be willing to pay for surgery as long as it is not priced at more than $25,000. At $25,000, the consumer would pay $2,500 and the insurance company would pay $22,500. However, if the same consumer has a 20% co-insurance rate, he will not elect surgery once the price rises above $12,500 because the cost to the consumer would be more than the consumer's $2,500 limit. For example, if the surgery cost $15,000, the consumer would owe $3,000 and the insurance company would cover the other $12,000.

The problem of moral hazard is particularly relevant in health care because consumers have an incentive to seek out more medical care—they think it will make them feel better. And, as noted earlier, an insured consumer is more likely to purchase a desirable health care good or service because the presence of insurance reduces her cost. The same cannot be said of owning home or auto insurance. Although consumers may be a little less careful because of the protection fire or car insurance affords them, it is unlikely that people will seek out a car accident or intentionally burn down their house just because they are insured.

ECONOMIC BASICS: SUPPLY

Supply is the amount of goods and services that producers are able and willing to sell at a given price over a given period of time. As with demand, the price of a product is a key factor in determining the level of supply. However, unlike demand, where there is often an inverse relationship between price and demand, an increase in the price a good is sold for usually leads to an increase in quantity supplied. Conversely, as the price consumers will pay for a product decreases, supply will often decrease as well. As with demand, there are many factors that affect the quantity of a good or service being supplied.

Costs

Costs are a key factor in determining the level of supply. Costs refer to what inputs are needed to produce a good or service. For example, the price of cotton may impact the cost of producing medical scrubs or bed linens made out of cotton. The price of steel may affect the cost of producing an autoclave or X-ray machine made with steel. As the cost of these inputs increases, the cost of producing the final good increases as well. If the price for a good or service does not increase as the cost of inputs increases, the quantity supplied is likely to decrease. Thus, if it costs a manufacturer $100 more to build an X-ray machine because the cost of steel has risen, it is likely that the manufacturer will pass that production cost increase on to the consumer by raising the purchase price of the X-ray machine. Or, the manufacturer may choose to absorb the $100 cost increase and not raise the purchase price, which will lead the manufacturer to supply fewer X-ray machines, find a way to produce the good more cheaply using the same method, or find a different way to produce the good.

Costs are counted in many different ways. We focus here on *average costs* and *marginal costs*.

- *Average cost* is the cost of producing one product over a specific period of time. For example, if it costs a manufacturer $2 million to produce 2,000 hospital beds in one year, the average cost is $1,000 per bed during that year.

  Average Cost = Total Cost/Quantity
  AC = $2,000,000/2,000 hospital beds
  AC = $1,000 per hospital bed

- *Marginal cost* refers to the price of producing one more unit of the output, or, in our example, one more hospital bed. Whatever additional labor, equipment, and supplies are needed to produce one more hospital bed is the marginal cost of production. As a general matter, the marginal cost increases as output increases.

Supply Shifters

Other factors in addition to sale price and cost can increase or decrease the supply of a product. Two common factors are:

- *Number of sellers:* As the number of sellers of a good increases, the supply of the good will increase as well because there are more companies producing the good. As long as the market is profitable, new sellers will be enticed to enter the market. This occurs until the market reaches equilibrium, where the quantity demanded equals the quantity supplied.
- *Change in technology:* New technology may mean a new way to produce a desired outcome, which may alter the supply of a good or service. For example, fiberglass has replaced plaster in most casts and the production of each material has shifted accordingly (fiberglass up, plaster down). New technology can also make a product more accessible than before. For example, many surgeries once handled on an inpatient basis may now be performed on an outpatient basis or in a physician's office due to new technology, such as arthroscopy. In addition, evolving technology has led to brand new fields, such as laser eye surgery. Technological improvements can increase demand for some services and reduce it for others, leading to a shift in the production of these goods and services.

Profit Maximization

Although consumers are driven by the desire to maximize their satisfaction, suppliers are driven by their desire to maximize revenues. For-profit companies seek to make profits to pass on to their shareholders, while not-for-profit companies face a variety of requirements regarding disposing of the revenue they generate in excess of expenses and the cost of acquiring capital to run the company. For ease of explanation, the term *profit* will be used here to discuss supplier incentives even though the health care field includes a large share of not-for-profit companies.

Profit is the price per unit sold less the production cost per unit. In a competitive market, profit is maximized at the level of output where the marginal cost equals the price. If a hospital bed costs $1,000 to produce and is sold for $1,500, the profit per bed is $500. If the marginal cost of producing one more bed is $1,400, the producer will make that additional bed because it can be sold for $1,500, a $100 profit. If the marginal cost of producing an additional bed is $1,600, the producer has no incentive to produce that additional bed because it can only be sold at a loss of $100. Due to the profit maximization goal, if the price of a product increases and a competitive market exists for the product, manufacturers will increase production of the product until the output level again reaches the point where the marginal cost equals the price.

When a profitable market exists, new producers will be drawn into the market so they can reap financial benefits. The new producer may price its hospital bed for less than $1,500 to attract consumers. Or, the new producer may think there is a niche for a higher-priced bed that has additional features. Assume the new producer chooses to market a similar bed as the $1,500 bed but sells it for $1,250. If a consumer can purchase the bed from the competing company for $1,250 with no additional opportunity costs, demand for the $1,500 hospital bed is likely to fall. The manufacturer of the $1,500 bed will have to lower its price or improve the product (or the perception of the product) to increase demand for a higher-priced bed. At the point where there is a balance between the quantity supplied and the quantity demanded and the price is set to the marginal cost of production, there is *equilibrium* in the market.

If such a balance does not occur, there is *disequilibrium* in the market. The disequilibrium could represent a surplus of a good or service due to excess supply or sudden drop in demand, or it could result from a product shortage due to inadequate supply or a sharp increase in demand. Surpluses occur when the market price in a competitive market is higher than the marginal cost of production. As a result, producers lower their prices to increase sales of their product. This will keep happening until market equilibrium is reached. For example, there could be a sudden drop in demand for a food product due to a news report that eating the product more than three times a week may put people's health at risk. Due to the sud-

den drop in demand, excess product will be available. Producers will in turn lower the price of the product until equilibrium is reached. Shortages occur when the market price is lower than the marginal cost of production. As a result of the shortage, consumers might be willing to pay more for the product, so producers increase their prices until demand stops increasing and market equilibrium is reached. If an opposite news story appeared, hailing the food product as improving health if eaten at least four times a week, there may be a sudden surge in demand. As a result, consumers will likely be willing to pay more for the product and producers will raise the price until equilibrium is reached. Because producers often cannot make significant changes to their production schedule or products in a short amount of time, market equilibrium positions may take some time to achieve.

Health Insurance and Supply

Just as the presence of health insurance affects a consumer's demand for medical goods and services, it also may impact a health care provider's willingness to supply goods and services. This is a complicated issue because, on the one hand, a provider is expected to act as her patient's agent and thus should act in her patient's best interests. If providers encourage only appropriate care, insurance is working in a positive way. On the other hand, providers may have financial incentive to encourage or discourage the consumption of health care goods and services. Providers could recommend against treatment because of financial incentives resulting from the presence or absence of health insurance. For example, financial incentives found in managed care may discourage providers from recommending a particular treatment. Additionally, if a patient is both uninsured and unable to pay for services out-of-pocket, providers have a financial incentive not to provide potentially necessary services due to their inability to receive payment.

On the other hand, a provider may seek to increase her income by encouraging inappropriate or excessive care. This problem—the provider version of moral hazard—is referred to as *supplier-induced demand*. Supplier-induced demand is the level of demand that exists beyond what a well-informed consumer would have chosen. The theory behind supplier-induced demand is that instead of consumer demand leading to an increase in suppliers (health care providers), the suppliers create demand in the consumers (patients), often by relying on information only available to the supplier. However, economists debate whether supplier-induced demand actually exists because it is difficult to study empirically and because behavior consistent with supplier-induced demand may also be consistent with appropriate medical treatment.[7](pp237–242)

ECONOMIC BASICS: MARKETS

To this point, we have reviewed many basic aspects of economic theory—how consumers behave, how suppliers behave, what drives and shifts demand, and what drives and shifts supply. To understand how these theories work in the health care industry, it is necessary to explore how health insurance affects markets, what kind of market exists for health care, how market structure relates to the production and distribution of goods and services, and why markets fail and what can be done to alleviate the problems associated with market failure.

Health Insurance and Markets

Before delving into the basics of economic markets, it is necessary to highlight how the presence of health insurance alters the dynamics of a standard economic transaction. In a typical market transaction such as buying food at the grocery store, there are only two parties involved—the consumer who buys the food and the supplier who sells the food. The cost to the consumer is the cost of the food; the consumer bears full responsibility for paying that cost and pays that cost directly to the supplier, the grocery store.

The typical medical transaction, however, does not follow these rules, both because of the types of events that lead to a medical transaction and the presence of health insurance. In health care, there are both routine and expected events (e.g., an annual physical) and unanticipated needs due to an unpredictable illness or injury. The exact diagnosis and treatment are often unknown initially and the patient's response to treatment is not guaranteed, resulting in an inability to predict exactly what resources will be needed. Without knowing what goods and services are required, it is impossible to estimate the cost to be incurred. This makes it very difficult for the consumer to weigh her preferences for medical care as compared to other goods and services, and makes it difficult for suppliers to know which goods and services will be demanded and at what price they can sell their goods and services.

Another reason health care transactions often do not follow the typical market exchange is because the presence of health insurance means that health care transactions involve three players, instead of two. These three players are (1) patients (the consumer), (2) health care providers (the supplier), and (3) insurers (who are often proxies for employers). Insurers are also known as "third-party payers" because they are the third party involved in addition to the two customary parties.[b] In the public insurance system the third-party payer is the government, whereas in the private sector the third-party payers are private health insurance companies. Having the health insurance carrier as a third party means that consumers do not pay the full cost of health care resources used and therefore may be less likely to choose the most cost-effective treatment option, to reduce the information gap between them and providers, or be as vigilant against supplier-induced demand as they might in other circumstances.

Market Structure

Understanding markets begins with the notion of a *perfectly competitive* market, because in economic theory a perfectly competitive market serves society by efficiently allocating the finite resources available. Due to specific market conditions that make up a perfectly competitive market, a competitive equilibrium is reached once quantities supplied equal the quantities demanded.

There are numerous types of market structures, ranging from perfectly competitive markets with many buyers and sellers to *monopolistic* markets with a single seller controlling the market, and many others in between. Based on the market structure, consumers and producers have varying degrees of power in terms of setting prices, choosing among products, and deciding whether to participate in the market. Table 5-1 reviews the characteristics of three market structures that are most useful to understanding health care markets: perfectly competitive markets, monopolistic markets, and monopolistically competitive markets.[c]

You know from the discussion of supply and demand that the health care market cannot be perfectly competitive based on the description in Table 5-1. (In fact, no markets are truly perfectly competitive.) Some consumers, such as the federal government, may have extensive market power as well as the ability to set prices. Producers of patent-protected health care products are provided with supply power for a limited period of time, which gives them an ability to control prices. Consumers do not have perfect information regarding health care needs and health care costs, and providers and insurers do not have perfect information regarding patient illnesses. Given the presence of health insurance, consumers do not bear all the cost of using health care services. With these characteristics, the health care market is monopolistically competitive. In many areas of the health care market, there are a few dominant firms with a lot of market power and many smaller firms who participate in the market, but the smaller firms do not have the power to shape market conditions.[d]

Market Failure

A *market failure* means that resources are not produced or allocated efficiently. As you recall, we defined efficiency generally as the state of least cost production where the resource distribution cannot be changed to make someone better off without making someone else worse off, and we also described

TABLE 5-1 Characteristics of Key Market Structures

	Perfectly Competitive	Monopoly	Monopolistically Competitive
Number of Firms	Many.	One (in a pure monopoly).	Many.
Market Share	No dominant firms.	One firm has all of the market share and controls price and output.	There may be many firms with market share or a few dominant firms. Firms can set price because of product differentiation.
Barriers to Entry for New Firms into Market	No.	Yes. Absolute barriers, no new firms may enter market.	Some barriers, due to differentiation of product, licensure, etc.
Product Differentiation	No. Products are substitutes for each other.	No. Only one product, no substitutes available.	Yes. Many products; they are not substitutes for each other (brand loyalty).
Access to Information and Resources	Consumers and producers have perfect information.	One firm controls all information (asymmetric information).	All firms have equal access to resources and technology unless there are a few dominant firms with more access and resources.
Cost of Transaction	Consumers bear cost of consumption and producers bear cost of production.	Higher price to consumer because firm has ability to reduce quantity, retain excess profits.	Blend of costs in perfectly competitive market and monopoly market.

a few specific types of efficiency. When something about the structure of the market prohibits it from being efficient, it is referred to as market failure; the question then becomes what interventions in the market, if any, should occur in an attempt to alleviate the market failure.

Before we turn to why markets fail, we must address one additional issue: Does an inequitable distribution of resources constitute a market failure? Under the traditional economic school of thought, the answer is no; a market failure refers to inefficiency, and concerns about equity are not part of the efficiency calculation. However, some economists consider equity a valid factor when evaluating the functioning of a market. Regardless, whether an inequitable distribution of resources fits under the economic designation of "market failure" is not as important as whether policymakers choose to intervene in a market based on equity concerns.

Some of the most salient reasons that market failures occur in health care include concentration of market power, imperfect information (producers or consumer not having complete and accurate information), the consumption of *public goods*, and the presence of *externalities*. We have already discussed concentration of market power and imperfect information; the next sections focus on public goods and externalities.

Public Goods

Public goods have two main features. First, public goods are *nonrival*, meaning that more than one person can enjoy the good simultaneously. An example of a rival private good would be a single pen. Two people may not use the same pen at the same time. Second, a public good is *nonexclusive* because it is too costly to try to exclude nonpaying individuals from enjoying public goods.[3(p230)]

Classic examples of public goods are national defense measures and lighthouses. Everyone simultaneously benefits from national defense and it is not economically feasible to exclude nonpaying individuals (e.g., tax evaders) from enjoying the benefits. In the same way, multiple ships may benefit at the same time from a warning provided by a lighthouse and it would be very difficult to exclude a particular ship from enjoying the benefit. In the health field, examples of local public goods include clean water in a public swimming area or a public health awareness campaign on city streets. Everyone enjoys the clean water (at least until it is over-crowded) and it would be costly to exclude nonpayers. Similarly, multiple people can benefit from a public health campaign simultaneously, and exclusion of nonpayers would be impossible or quite costly.

Public goods can be transformed into other types of goods. For example, a public good could be made exclusive by charging a fee. These are called *toll goods*.[8(p81)] The public swimming water could be fenced off and a fee charged for admission; or the public health campaign could be placed in the subway, which would exclude those who could not afford the fare. Once public goods are transformed into toll goods, concerns arise about whether the price is set at the most efficient level. Toll goods may still lead to market failure if the cost of using the good excludes users who would gain more from enjoying the good than they would cost society by consuming the good.[8(pp81–82)]

In addition, goods provided by local, state, and federal governments may be, but are not necessarily, public goods in the economic sense. For example, if a state funds a free health care clinic it is not funding a public good. Even though non-payers are, by definition, included, the benefits generally inure to the individual[e] and more than one individual cannot enjoy the same health care good or service.

Public goods also create the *free rider* problem, making it unprofitable for private firms to produce and sell goods due to the high cost of excluding nonpayers.[3(p230)] The free rider is one who enjoys the benefit of the good without paying for the cost of producing the good. Because it is impossible to exclude users or force consumers to reveal their true demand for the public good, they do not have incentive to pay for the units of the good they use.[8(p86)] For example, an individual cannot be prevented from gaining knowledge from a public health awareness campaign, so if a private company were responsible for providing the education campaign it could not force a consumer to pay for it. Eventually, even though many people would like to take advantage of clean air or health education, the lack of people paying for it would result in an underproduction of these services unless some action was taken to alter the market dynamics.

Externalities

Externalities are much more common than public goods in the health care market. "An *externality* is any valued impact (positive or negative) resulting from any action (whether related to production or consumption) that affects someone who did not fully consent to it through participation in a voluntary exchange."[8(p94)] In a typical economic transaction, the costs and benefits associated with a transaction impact only those involved in the transaction. For example, remember our consumer buying food at the grocery store? The only two people affected by that transaction are the consumer who pays money and receives food, and the grocer who provides food and receives money. Situations with externalities, however, are different. Externalities exist when the action of one party impacts another party *who is not part of the transaction*. In other words, the parties to the transaction will find there is an "unpriced byproduct" of producing or consuming a good or service.[3(p231)]

Externalities may be positive or negative. An example of a positive externality is when one person gets vaccinated against the chicken pox and other people benefit because chicken pox is less likely to be transmitted in that community. If enough people get vaccinated, "herd immunity" will exist in the community.[f] In this case, the positive unpriced byproduct is the additional protection received by others who were not vaccinated. An example of a negative externality is represented by illegal hazardous waste disposal. Say a hospital dumps biological waste such as blood, syringes, gauze with infected material on it, and the like into a public water source. The unpriced byproduct is paid by the general public, who face an increased risk of illness from using the contaminated water source. The costs to the general public may not have been included in the hospital's cost/benefit analysis when it decided to dump the biological waste.

With both positive and negative externalities, the cost and benefits of production or consumption are borne by individuals who do not participate in the transaction. Due to the un-priced byproducts, there are external costs and benefits that are not considered when deciding whether to make the transaction, leading to an under- or over-production of the resource from society's perspective.

Government Intervention

When market failures occur, the government may intervene to promote efficiency or to promote equity (of course, it may also choose not to intervene at all). Some examples of government interventions include financing or directly providing public goods, creating incentives through tax breaks and subsidies, imposing mandates through regulation, prohibiting activities, and redistributing income. We discuss these options in the following sections.

GOVERNMENT FINANCES OR DIRECTLY PROVIDES PUBLIC GOODS.   When market failure occurs, the government may choose to finance or provide a good or service directly instead of attempting to influence the actions of private producers. For example, if the government wanted to increase access to health care, it could create new government-run health centers or provide financing to privately run health centers.

These are two different paths—direct provision or financing—with different sets of issues. The main difference when the government provides or finances care instead of a private actor is the lack of profit motive on the part of the government.[3(p252)] Instead of focusing on the financial bottom line, public providers may focus on other goals such as equity or assuring the presence of a particular good or service for everyone or for specific populations.

When the government creates or expands a public program, there is concern that *crowd out* may occur. Whenever a program is established or expanded, the program has a particular goal and targets a particular audience. For example, the government may try to reduce the number of people without insurance by expanding an existing public program such as Medicaid. Crowd out occurs when instead of only reaching the target audience (in this case, the uninsured), the public program also creates an incentive for other individuals (in this case, privately insured people) to participate in the public program. Because the program has a finite amount of resources, some of the target audience (the uninsured) may be crowded out from participating in the program by the presence of the other, nontargeted individuals (the privately insured). This prevents programs from maximizing cost-effectiveness because instead of obtaining the largest change (in this case, the reduction in the number of uninsured) for the public dollar, some of the change is simply a result of a cost shift from a private payer (the privately insured) to a public payer (the expanded program). Crowd out may also change incentives for other providers of services. In this example, the presence of the new or expanded government program may reduce the incentive for private employers to provide the same good or service (in this case, health insurance).

GOVERNMENT INCREASES TAXES, TAX DEDUCTIONS, OR SUBSIDIES. Taxes and subsidies can be used to alter the price, production, or consumption of goods in an effort to fix a market failure. For example, increasing a tax on a good raises the price of that good and discourages consumption. This strategy is often employed to discourage consumption of harmful products, such as cigarettes. Similarly, the government could choose to tax cigarette producers as a way to encourage them to produce less of the harmful product or leave the market altogether.

Conversely, the government could subsidize a good, directly or through a tax deduction, when it wants to encourage the consumption and production of the good. For example, if the government wanted more low-income individuals to purchase health insurance, it could choose to subsidize their insurance premiums or allow individuals to take a tax deduction or receive a tax rebate to cover the cost of paying the premiums. Similarly, if the government wants to encourage vaccine manufacturers to produce more vaccine doses, it could accomplish this goal through direct subsidies to or tax deductions for the manufacturers.

Note that the government has an economic incentive to tax goods that are price inelastic. This incentive exists because the amount purchased declines by a smaller percentage than the price increase. For example, if cigarettes are price inelastic, a 10% cigarette tax increase will result in less than a 10% decrease in cigarette consumption, meaning the cigarette tax will be a good revenue producer for the government because consumers will continue to purchase cigarettes despite the tax. However, taxing price-inelastic goods is less effective as a public health tool for the same reason. If the government desires a 10% reduction in cigarette consumption, the tax must be much higher than 10% if cigarettes are price inelastic. Of course, the government may choose to impose a higher cigarette tax, but it is likely that for political reasons a higher tax increase will be harder to obtain than a smaller one.

GOVERNMENT ISSUES REGULATORY MANDATES. Regulations may be used to fix a market failure by controlling the price, quantity, or quality of goods and services, or the entry of new firms into the market.[3(p241)] For example, in Chapter 4 we described how health care consumers often have imperfect information when making their health care decisions. As a result, the government may choose to create a requirement that a type of provider, such as nursing homes, supply information to the public about the quality of care in their facilities to aid in consumers' decision making. The government may also promulgate regulations that restrict entry of new firms into a market and regulate prices because it is cheaper for one or a few firms to produce a high level of output. Of course, government regulations could also be used to achieve a policy goal like reducing the number of uninsured, by mandating that all employers offer health insurance or that all residents purchase health insurance.

The government could also set a cap on the price of a good and prohibit producers from selling that good above the set price. This will keep the good at a price the government deems socially acceptable. However, if the price is set below the market price, some unfavorable market consequences may occur because it is no longer profitable for the producer to supply the product. Possible consequences include:

- Suppliers exiting the market or reducing the quantity of the good supplied, resulting in a shortage
- Suppliers reducing the quality of the good by making cheaper products or providing less care
- Suppliers shifting cost from one product to another
- Suppliers engaging in unethical behavior because some consumers will be willing to pay more than the government price ceiling

Furthermore, regulations aimed at increasing the quality of a good or service will likely impose additional costs on producers of the good. As the cost of inputs rise, the price charged to consumers is likely to rise as well. As a result, some consumers will be priced out of the market for that good or service.

GOVERNMENT PROHIBITIONS.   Prohibiting the production of goods and services often is ineffective and leads to a "black market" for such services. Because the prohibited goods or services are not available legally, consumers are not protected by price or quality controls. This situation may occur with the use of non-FDA-approved drugs or supplements, including unapproved drugs from other countries entering the U.S. via the Internet or other sources. In addition, because other countries are producing the good or service, the U.S. may be at a competitive disadvantage. For example, if stem cell research is permitted abroad but not in this country, some scientists may leave the U.S. to work abroad and domestic companies may not remain competitive in certain fields.

REDISTRIBUTION OF INCOME.   In the case of market failure, the government may also act to redistribute income. Remember, efficient allocation of resources is not the same as equitable allocation of resources. A government may decide that every member of society should obtain a certain minimum level of income or resources or health status. Redistributing income may occur by taxing the wealthier members of society and using the revenue to provide resources to poorer members of society. If the government sought to create more market equity through voluntary donations, it is likely that a free rider problem would exist because some citizens would volunteer to contribute resources while others would not, but the latter would still receive a benefit from the redistribution. For example, wealthier citizens who should be in the "donor group" but do not contribute may benefit from the donations given by other wealthy citizens that lead to increased productivity and welfare of those in the recipient group. Both the notion of income redistribution and the decisions as to who should be providing versus receiving resources is open to debate. In addition, it is important to remember that income redistribution may reduce efficiency or have other undesirable market effects.

Box 5-2
Discussion Questions

Some people argue that the government should not intervene in the case of a market failure because the government itself is inefficient and will simply create new problems to replace the ones it is trying to fix. In addition, critics contend that the government is usually less efficient than private actors. Do you think the government is less efficient than the private sector? Does it depend on the issue involved? If you think it is inefficient in a particular area, does that lead you to recommend against government intervention or is there a reason that you would still support government intervention? If you think the government should intervene, which intervention options do you prefer and why?

CONCLUSION

This introduction to economic concepts illustrates why health policy analysts and decision makers must understand how economists analyze health care problems. We have taken a broad look at the issues of supply, demand, and market structure with a focus on concerns that are relevant in the health policy field. In particular, it is essential to understand how health insurance affects both consumer and producer decisions. Although we only scratched the surface of health care economics in this chapter, you should now realize that without understanding the economic ramifications of a policy decision, a health policy analyst cannot know, for example, whether to recommend addressing a problem through a government-run program, subsidy, or the like, or if it would be better to let the free market set the production level and price of a resource.

REFERENCES

1. Pindyck RS, Rubinfeld DL. *Microeconomics*, 5th ed. Upper Saddle River, N.J.: Prentice Hall; 2003.

2. Penner SJ. *Introduction to Health Care Economics and Financial Management: Fundamental Concepts with Practical Applications*. Philadelphia: Lippincott Williams & Wilkins; 2004.

3. Santerre RE, Neun SP. *Health Economics: Theories, Insights, and Industry Studies*, 3rd ed. Mason, OH: Thomas South-Western; 2004.

4. Feldstein P. *Health Care Economics*, 6th ed. Clifton Park, NY : Thomson Delmar Learning; 2005.

5. Kaiser Family Foundation. *Trends and Indicators in the Changing Health Care Market Place*. Menlo Park, Calif.: Kaiser Family Foundation. Available at: http://www.kff.org/insurance/7031/ti2004-1-1.cfm. Accessed August 1, 2006.

6. Heffler S, Smith S, Keehan S et al. U.S. health spending projections for 2004–2014. *Health Affairs*. 2005; Web Exclusive :W574–W585; http://content. healthaffairs.org/cgi/reprint/hlthaff.w5.74v1?maxtoshow=&HITS=10&hits=10 &RESULTFORMAT=&author1=heffler&andorexactfulltext=and&searchid=1 &FIRSTINDEX=0&resourcetype=HWCIT. Accessed August 1, 2006.

7. Phelps CE. *Health Economics*. 3d ed. Boston: Addison-Wesley, 2003.

8. Weimer D, Vining A. *Policy Analysis: Concepts and Practice*, 3rd ed. Upper Saddle River, N.J.: Prentice-Hall; 1999.

9. Gordis L. *Epidemiology*, 2nd ed. Philadelphia: WB Saunders; 2000.

ENDNOTES

a. This notion of efficiency in exchange is also referred to as Pareto-efficient, named after the Italian economist Vilfredo Pareto, who developed the concept.

b. As discussed in the previous chapter, managed care organizations combine the provision of care with the payment for care. Even under managed care, however, for the purposes of an economic transaction, the market still functions as if there are three parties to the transaction instead of two; patients receive their services from a health care provider but are billed separately by the insurance company, and the provider and the insurance company set the negotiated fee for a good or service without consulting the patient.

c. Other common market structures include oligopolies, which have a few dominant firms and substantial but not complete barriers to entry, and monopsonies, which have a limited number of consumers who control the price paid to suppliers.

d. For example, although most local areas are dominated by a couple of insurance companies, there may be a few local plans available as well. For example, in a particular state Blue Cross Blue Shield could be the dominant market player, with plans such as Humana, United Health Care, or WellPoint also holding small market shares.

e. This is not always true. For example, if someone stops smoking that person gains the health benefits of not smoking and those around the individual gain the health benefits of not being exposed to second-hand smoke.

f. *Herd immunity* is "the resistance of a group to an attack by a disease to which a large proportion of the members of the group are immune."[9(p19)] Once a certain portion of the group is immune, there is only a small chance that an infected person will find a susceptible person to whom the disease may be transmitted.

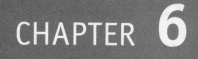

CHAPTER 6

Government Health Insurance Programs: Medicaid, SCHIP, and Medicare

LEARNING OBJECTIVES

By the end of this chapter you will be able to:

- Describe the basic structure, administration, financing, and eligibility rules for Medicaid
- Describe the basic structure, administration, financing, and eligibility rules for the State Children's Health Insurance Program (SCHIP)
- Describe the basic structure, administration, financing, and eligibility rules for Medicare
- Discuss key health policy questions and themes relating to each of these public programs

INTRODUCTION

Prior chapters discussed the significant role of employer-sponsored health insurance in financing health care, the flexibility that private insurers have in designing health insurance coverage and selecting who they will cover, why private insurers do not have incentive to cover high-risk populations, and a variety of ways government can intervene when the private marketplace is not performing in a way that meets a particular policy goal. Medicaid, the State Children's Health Insurance Program (SCHIP), and Medicare were established in part because the private health insurance market was not developing affordable, comprehensive health insurance products for society's low-income, elderly, and disabled populations. Federal and state governments chose to fill some of those gaps through

VIGNETTE

It is 2020 and health care spending has reached unsustainable levels. President Manha was recently elected on a platform that included reforming the health care system, beginning with the Medicaid and Medicare programs. She began to grapple with the following questions. How could it be possible that in a single family one child could be covered by Medicaid while another is not? Or that a family could have significantly better coverage in one state than another? Why did the country design a health care program for its elderly that did not include nursing home care, one of the biggest expenses they incur? Why has the health care system, including the Medicaid program, embraced managed care as a way to reduce health care costs, yet most Medicare beneficiaries remain in an expensive and inefficient fee-for-service system? Before the president can propose major reform, she must understand the answers to these, and many other, questions.

Medicaid, SCHIP, and Medicare. The gaps were substantial, as shown by the over 80 million beneficiaries served by these three programs today. Due to the needs of vulnerable populations and the requirements necessary to make health insurance coverage for them viable, these programs are quite different from the standard private health insurance plans described in Chapter 4.

Of course, there are numerous other important health insurance and direct service programs funded by federal, state, and local governments. Just a few examples include the Ryan White Care Act, which provides HIV/AIDS services to infected individuals and their families; the Women, Infants and Children Supplemental Nutrition Program, which provides nutritional supplements and education to poor women and their children; and the Indian Health Service, which provides federal health services to American Indians and Alaska Natives. Although these and many other health programs are vital to the health of our population, this chapter focuses only on the three major government health insurance programs in this country because in addition to providing health insurance to millions, these programs are also influential in terms of setting health care policy. For example, when Medicare, a program serving over 40 million people, makes a decision to cover a certain treatment, private insurance companies often follow suit, establishing a new standard for generally accepted practice in the insurance industry. Conversely, states may decide to try health care innovations with their Medicaid programs that, if successful, may become commonplace across the country. Thus, understanding these three major programs is essential in terms of both how this country finances and delivers health care and how it makes health policy decisions.

As you learn about specific rules for each program, keep in mind the numerous tensions that are present throughout the health care system as policymakers decide how to design and implement public insurance programs. This chapter touches on several recurring themes relating to these tensions: choosing between state flexibility and national uniformity; determining the appropriate role for government, the private sector, and individuals in health care financing and delivery; defining a primary decision-making goal (fiscal restraint, equity/social justice, improved health outcomes, uniformity, etc.); and settling on the appropriate scope of coverage to offer beneficiaries.

Before delving into the details of each program, it is necessary to explain the difference between entitlement and block grant programs. Medicaid and Medicare are *entitlement* programs whereas SCHIP is a *block grant* program. Some of the themes listed earlier, such as the appropriate role of government and primary decision-making goals, are implicated in the decision of whether to establish a program as an entitlement or a block grant.

In an *entitlement* program, everyone who is eligible for and enrolled in the program is legally entitled to receive benefits from the program. In other words, the federal or state governments cannot refuse to provide program beneficiaries all medically necessary and covered services due to lack of funds or for other reasons. Because everyone who is enrolled has a legal right to receive services, there cannot be a cap on spending. The absence of a spending cap has the advantage of allowing funds to be available to meet rising health care costs and unexpected needs, such as increased enrollment and use of services during recessions or natural or man-made disasters.

Opponents of entitlement programs focus on the open-ended budget obligation entitlements create. With health care costs straining federal and state budgets, critics would prefer to establish a cap on the funds spent on entitlement programs such as Medicaid. It is impossible to determine how many people will enroll in the program or how many and what kind of health care services they will use in any given year, so governments cannot establish exact budgets for their Medicaid program. In addition to these fiscal objections, many opponents reject the notion that government should play a large role in providing health insurance, preferring to leave that function to the private market.

Entitlement programs are often contrasted with *block grant* programs such as SCHIP. A block grant is a defined sum of money that is allocated for a particular program (often, but not always, from the federal government to the states) over a certain amount of time. If program costs exceed available funds, additional money will not be made available and program changes have to be made. Such changes could include terminating the program, capping enrollment in the program, reducing program benefits, or finding additional resources. Unlike entitlement programs, individuals who qualify for block grant programs may be denied services or receive reduced services due to lack of funds.

The arguments for and against block grant programs are similar to those found with entitlement programs. Proponents of block grant programs laud the limited and certain fiscal obligation and reduced role of government in providing health insurance. Opponents of block grant programs object to the lack of legal entitlement to services and the finite amount of funds available to provide health insurance.

MEDICAID[a]

Medicaid is the country's federal-state public health insurance program for the indigent. In this section, we discuss fundamental aspects of the Medicaid program, including its struc-

Box 6-1
Discussion Questions

Do you think it makes more sense to structure government health care programs as entitlements or block grants? What are the economic and health care risks and benefits of each approach? Does your answer depend on who is paying for the program? Who the program serves? What kinds of benefits the program provides? Do you think various stakeholders would answer these questions differently? How might the answers change if you ask a member of the federal government, a governor, a state legislator, an advocate, or a tax-paying citizen who is not eligible for benefits under the program?

ture, eligibility, benefits, and financing. Unlike private health insurance plans, which are based on actuarial risk, the Medicaid program is designed to ensure that funds are available to provide health care services to a poorer and generally less healthy group of beneficiaries; in order to do so, Medicaid has several features not found in private health insurance plans.

Program Administration

Medicaid is jointly designed and operated by the federal and state governments. The Center for Medicare and Medicaid Services is the federal agency in charge of administering the Medicaid program. Each state, the District of Columbia, and certain U.S. Territories,[b] as defined in the statute,[c] have the option to participate in the Medicaid program, and all have chosen to do so. The federal government sets certain requirements and policies for the Medicaid program though statute,[d] regulations,[e] a *State Medicaid Manual*,[f] and policy guidance such as letters to state Medicaid directors.[1] Each state has its own Medicaid agency that is responsible for implementing the program in the state. States file a Medicaid State Plan with the federal government outlining the state's own eligibility rules, benefits, and other program requirements;[g] this plan is effectively a contract between states and the federal government and between states and program beneficiaries.

The federal and state governments jointly set rules concerning who is covered and what services are provided by Medicaid. The federal government outlines which populations must be covered (*mandatory populations*) and which ones may be covered (*optional populations*), as well as which benefits must be covered (*mandatory benefits*) and which ones may be covered (*optional benefits*). Between these floors and ceilings, states have significant flexibility to determine how Medicaid will operate in

their particular state. In general, states must cover mandatory populations and they may choose to cover any combination of optional populations or benefits, including the choice not to offer any optional coverage at all. In addition, states may seek a waiver from federal rules, allowing states to experiment with coverage and benefit design while still drawing down federal funds to operate their program. Given all of these possible permutations, it is often said that "if you have seen one Medicaid program, you have seen one Medicaid program." In other words, within the broad federal parameters, every state (and territory) has a unique Medicaid structure—no two programs are exactly alike. As a result, similarly situated individuals in different states may have very different experiences in terms of the generosity of benefits they are entitled to or even if they are eligible for the program at all.

Eligibility

A variety of low-income populations are eligible for Medicaid. Generally, Medicaid covers low-income pregnant women, children, adults in families with dependent children, individuals with disabilities, and elderly. About half of all Medicaid beneficiaries are children, while adults account for another 25% of enrollees and the disabled and elderly make up the remaining quarter.[2] Approximately 7.4 million people are called *dual enrollee* or *dual eligible* elderly, meaning they qualify for both Medicaid and Medicare.[3] Although most dual enrollees are eligible for full Medicaid benefits, a small portion of them receive only premium and/or cost-sharing assistance to help them pay for Medicare, not full Medicaid benefits.[3]

Among all people with health insurance, members of ethnic or minority groups are more likely than Caucasians to have coverage through Medicaid. As shown in Figure 6-1, however, Medicaid beneficiaries are split almost evenly between white, non-Hispanic beneficiaries and beneficiaries who are

Box 6-2
Discussion Questions

What are the benefits and drawbacks of having a health program that varies by state versus having one that is uniform across the country? Do you find that the positives of state flexibility outweigh the negatives, or vice versa? Does your analysis change depending on what populations are served? Does your analysis change depending on whose point of view you consider? Is it fair that similarly situated individuals may be treated differently in different states? Does this occur in other aspects of society?

members of ethnic or minority groups. Figure 6-2 indicates that overall, Medicaid beneficiaries are more likely to be in poorer health than privately insured individuals.

Overall, 81% of nonelderly Medicaid enrollees are either poor (meaning they earn less than 100% of the Federal Poverty Level [FPL])[h] or near-poor (meaning they earn between 100% and 200% of the FPL).[4] Yet, not all low-income individuals are covered by the program, and nearly 30 million low-income Americans remain uninsured.[5] Left out of the program are low-income adults without disabilities, women who are not pregnant, and the near-poor who earn too much money to qualify for Medicaid.

Eligibility Requirements

To be eligible for Medicaid, one must meet *all five* of the following requirements:

1. Categorical
   • An individual must fit within a category (e.g., pregnant women) covered by the program.
2. Income
   • An individual/family must earn no more than the relevant income limits, which are expressed as an FPL percentage (e.g., 133% of the FPL).
3. Resources[i]
   • An individual/family must not have non-wage assets (e.g., car, household goods) that exceed eligibility limits.
4. Residency
   • An individual must be a U.S. resident and state resident.
5. Immigration status
   • Immigrants must meet certain requirements, including having been in the country for at least five years (for most immigrants).

As shown in Table 6-1, it is necessary to consider both categorical eligibility and income limits to understand who is covered by Medicaid and which populations are mandatory and

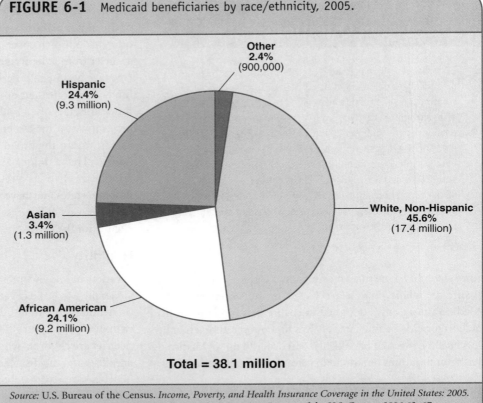

FIGURE 6-1   Medicaid beneficiaries by race/ethnicity, 2005.

Other
2.4%
(900,000)

Hispanic
24.4%
(9.3 million)

White, Non-Hispanic
45.6%
(17.4 million)

Asian
3.4%
(1.3 million)

African American
24.1%
(9.2 million)

Total = 38.1 million

Source: U.S. Bureau of the Census. *Income, Poverty, and Health Insurance Coverage in the United States: 2005.* Washington, D.C.: Economics and Statistics Administration. Bureau of the U.S. Census; 2006:62–67.

which are optional. The groups in Table 6-1 represent some of the larger and more frequently mentioned categories of Medicaid beneficiaries, but it is not an exhaustive list. There are approximately 50 categories of mandatory and optional populations in the Medicaid program, with each state picking and choosing which optional populations to include and at what income level. About two-thirds of beneficiaries qualify as part of a mandatory population, whereas one-third are part of an optional group. Among children, almost 80% are part of a mandatory group, whereas almost half of all elderly beneficiaries qualify in an optional category.[6]

Medically Needy

Medicaid's *medically needy* category is an option that has been picked up by 34 states as of 2001.[7] As its name implies, this category is intended to cover individuals who have extremely high medical expenses. These individuals fit within a covered category, but earn too much money to be otherwise eligible for Medicaid. Medically needy programs have both income and asset requirements. In terms of income requirements, states subtract the costs of individuals' medical expenses from their income level. States have the choice of deducting the medical expenses as they are incurred each month, every six months, or any time in between. As soon as otherwise qualified individuals "spend down" enough money on medical expenses, they are eligible for Medicaid through the medically needy option based on their reduced income level for the remainder of the period.

The following is a simplified example of how the "spend down" process works. Let's say a state calculates incurred medical expenses every three months to determine eligibility for the medically needy option, and in this state an individual (who we'll call Peter) must earn no more than $8,500 a year to qualify

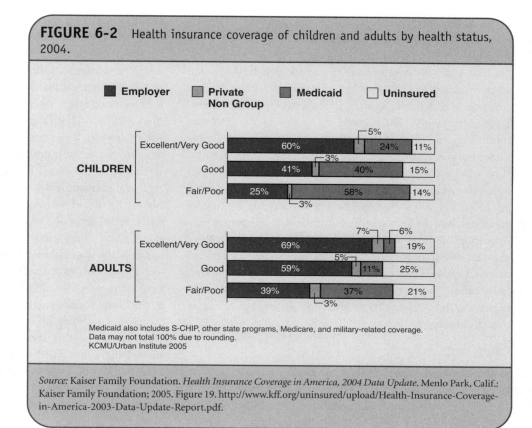

FIGURE 6-2 Health insurance coverage of children and adults by health status, 2004.

Medicaid also includes S-CHIP, other state programs, Medicare, and military-related coverage.
Data may not total 100% due to rounding.
KCMU/Urban Institute 2005

Source: Kaiser Family Foundation. *Health Insurance Coverage in America, 2004 Data Update.* Menlo Park, Calif.: Kaiser Family Foundation; 2005. Figure 19. http://www.kff.org/uninsured/upload/Health-Insurance-Coverage-in-America-2003-Data-Update-Report.pdf.

TABLE 6-1 Select Medicaid Mandatory and Optional Eligibility Groups and Income Requirements

Eligibility Category	Mandatory Coverage	Optional Coverage
Infants under 1	≤133% FPL	≤185% FPL
Children 1–5	≤133% FPL	> 133% FPL
Children 6–19	≤100% FPL	> 100% FPL
Pregnant women	≤133% FPL	≤185% FPL
Parents	Below state's 1996 AFDC* limit	May use income level above state's 1996 AFDC limit
Parents in welfare-to-work families (Transitional Medical Assistance)	≤185% FPL for at least six months and up to 12 months of coverage	N/A for income requirements, but may extend eligibility period beyond 12 months
Elderly and disabled SSI** beneficiaries	SSI income limits	Above SSI limits, below 100% FPL
Certain working disabled	May not exceed specified amount	Variable, SSI level to 250% FPL
Elderly—Medicare assistance only***	Variable, up to 175% FPL	Variable up to 175% FPL
Nursing home residents	SSI income limits	Above SSI limits, below 300% SSI
Medically needy	N/A	"Spend down" medical expenses to state set income level

* AFDC = Aid to Families with Dependent Children.

**SSI = Supplemental Security Income, a federal program that provides cash assistance to the aged, blind, and disabled who meet certain income and resource requirements

*** Medicare Assistance only = payment for Medicare cost-sharing requirements

as medically needy. Peter earns $11,000 per year and has $6,000 each year in medical expenses, incurred at a rate of $500 per month. After 3 months Peter has spent $1,500 on medical expenses. Instead of considering the income level to be the annual amount earned ($11,000), the state subtracts Peter's medical expenses as they occur. So after three months the state considers Peter to earn $9,500 annually ($11,000 − $1,500). Because this amount is still over the $8,500 limit, Peter is not eligible under the medically needy option. In another three months, Peter will have spent $3,000 in medical expenses over the past 6 months. At that time the state considers Peter to earn $8,000 annually ($11,000 − $3,000), making him eligible because he earns less than the $8,500 limit. For the rest of this period (i.e., three months), Peter is eligible for Medicaid. After another three months, the state recalculates his earnings and medical expenses. Each year, this entire calculation starts over. In the end, Peter will not be eligible for Medicaid for the first six months of the year, but will be eligible for Medicaid for the second six months of the year.

Immigrants

Before leaving the topic of Medicaid eligibility, we discuss the rules relating to immigrants. The Personal Responsibility and Work Opportunity Reconciliation Act of 1996 (PRWORA)[j] severely restricted immigrant eligibility for Medicaid (and most

---

Box 6-3
Discussion Questions

Does the medically needy category make sense to you? Do you think it is a good idea to discount medical expenses of high-need individuals so they can access the health care services they need through Medicaid? If so, is the process described above cumbersome and likely to result in people being on and off Medicaid (and therefore likely on and off treatment) because their eligibility is based on their spending patterns? Why should individuals with high medical needs have an avenue to Medicaid eligibility that is not available to other low-income people who have other high expenses, such as child care or transportation costs? Would it make more sense to simply raise the eligibility level for Medicaid so more low-income people are eligible for the program? Politically, which option would likely have more support? Does your view about the medically needy category vary depending on your primary decision-making goal (fiscal restraint, equity, improved health outcomes, etc.)?

---

of the same rules in PRWORA were later applied to SCHIP eligibility in 1997). Prior to PRWORA, legal immigrants followed the same Medicaid eligibility rules as everyone else, but undocumented immigrants were not eligible at all. PRWORA instituted a five-year bar, meaning that most immigrants[k] who come to the United States after August 22, 1996, are not eligible for Medicaid (or SCHIP) for the first five years after their arrival. After five years, legal immigrants are eligible on the same basis as U.S. citizens, while undocumented immigrants remain ineligible for full Medicaid (or SCHIP) benefits. However, both legal and undocumented immigrants who are otherwise eligible for Medicaid may receive emergency Medicaid benefits without any temporal restrictions. Finally, SCHIP funds, but not Medicaid funds, may be used to provide prenatal care regardless of a woman's immigration status.

Proponents of the immigrant restrictions believe they discourage people who cannot support themselves from coming to the United States and prevent immigrants from taking advantage of publicly funded programs they did not support through taxes before their arrival. In addition, some proponents believe that health care resources should go first to U.S. citizens, not non-citizens. Opponents of the restrictions assert that most immigrants pay taxes once they arrive in this country and therefore deserve to receive the full benefits of those taxes.[8(p15)] They also find the restriction ill-suited as a deterrent because immigrants often come to the U.S. for economic opportunities, not social benefits.[9] Furthermore, restricting immigrants' access to health care may be a public health hazard for all members of the community because contagious diseases do not discriminate by immigration status. Finally, opponents contend that having higher numbers of uninsured individuals in the U.S. will further strain the ability of providers to care for all vulnerable populations in a community and lead to rising health care costs, because uninsured immigrants are much less likely to obtain preventive care or early treatment for illnesses or injuries.[8(p15)] As a result, 23 states have decided to use state-only funds[l] to provide Medicaid or SCHIP services to some or all individuals who are otherwise ineligible due to their immigration status.[8(p16)] Five of these 23 states—plus two additional states—also have picked up the SCHIP option to provide prenatal care regardless of immigration status.[8(p16)] Even so, immigrants are still less likely to be insured or have access to care than native citizens.[8(pp1–6)]

Benefits

Medicaid benefits are structured in the same way as Medicaid eligibility—some are mandatory and some are optional. Again, this means that no two Medicaid programs are alike, as each state picks its own menu of optional benefits to provide.

Box 6-4
Discussion Questions

Looking at the eligibility rules overall, you see numerous value/policy judgments—pregnant women and children are favored over childless adults, the medically needy are favored over other low-income individuals with high costs, nonimmigrants are favored over immigrants. Can you find any other distinctions in the eligibility groups? Why were these eligibility decisions made? Assuming the resources are not available to cover all low-income individuals, how should these choices be made and who should make them? Or should we decide that for some populations the government should step in and provide coverage regardless of the cost? In other words, is there a point where equity trumps financial constraints? Should that coverage be uniform among all poor people instead of making categorical distinctions?

Historically, Medicaid programs have offered a rich array of benefits, including preventive services, behavioral health services, long-term care services, supportive services that allow people with disabilities to work, institutional services, family planning services, and more. In fact, the coverage provided by Medicaid generally has been more generous than the typical private insurance plan, particularly in the case of children.

Recent policy decisions may result in widespread reductions in the availability and affordability of Medicaid benefits. In February 2006, Congress passed and President Bush signed the Deficit Reduction Act of 2005 (DRA),[m] which contained, among other things, significant new changes to Medicaid benefit and cost-sharing options. Because the law is new at the time of this writing, there are numerous areas of uncertainty. Even so, it is clear that if states choose to pick up on the options provided in the DRA (and some appear poised to do so), Medicaid benefits may be severely curtailed. As a point of reference, we describe Medicaid benefit options as they existed prior to the DRA in Table 6-2.

Before addressing the DRA's benefit changes, we discuss the traditional Medicaid benefit package. All states provide the mandatory services listed on the left side of Table 6-2, and may provide the optional services listed on the right side.[n] In addition to requiring a wide array of services, Medicaid also defines many service categories quite broadly. For example, under the category of medical or remedial services, a state may pay for diagnostic, screening, or preventive services provided in any settings that are recommended by a licensed practitioner "for the maximum reduction of physical or mental disability and restoration of an individual to the best possible functional level."[o]

One of the broadest service categories is the early periodic screening, diagnosis, and treatment (EPSDT) package of services for beneficiaries under age 21. As the *E* in EPSDT indicates, this package of benefits provides preventive care to children to catch problems before they advance, and offers early treatment to promote healthy growth and development. EPSDT benefits include periodic and as-needed screening services, comprehensive health exams (to detect both physical and mental health conditions), immunizations, lab tests, health education, vision services, hearing services, dental services, *and* any other measure to "correct or ameliorate" physical or mental defects found during a screening, *whether or not those services are covered under a state plan*. In addition to these benefits, EPSDT also requires states to inform families about the importance of preventive care, seek out children in need of comprehensive care, and offer families assistance in securing care.

The "correct or ameliorate" standard is very different from the "medical necessity" standard that is used for adults in Medicaid and is commonly found in private health insurance plans. Typically, medically necessary services are those that restore "normal" function after an illness or injury. Not only does this standard generally preclude care before a diagnosis is made, but if recovery is not possible (say, as a result of blindness), services that improve the quality of life or prevent deterioration of a condition may be denied. By contrast, the EPSDT correct or ameliorate standard means a state must provide coverage for preventive and developmental treatment as well as for services needed to treat a specific diagnosis. Combined with the requirement to provide services regardless of state plan limitations, the correct or ameliorate standard means that almost any accepted treatment should be covered under EPSDT.

As shown in Box 6-5, the DRA gives states the option to choose a "benchmark" or "benchmark-equivalent" package of services for certain population groups, instead of following the mandatory and optional list of services identified in Table 6-2.[p] There are three benchmark packages: (1) the Federal Employee Health Benefits Plan (FEHBP), (2) a state's health plan for its own employees, and (3) the state's largest commercial non-Medicaid health maintenance organization (HMO) plan. In addition, the DRA allows the secretary of HHS to approve a plan as a benchmark. Benchmarks provide a state with a standard to follow when designing its Medicaid package of benefits—it does not mean that Medicaid beneficiaries are enrolled in the plans identified as benchmarks. Furthermore, a state may instead choose to offer "benchmark-equivalent" coverage that includes certain basic services as shown in Box 6-5. These services must have the same actuarial value as the services provided by one of

TABLE 6-2 Pre-DRA Medicaid Benefits

Mandatory	Optional
Acute Care Benefits	***Acute Care Benefits***
• Physician services	• Prescription drugs
• Laboratory and X-ray services	• Medical care or remedial care furnished by non-physician
• Inpatient hospital services	licensed practitioners
• Outpatient hospital services	• Rehabilitation and other therapies
• Early periodic screening, diagnosis, and treatment (EPSDT)	• Clinic services
services for beneficiaries under 21	• Dental services, including dentures
• Family planning services and supplies	• Prosthetic devices, eyeglasses, and durable medical equipment
• Federally qualified health center (FQHC) services	• Primary care case management
• Rural health clinic services	• Tuberculosis-related services
• Nurse midwife services	• Other specified medical or remedial care
• Certified pediatric and family nurse practitioner services	
Long-Term Care Benefits	***Long-Term Care Benefits***
• Nursing facility services for individuals 21 and over	• Intermediate care facility services for the mentally retarded
• Home health care services for individuals entitled to nursing	(ICF/MR)
facility care	• Inpatient/nursing facility services for individuals 65 and over in
	an institution for mental disease
	• Inpatient psychiatric hospital services for individuals under 21
	• Home- and community-based waiver services
	• Other home health care
	• Targeted case management
	• Respiratory care services for ventilator-dependent individuals
	• Personal care services
	• Hospice services
	• Services furnished under a Program of All-inclusive Care for
	the Elderly (PACE program)

Source: 42 U.S.C. § 1396d; 42 CFR Parts 430-498.

the three benchmarks listed above (i.e., the value of the services must be similar). States may choose to supplement their benchmark-equivalent plans with additional services, as listed in Box 6-5. These additional services are required to be worth only 75% of the actuarial value of the same service provided in a benchmark plan. Finally, it appears the DRA still guarantees the same set of EPSDT services for children under 19 by requiring states to provide "wrap-around" benefits that consist of the full array of EPSDT services in addition to the benchmark or benchmark-equivalent coverage selected by a state.[q]

The benefit changes allowed by the DRA may only be applied to certain populations, and these groups had to be part of a state plan prior to the law's enactment to receive the new benefits package. DRA-eligible populations include most categorically needy children, and parents and caretakers who receive Medicaid but not Temporary Assistance to Needy Families (the new welfare program created by

PRWORA). The list of populations excluded from the DRA is quite lengthy and includes beneficiary groups with high expenditures, such as the disabled, dual eligibles, and terminally ill hospice patients.[r]

Amount, Duration, and Scope, and Reasonableness Requirements

Although states have a great deal of flexibility in designing their Medicaid benefit packages, states had to follow several federal requirements prior to the DRA. These rules, collectively referred to as "amount, duration, and scope" and "reasonableness" requirements, were intended to ensure that all Medicaid beneficiaries in a state received adequate, comparable, and nondiscriminatory coverage. As discussed below, some of these rules have changed under the DRA.

You learned in Chapter 4 that private insurers typically are not drawn to Medicaid's population because of the likeli-

Box 6-5
DRA Benefit Options

Benchmark Plans
- Federal Employee Health Benefits Plan
- State employee health plan
- Largest commercial non-Medicaid HMO in the state
- HHS secretary–approved plan

Benchmark-Equivalent Plan
Full actuarial value for the following services:
- Inpatient and outpatient hospital
- Physician surgical and medical
- Laboratory and X-ray
- Well-baby and well-child
- Other appropriate preventive services (defined by HHS secretary)

Additional Optional Benchmark-Equivalent Services
75% actuarial value for the following services:
- Prescription drugs
- Mental heath
- Vision
- Hearing

Note: States must wrap around EPSDT coverage as necessary.

Box 6-6
Discussion Questions

Supporters of the Deficit Reduction Act (DRA) assert that states now have more flexibility to choose benefit packages tailored to the needs of different beneficiaries, provide Medicaid beneficiaries with the same coverage that large private plans provide, and give states additional needed flexibility to control state Medicaid budgets. Are these arguments convincing? Why or why not? If you agree, why do you think so many populations are exempt from DRA changes? Also, the beneficiaries who are excluded are often the most costly groups of patients. Does that make sense in terms of budget reduction or equity? What do you think was the primary decision-making goal by those supporting the DRA?

hood that the insureds would have relatively high health care needs. In addition, private insurers use a variety of tools (such as limited open-enrollment periods, experience rating, medical condition–based limitations, and narrow medical necessity standards) to limit their financial exposure. Medicaid, on the other hand, was designed as a health care entitlement program with the goal to provide services to a needy population that would otherwise be uninsurable through commercial plans.[10] Table 6-3 identifies some of the requirements that help the Medicaid program achieve this goal, as well as any changes to them found in the DRA.

Medicaid Spending

Health policymakers are concerned with not only how much money Medicaid costs, but also the distribution of program spending. In 2004, Medicaid spent $291 billion, accounting for approximately 15% of total personal health care spending in the United States.[11(p190)] Understanding which populations utilize the most services, which services are utilized most frequently,

TABLE 6-3	"Reasonableness" and "Amount, Duration, and Scope" Requirements in Medicaid	
Requirement	**Requirement Purpose**	**DRA Changes to the Requirement**
Reasonableness	State must provide all services to categorically needy beneficiaries in sufficient amount, duration, and scope to achieve its purpose.	States only have to meet amount, duration, and scope requirements found in the named benchmark or benchmark-equivalent plan.
Comparability	All categorically needy beneficiaries in the state are entitled to receive the same benefit package in content, amount, duration, and scope.	States may apply benchmark or benchmark-equivalent packages to some, but not all, populations.
Statewideness	In most cases, states must provide the same benefit package in all parts of the state.	States may apply benchmark or benchmark-equivalent packages to some, but not all, populations.
Nondiscrimination	States may not discriminate against a beneficiary based on diagnosis, illness, or type of condition by limiting or denying a mandatory service.	Unclear—some read the DRA as allowing individual-specific benefit packages.

and which services and populations are most costly helps policymakers decide if they need to change the Medicaid program and, if so, what changes should be made.

As you can see from Figures 6-3, 6-4, and 6-5, not all populations and services are equal when it comes to cost. Generally, children and adults are fairly inexpensive to cover whereas elderly and disabled beneficiaries use more services and more expensive services. In addition, 60% of Medicaid expenditures are for optional benefits or for mandatory benefits for optional populations. One of the biggest reasons the elderly and disabled account for a high proportion of Medicaid expenditures is their use of long-term care services, such as nursing homes and home- and community-based services. In addition, they are heavy users of prescription drugs and are relatively more likely to be hospitalized. As illustrated in Figure 6-5, over half of all Medicaid spending is for acute care services, and long-term care services account for over one-third of Medicaid expenditures.

Medicaid Financing

The Medicaid program is jointly financed by the federal and state governments, with about 57% of the total program costs paid for by the federal government and the rest by the states. In fact, Medicaid is the largest federal grant program that provides money to the states, accounting for 43% of all federal funds received by states.[12] Even with the federal government

Box 6-7
Discussion Questions

States have enormous flexibility in designing their Medicaid programs. Most state Medicaid expenditures are on optional services or mandatory services for optional populations. Yet, states complain that Medicaid expenditures are unsustainable and that significant reform, such as the DRA, is needed. If states have the ability to reduce Medicaid spending without any reforms, why do you think state politicians are focused on reforming the program? Why might states choose not to reduce their Medicaid program to cover only mandatory services and populations? Politically, what do you think is the most feasible way for states to reduce their Medicaid budgets?

picking up over half the tab, states have found their share of Medicaid costs to be increasingly burdensome, accounting for 17% of state budgets nationally.[12]

Program financing occurs through a matching payment system that divides the amount paid by the federal and state governments. The matching rate for most medical services, called the Federal Medical Assistance Percentage (FMAP), is determined by a formula that is tied to each state's per capita income. Poorer states—those with lower per capita incomes—receive more federal money for every state dollar spent on Medicaid, and the wealthier states receive less federal money for every state dollar spent. However, the FMAP rate may not be lower than 50% for any state, meaning that the costliest scenario for a state government is that it splits program costs evenly with the federal government. FMAP rates range from 50% to 76%, with an average rate of 60%.[13(pp82–83)] Given the variation in matching rates and state programs' size, federal funds are not distributed evenly among the states. In fact, 4 states[s] account for over

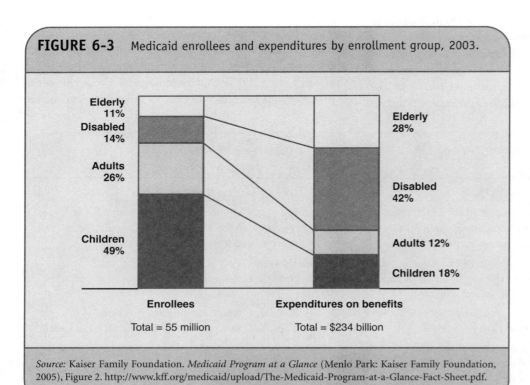

FIGURE 6-3 Medicaid enrollees and expenditures by enrollment group, 2003.

Elderly 11%
Disabled 14%
Adults 26%
Children 49%

Elderly 28%
Disabled 42%
Adults 12%
Children 18%

Enrollees
Total = 55 million

Expenditures on benefits
Total = $234 billion

Source: Kaiser Family Foundation. *Medicaid Program at a Glance* (Menlo Park: Kaiser Family Foundation, 2005), Figure 2. http://www.kff.org/medicaid/upload/The-Medicaid-Program-at-a-Glance-Fact-Sheet.pdf.

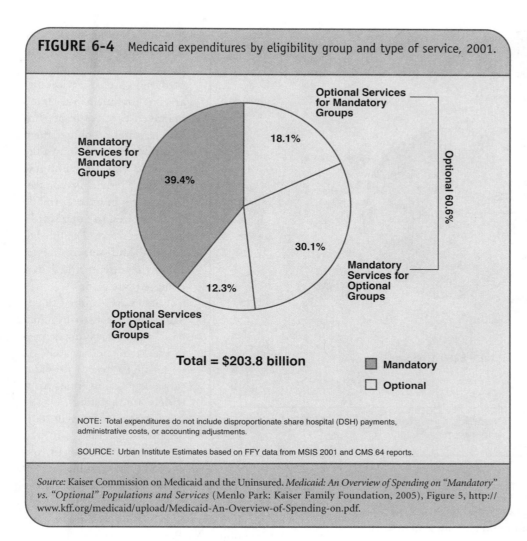

FIGURE 6-4 Medicaid expenditures by eligibility group and type of service, 2001.

Optional Services for Mandatory Groups

18.1%

Mandatory Services for Mandatory Groups

39.4%

Optional 60.6%

30.1%

Mandatory Services for Optional Groups

12.3%

Optional Services for Optical Groups

Total = $203.8 billion

☐ (shaded) Mandatory
☐ Optional

NOTE: Total expenditures do not include disproportionate share hospital (DSH) payments, administrative costs, or accounting adjustments.

SOURCE: Urban Institute Estimates based on FFY data from MSIS 2001 and CMS 64 reports.

Source: Kaiser Commission on Medicaid and the Uninsured. *Medicaid: An Overview of Spending on "Mandatory" vs. "Optional" Populations and Services* (Menlo Park: Kaiser Family Foundation, 2005), Figure 5, http://www.kff.org/medicaid/upload/Medicaid-An-Overview-of-Spending-on.pdf.

not pay the requisite amount. States may now charge Medicaid families earning between 100% and 150% FPL up to 10% of the cost of services, and may charge families earning above 150% FPL both premiums and up to 20% of the cost of services.[v] The aggregate of these cost-sharing requirements may not exceed 5% of a family's income. The statute is silent regarding cost sharing for families earning less than 100% FPL. Furthermore, the DRA permits higher cost sharing for prescription drugs and the use of emergency departments for non-emergency services. As with the DRA benefit changes, many groups and services are excluded from the new cost-sharing options.

Medicaid Provider Reimbursement

Medicaid's complex design also extends to its provider reimbursement methodology. States have broad discretion in setting provider rates. Not only do reimbursement rates vary by state, but they also vary by whether services are provided in a fee-for-service or managed care setting and by which type of provider (e.g., physicians, hospitals) renders a service.[w]

Fee-for-Service Reimbursement

When reimbursing fee-for-service care under Medicaid, states are required to set their payment rates to physicians at levels that are "sufficient" to ensure Medicaid patients have "equal access" to providers compared to the general population.[x] Despite this language, Medicaid reimbursement is much lower than both Medicare and private practice rates. Low reimbursement is one reason that many providers are wary of treating Medicaid patients. In 2001, one study found that approximately 20% of physicians were not accepting *any* new Medicaid patients compared to the 70% of physicians who were accepting *all* new Medicare and privately insured patients.[15]

one-third of all federal Medicaid spending, and 10 states[t] account for over half.[14]

Medicaid is also partially financed through beneficiary co-payments, co-insurance, and premiums. Prior to the DRA, Medicaid cost sharing was extremely limited, but the DRA included drastic changes to Medicaid's cost-sharing rules. In most cases, states historically could only charge "nominal" cost sharing such as $2 per month per family, or $.50 to $3.00 per service, or 5% of the state's payment rate.[u] In addition, pre-DRA, states were prohibited from charging any cost sharing to some beneficiaries and for some services. Furthermore, cost-sharing requirements were "unenforceable," meaning health professionals could not refuse to provide services if a beneficiary did not pay a required cost-share amount.

Under the DRA, however, states have options to impose much higher cost-sharing requirements and to make these requirements enforceable, meaning a provider may refuse service or beneficiaries may be disenrolled from Medicaid if they do

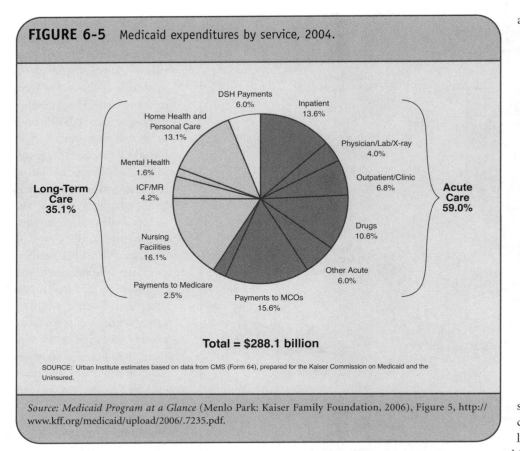

FIGURE 6-5 Medicaid expenditures by service, 2004.

Long-Term Care 35.1%

DSH Payments 6.0%
Home Health and Personal Care 13.1%
Mental Health 1.6%
ICF/MR 4.2%
Nursing Facilities 16.1%
Payments to Medicare 2.5%
Payments to MCOs 15.6%
Other Acute 6.0%
Drugs 10.6%
Outpatient/Clinic 6.8%
Physician/Lab/X-ray 4.0%
Inpatient 13.6%

Acute Care 59.0%

Total = $288.1 billion

SOURCE: Urban Institute estimates based on data from CMS (Form 64), prepared for the Kaiser Commission on Medicaid and the Uninsured.

Source: Medicaid Program at a Glance (Menlo Park: Kaiser Family Foundation, 2006), Figure 5, http://www.kff.org/medicaid/upload/2006/.7235.pdf.

Hospital fee-for-service services are reimbursed at a rate that is "consistent with efficiency, economy, and quality of care."[y] However, there is no specified minimum reimbursement level that states are required to meet, resulting in rates that are lower than what hospitals receive from Medicare and private insurance. Hospitals that serve a high number of low-income patients may receive additional Medicaid payments called disproportionate share hospital (DSH) payments.

Managed Care Reimbursement

As with the rest of the health care system, managed care has become an increasingly important part of the Medicaid program. About 28 million patients—63% of all Medicaid patients—were in Medicaid managed care plans in 2005.[16] All states except Alaska and Wyoming enroll some Medicaid beneficiaries in managed care, with 17 states enrolling over 80% of their beneficiaries in managed care plans.[17] States may require managed care enrollment for all beneficiaries except children with special health care needs, Native Americans, and Medicare recipients.[z]

Managed care organizations (MCOs) that enroll Medicaid beneficiaries receive a monthly capitated rate per member and assume financial risk for providing services. States and MCOs agree upon a set of services the MCOs will provide for the capitated rate. If there are any Medicaid-covered services that are not included in a state's managed care contract with MCOs, states reimburse them an amount in addition to the capitated rate or reimburse non-MCO providers on a fee-for-service basis to provide those services. In other words, beneficiaries are still entitled to all Medicaid services, even when they are enrolled in a managed care plan.

States are required to pay MCOs on an "actuarially sound basis," a term that is not defined in the Medicaid statute.[aa] As with other types of provider rates, capitation rates vary widely among states. Of the states that reported data in 2001, capitation rates ranged from a low of $105 in Michigan to a high of $149 in Washington.[18,bb] In general, states with higher fee-for-service rates also have higher capitation rates for their managed care plans.[13] However, it is difficult to compare capitation rates across states because of the variation in Medicaid programs generally and in the types of services and populations covered by the managed care contracts.

Box 6-8
Discussion Questions

Is higher Medicaid cost-sharing a good idea? What are the strongest arguments you can make for and against higher cost-sharing? Should Medicaid beneficiaries have the same cost-sharing responsibilities as privately insured individuals, or should the government bear more of the cost because Medicaid beneficiaries are low-income individuals? What is the primary decision-making goal that led to the exclusion of so many populations and services from the new cost-sharing options?

Box 6-9
Discussion Questions

Who should determine Medicaid provider reimbursement rates and how should they compare to other insurance programs or plans? Should the federal government play a stronger role in setting provider rates? Is this an area where it is better to have state variation or national uniformity? Should the federal or state governments be required to ensure that Medicaid reimbursement rates match private insurance reimbursement rates? What might occur if poorer states were required to provide higher reimbursement rates? What is the risk if reimbursement rates are very low?

Medicaid Waivers

Much of the previous discussion about Medicaid highlighted both the numerous requirements placed on states and the enormous amount of flexibility states have in operating their program. Medicaid *waivers* provide still another level of flexibility for states. There are several different types of waivers under Medicaid; here, we focus only on the broadest one—the "section 1115" waiver. Under section 1115 of the Social Security Act, states may apply to the secretary of HHS to waive requirements of health and welfare programs under the Social Security Act, including both Medicaid and SCHIP. The secretary may grant section 1115 waivers, also called demonstration projects, as long as the proposal "assists in promoting the objectives" of the federal program.[cc] This broad standard has not been defined and leaves the secretary with enormous discretion to approve or reject waiver applications. One of the most important aspects of a waiver is the "budget neutrality" requirement. A state must show that the waiver project will not cost the federal government more money over a five-year period than if the waiver had not been granted. Although the amount of money spent remains the same, by seeking a waiver a state is agreeing to use itself as a "policy laboratory" in exchange for being able to operate its Medicaid program with fewer requirements. Ideally, other states and the federal government will learn from these demonstration projects and incorporate their positive aspects, while avoiding negative ones.

In 2001, the Bush administration created a specific type of section 1115 waiver called the Health Insurance Flexibility and Accountability (HIFA) demonstration. These waivers differ from traditional 1115 waivers in that they encourage integration of Medicaid and SCHIP with private insurance through premium assistance programs and other means. HIFA waivers also allow states to achieve budget neutrality by reducing the amount, duration, and scope of optional benefits and increasing cost-sharing requirements for optional eligibility groups (changes that may now be possible under the DRA without the need for a formal waiver). Although states may reduce optional benefits and populations under HIFA, mandatory populations must remain covered and mandatory benefits may not be reduced. Given these rules, HIFA waivers often involve a trade-off between covering more people with fewer services or fewer people with more services.

Between 2001 and 2005, HHS approved section 1115 waivers in 17 states, some of which were HIFA-1115 waivers.[19(pp5–6)] States are taking a variety of approaches to changing their Medicaid programs through these waivers. For example, several states have implemented tiered benefit systems, meaning that not all beneficiaries are entitled to the same benefits, in exchange for covering new populations.[19(pp3–6)] Other states have created premium assistance programs with limited or no cost-sharing as an alternative to direct coverage through Medicaid. Florida received a waiver that allows the state to provide certain beneficiaries with a specific amount of money—determined based on their health status—that they use to purchase health insurance from state-approved managed care plans, employer-sponsored plans, or individual health insurance plans.[20] Oklahoma is currently considering a similar change, possibly signaling a major shift from states viewing Medicaid as a defined benefit program (beneficiaries are entitled to a certain set of benefits) to a defined contribution program (beneficiaries are entitled to a certain amount of money).

The Future of Medicaid

Due to the high cost of the Medicaid program, the large federal deficit, other pressures on federal and state budgets, and ideological differences among policymakers, Medicaid reform has been a hot topic in recent years. Between 2002 and 2005, every state reduced its Medicaid provider reimbursement rates and instituted prescription drug cost controls, 38 states restricted program eligibility, and 34 states reduced program benefits.[13] As noted in the previous section, the DRA and Medicaid waivers permit large-scale changes in the way the Medicaid program is viewed and operated. Many policymakers appear to be moving away from viewing Medicaid as a social insurance program that provides a certain set of health care benefits and specific legal protections to vulnerable populations. Instead, they are fashioning Medicaid as a program that more closely mirrors private insurance plans in terms of their use of risk, cost-sharing, limited benefits, and lack of extra protections that ensure fairness and access to care. On

Box 6-10
Discussion Questions

What type of Medicaid reform or waivers, if any, do you support? Should Medicaid beneficiaries be treated like privately insured individuals, meaning increased cost-sharing requirements, fewer legal protections, and fewer guaranteed benefits than in the current Medicaid program? Is it fair to provide a more generous package of benefits to publicly insured individuals than most privately insured people receive? Can the country afford a more generous Medicaid program? Can it afford not to provide adequate health insurance and access to care to the poor and near poor? Is it best to let states experiment with new ideas? If you could design a new Medicaid program, what would be your primary decision-making goal?

an ever-larger scale, some policymakers are advocating for ending Medicaid as an entitlement program and transforming it into a block grant program in which the federal government will give states a set amount of funds for a specified period of time to run their Medicaid program as they see fit.

STATE CHILDREN'S HEALTH INSURANCE PROGRAM

Congress created the State Children's Health Insurance Program (SCHIP) in 1997 as a $40 billion, 10-year block grant program, codified as Title XXI of the Social Security Act.[dd] SCHIP is designed to provide health insurance to low-income children whose family income is above the eligibility level for Medicaid in their state. SCHIP has been successful at insuring low-income children, enrolling more than 4 million children at the end of 2005.[21] Nonetheless, over 8 million children remain uninsured as of 2005, and many of them live in low-income families.[22] SCHIP is due to be reauthorized in 2007, meaning Congress and the president are currently facing numerous policy decisions about the funding for and features of the SCHIP program.

SCHIP Structure and Financing

SCHIP is an optional program for the states, but all 50 have chosen to participate. States have three options regarding how their SCHIP program is structured:

1. States may incorporate SCHIP into their existing Medicaid program by using SCHIP children as an expansion population.
2. States may create an entirely separate SCHIP program.

3. States may create a hybrid program with lower-income children part of Medicaid and higher-income children in a separate SCHIP program.

In 2003, 14 states had a separate program, 16 states had a Medicaid expansion program, and 20 states had a hybrid program.[23]

As with Medicaid, federal SCHIP funds are disbursed on a matching basis, although the federal match is higher for SCHIP than for Medicaid. SCHIP matching rates range from 65% to 85%, compared to 50% to76% for Medicaid.[24] States receive their matching payments up to an annual limit or "allotment," based on state-specific estimates of the number of low-income uninsured children, the number of low-income children generally, and health care costs relative to other states.[25] Allotments are set on a three-year basis.

One very important difference between Medicaid and SCHIP is that whereas Medicaid is an entitlement program, SCHIP is a block grant. As mentioned earlier, as a block grant the federal matching funds are capped (through the allotments). Thus, a state is not entitled to limitless federal money under SCHIP, and children, even if eligible, are not legally entitled to services once the allotted money has been spent. If a state runs out of funds and operates its SCHIP separate from Medicaid, it will have to cut back its SCHIP program by eliminating benefits, lowering provider reimbursement rates, disenrolling beneficiaries, or wait-listing children who want to enroll in the program. A state with a Medicaid expansion SCHIP program or a hybrid structure would not receive new SCHIP money, but would continue to receive federal funds for Medicaid-eligible children as allowed under the Medicaid rules and at the Medicaid matching rate.

If states do not use all of their federal SCHIP allotments, the money reverts back to the federal treasury and may be used for any purpose chosen by Congress. There are a variety of reasons that state allotments are either more or less than the state needs to run its SCHIP program. States that have exceeded their allotments may have generous SCHIP programs in terms of eligibility and benefits, effective outreach to enroll children, higher provider payment rates, or insufficient allotments due to factors that are not reflected in the allotment formula. Some states have not used their full allotments because of incurring low costs during the initial start-up time due to a low number of enrollees, having a limited SCHIP program, using complicated enrollment procedures, or employing poor outreach strategies. Other states have not used their allotment because their Medicaid programs were so generous that most of the low-income children in the state were already insured when SCHIP was created.

Box 6-11
Discussion Questions

Why do you think that Medicaid was created as an entitlement program but SCHIP was established as a block grant? Both programs are federal-state insurance programs for low-income individuals, so does the distinction make sense? Does it matter that one program is for children and the other is broader? Should one program be changed so they are both either entitlements or block grants? Which structure do you prefer?

SCHIP Eligibility

Under SCHIP, most states may cover children up to 200% FPL, while those states with generous Medicaid programs may exceed that ceiling within certain limits.[ee] In general, states with separate SCHIP programs have set income eligibility levels that are the same for children of all ages in a state, unlike Medicaid, which is more generous with respect to younger children. Most states with separate SCHIP programs have income eligibility levels at or above 200% FPL, while there is more variation in income eligibility levels in Medicaid expansion programs. In addition, states may not exclude children based on preexisting conditions.

SCHIP Benefits and Beneficiary Safeguards

States must provide "basic" benefits in their SCHIP programs, including inpatient and outpatient hospital care, physician services (surgical and medical), laboratory and X-ray services, well-baby and well-child care, and age-appropriate immunizations. States may also choose to provide additional benefits such as prescription drug coverage, mental health services, vision services, hearing services, and other services needed by children.[ff]

Various standards may be used for a benefit package. Under a stand-alone SCHIP program, the benefit package may be the same as the state's Medicaid package or equal to one of the following benchmarks:

- The health insurance plan that is offered by the HMO that has the largest commercial non-Medicaid enrollment in the state.
- The standard Blue Cross Blue Shield preferred provider plan for federal employees.
- A health plan that is available to state employees.
- A package that is actuarially equivalent to one of the above plans.
- A coverage package that is approved by the HHS secretary.[gg]

Do these benchmark plans sound familiar? Clearly, the DRA changes to Medicaid were modeled on the existing SCHIP program. As a result, it is likely that states electing the DRA option will make similar decisions regarding their Medicaid program as they did when implementing their SCHIP programs. Unfortunately for Medicaid beneficiaries, states with separate SCHIP programs commonly create benefit packages that are less generous than the ones available in their Medicaid programs.[26]

In addition to the benefit package options, there are other areas where SCHIP provides states with more program flexibility and beneficiaries with less protection than is the case under Medicaid. SCHIP does not have the same standards regarding reasonableness, benefit definitions, medical necessity, or nondiscrimination coverage on the basis of illness (though, as noted earlier, states may opt out of or alter some of these protections in Medicaid under the DRA). Also like the new DRA cost-sharing option, states with separate SCHIP programs may impose cost-sharing requirements up to 5% of a family's annual income. In 2004, half of the states increased cost-sharing or imposed new cost-sharing requirements in their SCHIP programs, again indicating that similar changes

Box 6-12
Discussion Questions

When designing SCHIP, policymakers chose to follow the private insurance model instead of the Medicaid model. Although states have the choice to create a generous Medicaid expansion program for their SCHIP beneficiaries, they also have the choice to implement a more limited insurance program with fewer protections. Similar choices were made when the DRA options were created for Medicaid. These decisions raise essential questions about the role of government in public insurance programs. Does the government (federal or state) have a responsibility to provide additional benefits and protection to its low-income residents? Or, is the government satisfying any responsibility it has by providing insurance coverage that is equivalent to major private insurance plans? What if the standard for private insurance plans becomes lower, does that change your analysis? Is it fair for low-income individuals to receive more comprehensive health insurance coverage than other individuals? Is there a point where fiscal constraints trump equity or the likelihood of improved health outcomes when designing a public insurance program?

may be in store for Medicaid beneficiaries in states that adopt the DRA options.[27]

SCHIP and Private Insurance Coverage

In devising SCHIP, Congress was concerned that Medicaid-eligible children would enroll in SCHIP instead of Medicaid without reducing the overall number of uninsured children in a state. To avoid this outcome, SCHIP requires that all children be assessed for Medicaid eligibility and, if eligible, enrolled in Medicaid instead of SCHIP.[hh] In addition, Congress wanted to make sure that the government did not start funding health insurance coverage that was previously being paid for in the private sector. In other words, it did not want to give individuals or employers incentive to move privately insured children to the new public program. To avoid private insurance crowd out, Congress allowed states to institute enrollment waiting periods and impose cost-sharing requirements as a disincentive to switch to SCHIP.

SCHIP Waivers

As noted in the Medicaid section, states may apply to the secretary of HHS to waive SCHIP program requirements in exchange for experimenting with new ways to increase program eligibility or benefits. The most common use of SCHIP waivers is to expand eligibility for uncovered populations such as childless adults and parents and pregnant women who are not eligible under a state's Medicaid program. Using SCHIP funds to provide coverage for adult populations is controversial. Although no one disputes these groups need insurance coverage, critics contends that all of SCHIP's funds should be used to provide insurance coverage for children, because that was the reason the program was initially created.

In addition, a few states have used SCHIP waivers to create premium assistance programs. Premium assistance means that public subsidies (in this case, SCHIP funds) are available to help beneficiaries cover the cost of private health insurance premiums for employer-sponsored coverage or other health insurance plans that are available to them. States favor premium assistance programs as a way to reduce the state's cost of providing a child with health insurance. Premium assistance programs may also reduce crowd out by providing an incentive for people to keep their children in private coverage instead of enrolling them in SCHIP. States must abide by numerous rules when creating a premium assistance program under SCHIP, including requiring a reasonable employer contribution and ensuring that the benefit package and cost-sharing requirements are equivalent to the state's SCHIP package. Because of these rules and the high cost of private insurance, there has been low enrollment in SCHIP premium assistance programs in the few states that have initiated them.[28]

The Future of SCHIP

As you can see, policymakers have designed the Medicaid and SCHIP programs differently. These differences are highlighted in Table 6-4. SCHIP has proved to be an effective program for providing low-income children with health insurance and a popular program among policymakers. Politicians who support increasing health insurance for children and those who oppose entitlement programs found common ground with the SCHIP program. It is likely that the program will be reauthorized in 2007, though it is unknown whether the reauthorization bill will include new policies regarding financing, benefits, or eligibility.

MEDICARE

Medicare is the federally funded health insurance program for the elderly and some persons with disabilities. As a completely federally funded program with uniform national guidelines, Medicare's administration and financing is quite different from that found in Medicaid and SCHIP. This section reviews who Medicare serves, what benefits the program provides, how Medicare is financed, and how Medicare providers are reimbursed.

Medicare Eligibility

Medicare covers two main groups of people—the elderly and the disabled. In 2005, there were 35.4 million elderly and 6.3 million persons with disabilities or end-stage renal disease[ii] enrolled in Medicare.[29] To qualify for Medicare under the elderly category, individuals must be at least 65 years old and be eligible for Social Security payments by having worked and contributed to Social Security for at least 10 years. Individuals who are 65 but do not meet the work requirements may become eligible for Medicare on the basis of their spouse's eligibility. To qualify for Medicare as a person with disabilities,

Box 6-13
Discussion Questions

Although many Medicare beneficiaries are poor, there is no means test (income- or resource-specific eligibility level) to determine eligibility as there is with Medicaid and SCHIP. Is there a good public policy reason for this difference? What would be the basis for making this distinction? Does the government have a different role to play in providing health care based on the population involved?

TABLE 6-4 Comparing Key Features of Medicaid and SCHIP

Feature	Medicaid	SCHIP
Structure	Entitlement	10-year block grant
Financing	Federal-state match	Federal-state match at higher rate than Medicaid
Funds may be used for premium assistance	No (without a waiver)	Yes
Benefits	Federally defined, with option to use benchmark or benchmark-equivalent benefits package; broad EPSDT services for children	Benefits undefined; use benchmark package; limited "basic" services required
Cost-sharing	Limited or prohibited for some populations and services, higher amounts allowed for some populations and services	Cost-sharing permitted within limits, but prohibited for well-baby and well-child exams
Anti-discrimination provision	Yes	No

individuals must be totally and permanently disabled and receive Social Security Disability Insurance (SSDI) for at least 24 months, or have end-stage renal disease. These categories do not have an age requirement, so disabled Medicare beneficiaries may be under age 65. Unlike Medicaid and SCHIP, Medicare eligibility is not based on an income or asset test. In other words, individuals of any income level are eligible for Medicare if they meet the eligibility requirements.

Even though Medicare does not target low-income elderly and disabled, a significant portion of Medicare beneficiaries are indigent and in poor health. Almost 25% of Medicare beneficiaries are in families with annual incomes of $10,000 or less and just over half have incomes under 200% FPL.[29] These low-income beneficiaries are more likely to be female, in fair or poor health, part of a racial or ethnic minority group, and disabled than other beneficiaries.[29] In addition, about 87% of Medicare beneficiaries have one or more chronic conditions, 28% are in poor or fair health, and 26% have a cognitive impairment.[29] Even though approximately 80% of Medicare beneficiaries identify as non-Hispanic white, almost twice as many African-American and Hispanic beneficiaries report being in fair or poor health compared to non-Hispanic white beneficiaries.[29]

Medicare Benefits

Medicare is split into several parts, each covering a specified set of services. Beneficiaries are automatically entitled to Part A, also known as Hospital Insurance (HI). Part B services, also known as Supplemental Medical Insurance (SMI), covers physician, outpatient, and preventive services. Part B is voluntary for enrollees, but 95% of Part A beneficiaries also opt to have Part B. Beneficiaries may choose to receive their benefits through Part C, Medicare Advantage, which includes the Medicare managed care program and a few other types of plans. Part D is the new prescription drug benefit. Table 6-5 lists Medicare benefits by part. Although Medicare benefits are quite extensive, the list excludes services that one might expect to be covered in health insurance targeting the elderly, such as nursing home care.

There was rapid growth of Medicare managed care in the mid-to-late 1990s, but the number of managed care plans participating in Medicare has since fallen by half. In 2005, the 179 plans enrolled just 4.8 million beneficiaries (13% of all Medicare enrollees).[29] The remaining 87% of beneficiaries receive Medicare services through a traditional fee-for-service arrangement under Parts A and B. Future Medicare Advantage enrollment projections vary.[29] HHS estimates that close to one-third of Medicare beneficiaries will enroll in Medicare Advantage by 2013, whereas the Congressional Budget Office projects the rate will be just 16%.[30]

Although HMOs have participated in Medicare since the 1970s, Part C has evolved over the last decade to include a number of new insurance options. In 1997, Congress added private fee-for-service plans,[jj] medical savings accounts coupled with high-deductible plans, county-based preferred provider organizations (PPOs), and point-of-services plans.[30] Recently, as part of the Medicare Prescription Drug Improvement and Modernization Act of 2003 (MMA),[kk]

TABLE 6-5   Medicare Benefits

Part	Services Covered
A	Inpatient hospital, 100 days at skilled nursing facility (SNF), limited home health following hospital or SNF stay, and hospice care.
B	Physician, outpatient hospital, X-rays, laboratory, emergency room, other ambulatory services, medical equipment, limited preventive services including one preventive physical exam, mammography, pelvic exam, prostate exam, colorectal cancer screening, glaucoma screening for high-risk patients, prostate cancer screening, cardiovascular screening blood test, diabetes screening and outpatient self-management, bone-mass measurement for high-risk patients, hepatitis-B vaccine for high risk patients, pap smear, pneumococcal vaccine, and flu shot.
C	Managed care plans, private fee-for-service plans, special needs plans, and medical savings accounts. The plans provide all services in Part A and Part B and generally must offer additional benefits or services as well.
D	Prescription drug benefit.

Congress added regional PPOs and "special needs plans" for the institutionalized and for beneficiaries with severe and disabling conditions.

The MMA also created Part D, Medicare's prescription drug benefit. The drug benefit was made available to recipients beginning in 2006. Medicare contracts with private drug insurance plans in each of 34 regions. If at least two plans are not available in a region, the government contracts with a fallback plan (a private plan that is not an insurer) to serve that area. All plans must cover at least two drugs in each therapeutic class or category of Part D drugs. Dual enrollees (individuals enrolled in both Medicaid and Medicare) are no longer eligible for prescription drug coverage under Medicaid; they must receive their prescription drug benefit through Medicare.

To obtain prescription drugs through Medicare, beneficiaries have the choice of remaining in traditional fee-for-service Medicare under Parts A and B and enrolling in a separate private prescription drug plan, or enrolling in a Part C plan through Medicare Advantage that includes prescription drug coverage. As of 2006, Medicare Advantage plans are required to offer basic prescription drug benefits and may offer supple-

mental prescription drug benefits for an additional premium. Beneficiaries who currently have drug benefit coverage through a Medigap insurance policy[ll] must choose between keeping their current policy or enrolling in Part D. In the future, however, Medigap plans will not be allowed to issue insurance policies that include Part D coverage.[31,32] Some beneficiaries may also have access to employer-sponsored health insurance that includes prescription drug benefits. These beneficiaries may keep their employer coverage only, keep their employer coverage and enroll in Part D, or drop their employer coverage. Finally, beneficiaries may also choose not to obtain any prescription drug coverage. However, in certain circumstances a beneficiary who declines to enroll in Part D during the allotted enrollment period may pay increased premiums if he decides to enroll at a later date.

Medicare Spending

Provider payment reforms have limited Medicare's spending growth somewhat, and since 1970 the annual spending per beneficiary has been about 1 percentage point lower than per-person private health insurance spending.[11(p189),33] Even so, Medicare expenditures were expected to reach $325 billion in 2005 (final figures are not yet available for that year), which would account for 13% of the total federal budget.[32] Furthermore, with the new prescription drug benefit estimated to cost $724 billion between 2006 and 2015, the high number of enrollees expected when the Baby Boom generation begins to re-

Box 6-14
Discussion Questions

Lawmakers were concerned that adding a prescription drug benefit to Medicare would encourage employers to drop prescription drug coverage to the 11 million beneficiaries who receive prescription drugs through retiree health plans. In an effort to avoid a shift in elderly people who rely on public insurance instead of private insurance for their prescription drug coverage, Congress included in the MMA a tax-free subsidy to encourage employers to maintain prescription drug coverage. The amount of the subsidy is based on the prescription drug costs of individuals who remain with the employer's plan and do not enroll in Part D.

Is this subsidy a good idea? Is the proper role of government to pay private companies to maintain insurance coverage? If so, should it occur for other benefits? Do you have a preference between giving incentives for private entities to provide insurance coverage versus the government financing the coverage directly?

tire (it is projected that 78 million elderly will enroll in Medicare by 2030),[29] recent increases in payments for rural health providers and Medicare managed care plans, the use of new technology, and rising health care costs, Medicare is projected to constitute 20.8% of national health care expenditures by 2014.[33]

Not all Medicare beneficiaries cost the same amount to care for because of the disparities in the amount and type of services they require. Almost half (45%) of Medicare's expenditures pay for hospital services, while physician services account for another 17% of Medicare expenditures.[11(p189),33(p7)] A relatively few beneficiaries use a high proportion of these and other services. In 2001, 10% of all beneficiaries accounted for over 60% of Medicare expenditures.[34]

Medicare Financing

Medicare is a federally funded program. Unlike Medicaid and SCHIP, state governments do not generally contribute to Medicare spending and therefore a matching system is not required. Although Medicare financing is simpler than Medicaid financing in many respects, each Medicare part has its own financing rules, adding some complexity to the program. In addition, beneficiary contributions in the form of premiums, deductibles, and co-payments contribute to financing Medicare expenditures.

Part A (HI) benefits are paid from the HI Trust Fund, funded through a mandatory payroll tax. Employers and employees each pay a tax of 1.45% of a worker's earnings (self-employed persons pay both shares for a total tax of 2.9%), which is set aside for the Trust Fund.[mm] These payroll taxes accounted for 51% of funding for Medicare in 2003.[33(p5)] In addition, beneficiaries pay a deductible for each inpatient hospital episode, and co-insurance for hospital care beyond 60 days, skilled nursing care beyond 20 days, outpatient drugs, and inpatient respite care.

By relying on payroll taxes, Medicare Part A uses current workers and employers to pay for health benefits for the disabled and those over 65 years old, many of whom are already retired. This formula is problematic in the face of the looming retirement of those from the

Baby Boom generation; between 2010 and 2030, it is projected that a 10-million-person increase in the working population will have to support an increase of 30 million new elderly Medicare beneficiaries. To put it another way, in 2003 payroll taxes from almost four workers supported each Medicare beneficiary, but in 2030 it is expected that taxes on only 2.4 workers will be available to support each Medicare beneficiary.[33(p13)] Because of this and for other reasons, the 2005 Medicare Board of Trustees estimated that the Part A HI Trust Fund would be exhausted by 2020.[35]

Part B (SMI) is financed through general federal tax revenues and monthly premiums, deductibles, and cost-sharing paid by beneficiaries. Starting in 2007, beneficiaries with incomes over $80,000 (or $160,000 for a couple) will pay a higher income-related monthly premium than other beneficiaries. In addition to the monthly premium, beneficiaries pay an annual deductible for physician and medical services and have co-insurance requirements for outpatient hospital care, ambulatory surgical care, clinical diagnostic services, outpatient mental health services, and most preventive services.

Despite the federal government's and beneficiaries' investment in Medicare benefits, the program covers less than half of beneficiaries' actual health care expenses. As is shown in Figure 6-6, other insurance coverage and out-of-pocket expenses pay for the rest of these costs.[35]

Part C Medicare Advantage plans provide services from Parts A and B and receive their funding from the sources described

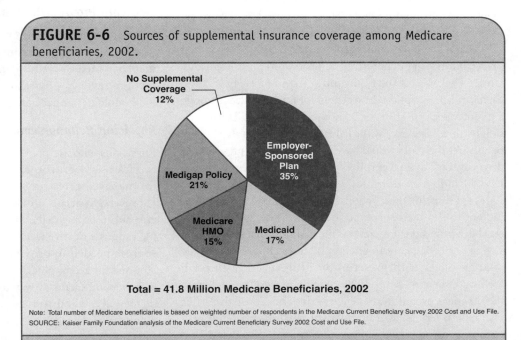

FIGURE 6-6 Sources of supplemental insurance coverage among Medicare beneficiaries, 2002.

No Supplemental Coverage 12%

Employer-Sponsored Plan 35%

Medigap Policy 21%

Medicare HMO 15%

Medicaid 17%

Total = 41.8 Million Medicare Beneficiaries, 2002

Note: Total number of Medicare beneficiaries is based on weighted number of respondents in the Medicare Current Beneficiary Survey 2002 Cost and Use File.
SOURCE: Kaiser Family Foundation analysis of the Medicare Current Beneficiary Survey 2002 Cost and Use File.

Source: Juliette Cubankski et al., *Medicare Chart Book*, 3rd ed. (Menlo Park: Kaiser Family Foundation, 2005), Figure 3.1. http://www.kff.org/medicare/upload/Medicare-Chart-Book-3rd-Edition-Summer-2005-Section-3.pdf.

above. The federal government contracts with private plans and pays them a capitated rate to provide Medicare benefits to program participants. The plans charge beneficiaries varying premiums and co-payments.

Part D, Medicare's prescription drug benefit, is financed through an annual deductible, monthly premiums, general revenues, and state payments for dual enrollees. The annual deductible was $250 in 2006. If the beneficiary spends between $250 and $2,250 on prescription drugs annually, Medicare covers 75% of prescription drug costs and beneficiaries cover the remaining 25%. If the beneficiary spends between $2,251 and $5,100, Medicare covers nothing; the beneficiary pays 100% of costs. (This gap in Medicare coverage is commonly referred to as the "doughnut hole" provision.) If a beneficiary spends over $5,100 on prescription drugs annually, Medicare pays 95% of the costs while the beneficiary picks up the remaining 5%.[31]

Under Part D, deductibles, premiums, benefit limits, and catastrophic thresholds are not fixed, but indexed to increase with the growth in per capita Medicare spending for Part D. For example, by 2014, the prescription drug monthly premium is projected to increase from $37 to almost $65, the annual deductible is expected to rise from $250 to $437, and the initial coverage limit (when the doughnut hole is implicated) is projected to start at $3,934 instead of $2,251. To offset these charges, the MMA includes provisions to assist low-income beneficiaries by reducing or eliminating cost-sharing requirements and the doughnut hole. There are three low-income assistance tiers for beneficiaries who earn up to 150% FPL.[29(p47)]

The MMA also requires that dual enrollees receive their prescription drug benefit through Medicare, not Medicaid. Under the MMA, states are now required to help fund Medicare's prescription drug benefit for dual enrollees through a maintenance-of-effort or "clawback" provision. This provision requires states to pay the federal government a share of expenditures the states would have made to provide prescription drug coverage to dual enrollees. The state share begins at 90% in 2006 and tapers down to 75% in 2015 and beyond. Many states are resisting these requirements and some are threatening not to pay their share. To the extent states adhere to the clawback provision, it represents the first time that states are assisting with Medicare financing. If states choose to provide dual enrollees with prescription drug coverage through Medicaid, states must use 100% of their own dollars to finance the coverage, even if the beneficiary does not enroll in Part D.

Table 6-6 provides a summary of Medicare financing provisions. Because Part C is financed by parts A and B and is an alternative to A and B, it is not included in the table. Whether beneficiaries have cost-sharing and other requirements under Part C depends on the specifics of each managed care plan.

Box 6-15
Discussion Questions

The clawback provision is controversial and highlights some of the tensions about state flexibility and national uniformity that policymakers face when designing public programs. The clawback seems to contradict the prior decision to provide states with flexibility and program design responsibilities under Medicaid. In addition, it changes the decision to use only federal funds to pay for Medicare. Given decisions made by states prior to the MMA, there are many variations among state prescription drug benefits that will be "frozen" in place with the clawback provision. At the same time, the MMA creates a uniform rule about how all states finance prescription drug funding in the future, which could impact state-level decisions about dual enrollee coverage.

Is the clawback provision a good idea? Should states help pay for federal prescription drug coverage? Is there a better design? Should states or the federal government control Medicaid prescription drug coverage that is provided to dual enrollees? Should dual enrollees be treated differently than other Medicaid beneficiaries?

Medicare Provider Reimbursement

Medicare's reimbursement rules vary by provider type and by whether care is provided through a fee-for-service arrangement or a Medicare Advantage (i.e., managed care) plan. This section reviews physician and hospital reimbursement methodologies under both payment systems.

Physician Reimbursement

Physicians who are paid by a managed care plan to provide Medicare services to beneficiaries follow the same general rules for managed care reimbursement discussed in Chapter 4. However, physicians providing care on a fee-for-service basis are paid according to the Medicare fee schedule. The fee schedule assigns a relative weight to every service to reflect the resources needed to provide the service. These weights are adjusted for geographic differences in costs and multiplied by a conversion factor (a way to convert the relative value that defines all medical services on the fee schedule into a dollar amount) to determine the final payment amount. Payment rates are changed through upward or downward shifts in the conversion factor. Overall, Medicare physician fees are about 81% of those provided by private insurers, but higher than reimbursement rates provided by Medicaid.[33(pp72–78)]

TABLE 6-6 Medicare Financing by Part

Medicare Part	Government Financing Scheme	Beneficiary Payment Requirements		
		Annual Deductible	*Monthly Premium*	*Cost Sharing*
A	Trust fund through mandated employer and employee payroll taxes	Yes	No, if meet Social Security work requirements	Yes
B	General federal tax revenue	Yes	Yes	Yes
D	General federal tax revenue and state clawback payments for dual enrollees	Yes—except some low-income beneficiaries	Yes—except some low-income beneficiaries	Yes—except some low-income beneficiaries

Hospital Reimbursement

Hospitals are paid for acute inpatient services on a prospective basis using "diagnostic related groups" (DRGs). DRGs sort patients into more than 500 groups based on their diagnoses. Various diagnoses are grouped together if they have similar clinical profiles and costs. Each DRG is assigned a relative weight based on charges for cases in that group as compared to the national average for all groups. In addition, the part of the DRG covering hospitals' cost of labor is adjusted by a wage index to account for different geographic costs.[33(p43)] Hospitals may also receive additional payments for providing high-cost outlier cases; incurring costs associated with use of new technology; incurring indirect medical education costs; serving a high proportion of low-income patients; or being a qualified sole community provider, a rural referral center, a small Medicare-dependent hospital, a rural hospital treating fewer than 200 admissions, or a critical access hospital (a qualified rural hospital that provides critical care services).[33(pp43–44)]

For outpatient care, hospitals are reimbursed by Medicare using a different prospective system. Each outpatient service is assigned to one of about 800 ambulatory payment classification (APC) groups. APCs have a relative weight based on the median cost of the service as compared to the national average. Again, a conversion factor is used to calculate the specific dollar amount per APC and the labor cost portion is adjusted based on a hospital wage index to account for geographic cost differences. APC payments may be adjusted when hospitals use new technologies or biologics, and when they treat unusually high-cost patients.[33(p44)]

Medicare Advantage Reimbursement

Medicare Advantage plans are paid a capitated rate by the federal government to provide Parts A, B, and D benefits to each enrollee in their plan. The rate is based on a contract between plans and the federal government that details the services the plan will provide and the premiums, deductibles, and cost sharing it will charge beneficiaries. Medicare is phasing in the use of risk adjustments (providing higher rates to plans that serve beneficiaries who are likely to need more costly care) when calculating capitation rates, with all plan payments to be risk-adjusted by 2007.

CONCLUSION

This chapter provided you with an overview of the three main public programs that provide health insurance coverage to approximately 80 million people in the United States, and raised a series of policy questions for your consideration. Based on the size of the programs, their costs to the federal and state governments, and their importance to millions of (often low-income) individuals, the role and structure of Medicaid, SCHIP, and Medicare are constantly being debated. Some people would like to see coverage expanded to ensure that everyone has adequate access to health insurance, others would like to dismantle the programs in the interest of eliminating government-funded entitlements, and still others suggest incremental changes to the programs. Each of these decisions, and many others, reflect the recurring themes that have been discussed throughout this chapter: choosing between state flexibility and national uniformity; determining the appropriate role for government, the private sector, and individuals in health care financing and delivery; defining a primary decision-making goal (fiscal restraint, equity/social justice, improved health outcomes, uniformity, etc.); and settling on the appropriate scope of coverage to offer beneficiaries. Given these programs' expected increase in beneficiaries and the complementary increase in their cost, it is likely that the debates over Medicaid, SCHIP, and Medicare will continue vigorously in the foreseeable future.

REFERENCES

1. Department of Health and Human Services. Medicaid program—letters to state officials. Center for Medicare and Medicaid Services. Available at: http://www.cms.hhs.gov/SMDL/. Accessed August 1, 2006.

2. Kaiser Commission on Medicaid and the Uninsured. *The Medicaid Program at a Glance*. Menlo Park, Calif.: Kaiser Family Foundation; 2005. Available at: http://www.kff.org/medicaid/upload/The-Medicaid-Program-at-a-Glance-Fact-Sheet.pdf. Accessed August 1, 2006.

3. Kaiser Family Foundation. Dual eligibles enrollment, 2003. State Health Facts. Available at: http://www.statehealthfacts.org/cgi-bin/healthfacts.cgi?action=compare&category=Medicaid+%26+SCHIP&subcategory=&topic=&link_category=Medicare&link_subcategory=Dual+Eligibles&link_topic=Dual+Eligibles+Enrollment&viewas=&showregions=0&sortby=&printer-friendly=0&datatype=number. Accessed August 1, 2006.

3. Department of Health and Human Services. The 2006 HHS poverty guidelines. Available at: http://aspe.hhs.gov/poverty/06poverty.shtml. Accessed August 1, 2006.

4. Kaiser Commission on Medicaid and the Uninsured. Distribution of the Nonelderly with Medicaid by Federal Poverty Level, U.S., 2005. State Health Facts. Available at: http://www.statehealthfacts.org/cgi-bin/healthfacts.cgi?action=compare&category=Medicaid+%26+SCHIP&link_category=Health+Coverage+%26+Uninsured&link_subcategory=Nonelderly+With+Medicaid&link_topic=Distribution+by+FPL Accessed October 25, 2006.

5. Kaiser Commission on Medicaid and the Uninsured. *Who Needs Medicaid?* Menlo Park, Calif.: Kaiser Family Foundation; 2006. Available at: http://www.kff.org/medicaid/upload/7496.pdf. Accessed August 1, 2006.

6. Kaiser Commission on Medicaid and the Uninsured. *Medicaid: An Overview of Spending on "Mandatory" vs. "Optional" Populations and Services*. Menlo Park, Calif.: Kaiser Family Foundation; 2005. Available at: http://www.kff.org/medicaid/upload/Medicaid-An-Overview-of-Spending-on.pdf. Accessed August 1, 2006.

7. Kaiser Family Foundation. Medically needy eligibility as a percent of federal poverty level, 2001. State Health Facts. Available at: http://www.statehealthfacts.org/cgi-bin/healthfacts.cgi?action=compare&category=Medicaid+%26+SCHIP&subcategory=Medicaid+Medically+Needy&topic=Medically+Needy+Eligibility. Accessed August 1, 2006.

8. Fremstad S, Cox L. *Covering New Americans: A Review of Federal and State Policies Related to Immigrants' Eligibility and Access to Publicly Funded Health Insurance*. Menlo Park, Calif.: Kaiser Family Foundation; 2004. Available at: http://www.kff.org/medicaid/upload/Covering-New-Americans-A-Review-of-Federal-and-State-Policies-Related-to-Immigrants-Eligibility-and-Access-to-Publicly-Funded-Health-Insurance-Report.pdf. Accessed August 1, 2006.

9. Passell JS. *Unauthorized Migrants: Numbers and Characteristics*. Washington, D.C.: Pew Hispanic Center; 2005. Available at: http://pewhispanic.org/files/reports/46.pdf. Accessed August 1, 2006.

10. Rosenbaum S. Health policy report: Medicaid. *N Engl J Med*. 2002;346:635–640.

11. Smith C, Cownan C, Heffler S, et al. National health spending in 2004: recent slowdown led by prescription drug spending. *Health Affairs*. 2006;25:186–196.

12. Kaiser Family Foundation. Tutorial—Medicaid: the basics. Figure 23 http://www.kaiseredu.org/tutorials/medicaidbasics/medicaid.html . Accessed October 25, 2003.

13. Kaiser, Medicaid Resource Book.[a]

14. Kaiser Commission on Medicaid and the Uninsured. Total Medicaid Spending, FY 2005. State Health Facts. Available at http://www.statehealthfacts.org/cgi-bin/healthfacts.cgi?action=compare&category=Medicaid+%26+SCHIP&subcategory=Medicaid+Spending&topic=Total+Medicaid+Spending%2c+FY2005, Accessed October 25, 2006.

15. Cunningham PJ. *Mounting Pressures: Physicians Servicing Medicaid Patients and the Uninsured, 1997–2001*. Center for Studying Health Systems Change, Community Tracking Study No. 6; 2002. Available at: http://www.hschange.com/CONTENT/505/. Accessed August 1, 2006.

16. Department of Health and Human Services. Medicaid managed care enrollment as of December 31, 2004. Center for Medicare and Medicaid Services. Available at: http://www.cms.hhs.gov/MedicaidDataSourcesGenInfo/Downloads/mmcpr04.pdf. Accessed August 1, 2006.

17. Kaiser Family Foundation. State health facts—Medicaid managed care enrollees as a percent of state Medicaid enrollees, as of December 31, 2004. Available at: http://www.statehealthfacts.org/cgi-bin/healthfacts.cgi?action=compare&category=Medicaid+%26+SCHIP&subcategory=Medicaid+Managed+Care&topic=MC+Enrollment+as+a+%25+of+Medicaid+Enrollment. Accessed August 1, 2006.

18. Kaiser Family Foundation. State health facts—statewide adjusted Medicaid managed care rates, 2001. Available at: http://www.statehealthfacts.org/cgi-bin/healthfacts.cgi?action=compare&category=Medicaid+%26+SCHIP&subcategory=Medicaid+Managed+Care&topic=Medicaid+Managed+Care+Capitation+Rates. Accessed August 1, 2006.

19. Artiga S, Mann C. *New Directions for Medicaid Section 1115 Waivers: Policy Implications of Recent Waiver Activity*. Menlo Park, Calif.: Kaiser Family Foundation; 2005. Available at: http://www.kff.org/medicaid/upload/New-Directions-for-Medicaid-Section-1115-Waivers-Policy-Implications-of-Recent-Waiver-Activity-Policy-Brief.pdf. Accessed August 1, 2006.

20. Kaiser Commission on Medicaid and the Uninsured. *Florida Medicaid Waiver: Key Program Changes and Issues*. Menlo Park, Calif.: Kaiser Family Foundation; 2005. Available at: http://www.kff.org/medicaid/upload/7443.pdf. Accessed August 1, 2006.

21. Center for Medicare and Medicaid Services. FY 2005 fourth quarter ever enrolled data by state—total SCHIP. Available at: http://www.cms.hhs.gov/NationalSCHIPPolicy/SCHIPER/itemdetail.asp?filterType=none&filterByDID=-99&sortByDID=2&sortOrder=ascending&itemID=CMS056615. Accessed August 1, 2006.

22. Hoffman C, Carbaugh A. *Health Coverage in America: 2003 Update*. Menlo Park, Calif.: Kaiser Family Foundation; 2004. Available at: http://www.kff.org/uninsured/upload/Health-Coverage-in-America-2004-Data-Update-Report.pdf. Accessed August 1, 2006.

23. Rosenbaum S, Markus A, Sonosky C. Public health insurance design for children: the evolution from Medicaid to SCHIP. *J Health Biomedical Law*. 2004;1:1–47.

24. Mann C, Rudowitz R. *Financing Health Coverage: The State Children's Health Insurance Program Experience*. Menlo Park, Calif.: Kaiser Family Foundation; Available at: http://www.kff.org/medicaid/7252.cfm. Accessed October 25, 2005.

25. Dubay L, Hill I, Kenney G. *Five Things Everyone Should Know about SCHIP*. Washington, D.C.: The Urban Institute; 2002:fn. 6. Available at: http://www.urban.org/Template.cfm?Section=ByTopic&NavMenuID=62&template=/TaggedContent/ViewPublication.cfm&PublicationID=7958. Accessed August 1, 2006.

26. Rosenbaum S, Markus A, Sonosky C, Respach L. *Policy Brief #2: State Benefit Design Choices under SCHIP: Implications for Pediatric Health Care*. Washington, D.C.: The George Washington University Center for Health Services Research and Policy; 2001. Available at: http://www.gwumc.edu/sphhs/healthpolicy/chsrp/downloads/SCHIP_brief2.pdf. Accessed August 1, 2006.

27. Hill I. Is the glass half full or half empty? State SCHIP policy responses to the economic downturn. National Conference of State Legislatures Webcast, March 10, 2004. Available at: http://www.ncsl.org/programs/health/IanHill_files/frame.htm#slide0310.htm. Accessed August 1, 2006.

28. Lutzky AW, Hill I. *Premium Assistance Program Under SCHIP: Not for the Faint of Heart?* Washington, D.C.: The Urban Institute; 2003. Available at: http://www.urban.org/Template.cfm?Section=ByTopic&NavMenuID=62&template=/TaggedContent/ViewPublication.cfm&PublicationID=8394. Accessed August 1, 2006.

29. Cubanksi J, Voris M, Kitchman M, et al. *Medicare Chart Book*, 3rd ed. Menlo Park, Calif.: Kaiser Family Foundation; 2005.

30. Kaiser Family Foundation. *Medicare Advantage*. Menlo Park, Calif.: Kaiser Family Foundation; 2005. Available at: http://www.kff.org/medicare/upload/Medicare-Advantage-April-2005-Fact-Sheet.pdf. Accessed August 1, 2006.

31. Kaiser Family Foundation. *The Medicare Prescription Drug Benefit.* Menlo Park, Calif.: Kaiser Family Foundation; 2005. Available at: http://www.kff.org/medicare/loader.cfm?url=/commonspot/security/getfile.cfm&PageID=33325. Accessed August 1, 2006.

32. Kaiser Family Foundation, *Medicare at a Glance.* Menlo Park, Calif: Kaiser Family Foundation; 2006. Available at http://www.kff.org/medicare/upload/1066-09.pdf. Accessed October 25, 2006.

33. Medicare Payment Advisory Committee. *Report to Congress: Medicare Payment Policy.* Washington, D.C.: Medicare Payment Advisory Committee; 2005.

34. Congressional Budget Office. *High-Cost Medicare Beneficiaries.* Washington D.C.: Congressional Budget Office; 2005.

35. Kaiser Family Foundation. *Medicare Spending and Financing.* Menlo Park, Calif.: Kaiser Family Foundation; 2005. Available at: http://www.kff.org/medicare/upload/7305.pdf. Accessed August 1, 2006.

ENDNOTES

a. For a comprehensive description of the Medicaid program, see Kaiser Commission on Medicaid and the Uninsured. *The Medicaid Resource Book* (Menlo Park: The Kaiser Family Foundation, 2002).

b. Puerto Rico, the U.S. Virgin Islands, Guam, Northern Mariana Islands, and American Samoa participate in Medicaid. However, financing rules are different in these territories than in the 50 states. Federal spending is capped and appropriated by Congress annually.

c. Social Security Act §§ 1108(f), (g) & 1905(b), 42 U.S.C. §§ 1308 & 1396d(b).

d. Title XIX of the Social Security Act, §§ 1901-1935; 42 U.S.C. §§ 1396-1396v.

e. 42 C.F.R. Parts 430-498.

f. The *State Medicaid Manual* is available on the CMS Web site, http://www.cms.gov/manuals/.

g. States may also issue regulations, create program manuals, and disseminate policy notices outlining program requirements.

h. The federal poverty guidelines are determined annually and calculated based on the number of individuals in a family. These guidelines are commonly referred to as the Federal Poverty Level, although HHS discourages the use of this term because the agency considers it ambiguous since the Census Bureau also calculates a figure referred to as the federal poverty thresholds. However, because the term Federal Poverty Level is still commonly used when discussing eligibility for federal and state programs, we use it here. According to the 2006 HHS Poverty Guidelines, an individual who earns $9,800 or less and a family of four that earns $20,000 or less are considered poor (i.e., at 100% of the federal poverty level). The poverty thresholds are somewhat higher for Alaska and Hawaii due to administrative procedures adopted by the Office of Economic Opportunity.[3]

i. In some states, some groups are exempt from the resource test.

j. Public Law 104-193.

k. The five-year ban does not apply to refugees and other humanitarian immigrants.

l. The immigration restrictions prevent the use of federal funds to provide service to immigrants, but states may use their own money to do so if they wish. We discuss Medicaid financing in more detail in the next section.

m. Public Law No. 109-362.

n. Federal Medicaid regulations prohibit very few services. Two areas of prohibition relate to abortion and substance abuse. Since 1977 Congress has prohibited the use of federal funds to pay for the costs of an abortion or Mifepristone (commonly known as RU-486), a drug that induces medical abortions. In addition, drug addiction or alcohol dependency may not be used to qualify someone as disabled under SSI (and therefore, under Medicaid), though if an individual is eligible for Medicaid for another reason, Medicaid programs may pay for substance abuse treatment.

o. 42 U.S.C. § 1396d(a)(13); 42 C.F.R. § 440.130.

p. DRA § 6044 *to be codified at* 42 U.S.C. § 1937.

q. 42 U.S.C. § 1937(a).

r. 42 U.S.C. § 1937(a)2.

s. New York, California, Texas, and Pennsylvania.

t. New York, California, Texas, Pennsylvania, Florida, Ohio, Illinois, Massachusetts, North Carolina, and Michigan.

u. 42 C.F.R. 447.50-.59.

v. 42 U.S.C. § 1916A.

w. Community health centers have their own per-visit prospective payment system for reimbursement under Medicaid. This methodology is described in Chapter 2.

x. 42 U.S.C. 1396a(a)(30)(A).

y. 42 U.S.C 1396a(a)(30)(A).

z. The provisions relating to managed care are found in §1932 of the Social Security Act (42. U.S.C. § 1936u-2). However, states may seek a waiver permitting them to enroll exempt populations. Medicaid waivers are discussed in the following section. The provisions relating to managed care are found in §1932 of the Social Security Act (42. U.S.C. § 1936u-2).

aa. 42 U.S.C 1396b(m)(2)(A)(iii). Federal regulations also cover managed care generally. These can be found at 42 C.F.R. 438.

bb. In 2001, 39 states had Medicaid managed care programs and 36 responded to the survey.

cc. Although federal law does not elaborate on the specifics of section 1115 waivers, other federal guidance does. In 1994, HHS prepared a nonbinding notice, "Demonstration Proposal Pursuant to Section 1115(a) of the Social Security Act," 59 Fed. Reg. 49249 (1994), and then the Health Care Financing Administration (now CMS) published a "Review Guide for Section 1115 Research and Demonstration Waiver Proposals for State Health Care Reform." The *State Medicaid Manual* also contains information relating to Section 1115 waivers.

dd. 42 U.S.C. §§ 1397aa-1397jj.

ee. If eligibility for a state's Medicaid program was already near or above 200% FPL, the state is allowed to cover children under SCHIP up to 50 percentage points above the limits in place at the end of March 1997. States may also disregard additional family income for institutionalized individuals as allowed under Section 1902(r)(2) of Medicaid.

ff. Title XXI, § 2103(c); 42 U.S.C. § 1397cc(c).

gg. 42 U.S.C. § 1397cc.

hh. Title XXI, § 2102(a); 42 U.S.C. § 1397bb(a).

ii. Patients with end-stage renal disease are also eligible for Medicare. It is the only disease-specific eligibility group in Medicare.

jj. Private fee-for-service plans, usually offered at the county level, provide the standard Medicare coverage, but beneficiaries may see only physicians who participate in the plan and must pay premiums and co-payments or co-insurance to the private plan instead of to individual providers. In return, the private plan may offer additional services not covered by Medicare.

kk. Public Law No. 108-173.

ll. Medigap policies are designed to cover payments required by Medicare, such as premiums and co-payments. In essence, beneficiaries buy additional coverage to protect themselves against the risk of having to pay high out-of-pocket amounts. In addition, some Medigap policies offer additional benefits. CMS has approved 12 standard Medigap policies (labeled A–K). Private insurance companies that sell Medigap policies do not have to offer all 12 policies, but they cannot deviate from the terms of Medigap policies set by CMS. Insurance companies may set their own prices for the policies, in accordance with federal and state laws.

mm. Beneficiaries who did no work for 40 quarters are required to pay a monthly premium, which was set at $375 in 2005 and is projected to reach $457 by 2010.

The Uninsured and Health Reform

LEARNING OBJECTIVES

By the end of this chapter you will be able to:

- Identify common characteristics of the uninsured
- Understand the effect of insurance on access to care and on health status
- Describe the types of providers who care for uninsured patients
- Describe previous national health reform attempts and recent state health reform activity
- Understand why national health reform has been difficult to achieve in the United States

INTRODUCTION

Most people in the United States have health insurance through a patchwork collection of private plans and public programs. Unfortunately, like Casey, there are also many people who are uninsured. Although the number of uninsured varies from year to year, over the last several decades the rate of uninsurance has consistently hovered between 12% and 16% of the population.[1(pp16–17)] In 2005, 46.6 million people in this country (15.9% of the population) did not have health insurance,[1(p18)] and most of them were without coverage for at least two years.[2(pp4–5)] An even greater number are uninsured at any given point during a calendar year because many people cycle on and off of insurance plans depending on their circumstances (job loss, relocation, marriage, etc.).[3] As we discuss in more detail

VIGNETTE

Casey is a recent college graduate with a degree in fine arts. She works in retail as a way to pay the bills until her career as an artist takes off. Her employer does not offer health insurance, but even if it did, Casey would rather spend her limited funds on art supplies than on health insurance. Despite her low income, Casey makes too much money to qualify for any of the public health insurance programs in her state. One evening when Casey was up late working on an art project, she cut a tendon in her hand with a sharp knife. She rushed to the emergency room, where she waited for 7 hours, due to the high volume of patients that night, before being treated. Doctors stitched up her hand, provided her with pain killers, and told her she would need physical therapy to ensure that she regained full function in her hand. Casey looked into private physical therapy programs but found them unaffordable. The public clinics in her area that provide free or reduced-cost care did not offer physical therapy services. Casey decided to forgo the physical therapy and rehabilitate her hand on her own. In addition, she received a $1,500 bill from the hospital, an amount equal to her savings.

later in this chapter, the uninsured have less access to care and poorer health status than the insured. Yet, even the insured have difficulties paying their medical expenses. Depending on the definition used, an estimated 10% to 25% of the insured are *under*insured, meaning they have an insurance plan that does not provide adequate financial protection.[4,5]

In the U.S., the persistent rate of uninsurance and concerns about the adequacy of insurance plans have led to numerous attempts to implement national health reform that provides comprehensive coverage for most or all residents. Yet, each attempt has failed due to a constellation of practical, political, and social factors. As a result of this national inaction, there also have been significant health coverage reform efforts on the state level. It is fair to say that the intractable problem of uninsurance is this country's biggest health policy problem today.

This chapter begins with an examination of the problem of the uninsured—who they are, why they are uninsured, who provides care for them, and the impact and cost of uninsurance on patients, providers, and society as a whole. It then moves to a discussion of national health reform by considering why it is so difficult to achieve broad reform and by examining the numerous failed attempts at national health reform over the last century. It ends with a discussion of state efforts that have emerged in the absence of national health reform. Throughout this chapter you will revisit the themes highlighted in Chapter 6: choosing between state flexibility and national uniformity; determining the appropriate role for government, the private sector, and individuals in health care financing and delivery; defining a primary decision-making goal (e.g., fiscal restraint, equity/social justice, improved health outcomes, uniformity, etc.); and settling on the appropriate scope of coverage to offer beneficiaries. Finally, the addendum at the end of this chapter includes a comprehensive time line of the political and social events that affected developments in health insurance and medical care in the U.S. between the late 1700s and the beginning of the 21st century.

CHARACTERISTICS OF THE UNINSURED

There are many myths relating to the uninsured. It is often assumed that the uninsured do not work or simply choose not to purchase health insurance even though it is available and affordable. Although this may be true in some cases, in most instances it is not. Furthermore, many people believe that all employers offer insurance or that those individuals without private insurance are always eligible for public programs. As you will see, these assumptions are also false.

Income Level

The primary reason people do not have health insurance is financial—available coverage is simply too expensive.[2(p6)] Two-thirds of the uninsured are individuals or families earning less than 200% of the Federal Poverty Level (FPL) (about $40,000 for a family of four in 2006).[6] About 37% of the uninsured are poor (earning 100% FPL or less) and another 28% are near-poor (earning between 101% and 199% FPL).[2(p4)] Given these data, it is not surprising that the uninsured rate among the poor is twice as high as the national average.[2(p4)]

Employment Status

Over 80% of the uninsured work or are in families with workers. Most of them (about 70%) have at least one full-time worker in the family, and a much smaller proportion have only part-time workers.[2(p4)] This pattern holds true even for the very poor. Over half of the poor uninsured have at least one worker in their family.[2(p4)]

Workers are uninsured because they cannot afford the insurance coverage offered by their employers or because they work in jobs that do not offer coverage.[7(p62)] Workers are more likely to be uninsured if they work in small firms, low-paying firms, non-unionized firms, retail/sales firms, or in the agricultural, forestry, fishing, mining, and construction sectors. In addition, self-employed individuals are often uninsured.[7(pp67–70)] Overall, families whose primary wage earner is a blue-collar worker are more likely to be uninsured than families whose primary wage earner is a white-collar worker.[7(p67)]

Because of the disparity in opportunities to obtain employer-sponsored insurance, it is not just overall income that determines whether a family is insured, but also the way a family earns money. It is more likely that one earner who makes $50,000 will have access to an affordable employer-sponsored health insurance policy than two workers who earn $25,000 each, due to the type of jobs the latter are likely to hold.[7(p65)]

Age

Because Medicaid and the State Children's Health Insurance Program (SCHIP) provide extensive coverage for low-income children, adults are more likely to be uninsured than children. In 2004, 8.3 million children (11.2% of the population) were uninsured, compared to 37.5 million adults (17% of the population).[1(pp16–18)] Approximately 31% of young adults ages 18–24 are uninsured, which is almost twice the rate of the general population.[1(p18)] This is a trend that has remained in place since the mid-1980s.[7(p72)]

As young adults transition from school to the workforce, they may become ineligible for their family's coverage for the first time, may have entry-level jobs earning too little income to afford a policy, or may work for an employer that does not offer health insurance. Although some young adults do not consider health insurance a priority expense because they are usually healthy, studies have shown that cost is the primary factor in whether people in this age bracket decide to obtain coverage.[7(pp73-74)]

Although adults ages 55–64 are more likely to be insured than the overall population, the 8% of uninsured who fall into this age group are a cause for concern because they are medically high risk and often have declining incomes.[7(p72)] These adults account for two-thirds of all deaths and one-third of all hospital days among non-elderly adults. In addition, they are more likely to report being in fair or poor health, having a chronic disease, or experiencing a disabling condition.[7(p74)] The disability provisions of Medicaid and Medicare and the availability of employer-based insurance keep the number of uninsured in this group relatively small, which is important because it would be very expensive for individuals in this demographic to purchase individual insurance policies in the private market. Figure 7-1 illustrates the characteristics of the uninsured by income, age, and work status.

Education Level

Education level is also an important factor in insurance status because it is easier, for example, for college graduates to earn higher incomes and obtain jobs that provide affordable employment-based insurance.[7(p74)] Over 25% of uninsured adults do not have a high school diploma and almost 40% of those who did not graduate from high school are uninsured.[7(p66–67)]

Race, Ethnicity, and Immigrant Status

Although approximately half of the people who are uninsured are white, a greater proportion of minorities are uninsured. About 11% of whites are uninsured, compared to 33% of Hispanics, 29% of American Indians and Alaskan Natives, 20% of African Americans, and 17% of Asian Americans.[1(pp17–18)] This difference is only partially explained by variations in income. Minorities also have lower rates of employment-based coverage, although this is partially offset by their higher rates of public insurance coverage.[7(p83)] Because eligibility for public coverage is generally less stable than for private coverage, this difference in type of coverage is a key public policy issue.[7(p89)]

Although most of the uninsured are native citizens, a higher proportion of immigrants are uninsured. Compared to the 13% of native-born citizens who are uninsured, 33% of foreign-born residents are uninsured.[1(pp18–19)] Of the foreign-born uninsured, 17% are naturalized and 44% are non-citizens.[1(pp18–19)] Some of the disparity in coverage rates among U.S. native and foreign-born individuals is because non-native residents have lower rates of employer-based coverage, higher rates of low-wage jobs, and higher rates of

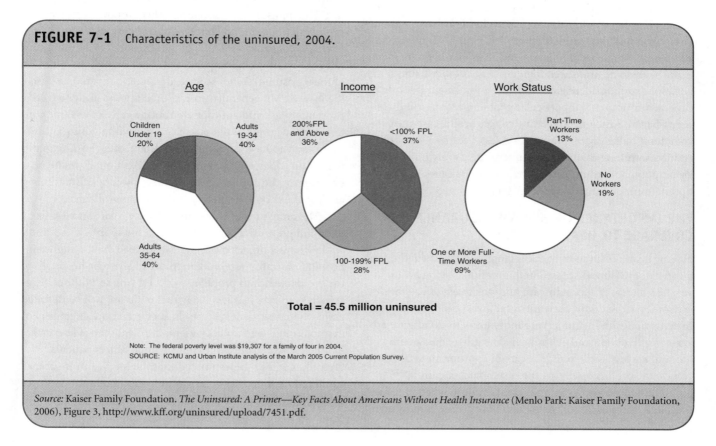

FIGURE 7-1   Characteristics of the uninsured, 2004.

Note: The federal poverty level was $19,307 for a family of four in 2004.
SOURCE: KCMU and Urban Institute analysis of the March 2005 Current Population Survey.

Source: Kaiser Family Foundation. *The Uninsured: A Primer—Key Facts About Americans Without Health Insurance* (Menlo Park: Kaiser Family Foundation, 2006), Figure 3, http://www.kff.org/uninsured/upload/7451.pdf.

employment in sectors that are less likely to provide insurance.[7(p81)] In addition, the restrictive eligibility rules pertaining to immigrants in public programs make it difficult for non-natives to obtain public coverage. For example, with a few exceptions, the national 1996 welfare reform law included provisions that bar legal immigrants from obtaining full Medicaid or SCHIP coverage for their first five years in the U.S.[7(pp82–83),a]

Gender

Gender variations exist in both rate of insurance and type of insurance coverage. In general, non-elderly men are more likely to be uninsured than non-elderly women. Yet, of those with insurance, men are more likely to have employer-based coverage and women are more likely to have public coverage, due to their lower average income level. This difference in public coverage rates is in large part due to the extensive coverage for low-income pregnant women under Medicaid.

Geography

Residents of the South and West are more likely to be uninsured than residents of the North and Midwest. These variations are based on numerous factors including racial/ethnic composition, other population characteristics, public program eligibility, and employment rates and sectors.[7(p90)] Although a greater number of uninsured residents live in urban areas, the likelihood of being uninsured is similar in both urban and rural areas. Residents of remote rural areas, however, are much more likely to be uninsured than residents of urban areas.[8] In addition, rural residents are uninsured for longer periods of time. Uninsurance is a particular problem among rural residents because they have relatively high health care needs—they tend to be older, poorer, and less healthy than urban residents. Among the insured, rural residents rely more heavily on public programs due to their lower incomes and fewer opportunities to obtain employer-based coverage.[8]

THE IMPORTANCE OF HEALTH INSURANCE COVERAGE TO HEALTH STATUS

Having health insurance provides tangible health benefits. For a variety of reasons discussed in this section, having health insurance increases access to care and positively affects health outcomes. Conversely, the uninsured, who do not enjoy the benefits of health insurance, are more likely to experience adverse health events and a diminished health-related quality of life, and are less likely to receive care in appropriate settings or receive the professionally accepted standard of care.[9(pp42–46)]

Health insurance is an important factor in whether someone has a "medical home," or consistent source of care. In turn,

> **Box 7-1   Discussion Questions**
>
> Are the characteristics just described interrelated, or should they be addressed separately from a policy perspective? If you are trying to reduce the number of uninsured, do you think the focus should be on altering insurance programs or changing the effect of having one or more of these characteristics? Whose responsibility is it to reduce the number of uninsured? Government? The private sector? Individuals?

having a consistent source of care is positively associated with better and timelier access to care, better chronic disease management, fewer emergency room visits, fewer lawsuits against emergency rooms, increased utilization rates, and increased cancer screenings for women.[10,11] Unfortunately, the uninsured are much less likely to have a usual source of care than are insured patients. About 42% of the uninsured do not have a usual source of care, compared to 9% of the insured. In addition, 20% of the uninsured consider the emergency room their usual source of care, compared to just 3% of the insured.[2(p6)]

The uninsured are also less likely to follow treatment recommendations due to concerns about cost (see Figure 7-2). Financial constraints led 37% of the uninsured to decide against filling a prescription, compared to 13% of the insured, and 47% of the uninsured did not seek needed care, compared to 15% of the insured.[2] In general, the uninsured are less likely to receive preventive care and appropriate routine care for chronic conditions.[2] One result of this is that children without insurance are more likely to have developmental delays, often leading to difficulties in education and employment. Also, quality of life may be lower for the uninsured due to their lower health status and anxiety about both monetary and medical problems.

The uninsured are more likely to forgo care and less likely to obtain preventive care or treatment for specific conditions, so they have a higher mortality rate overall, have a higher in-hospital mortality rate, and are more likely to be hospitalized for avoidable health problems.[12(p3)] Of course, without regular access to care it is less likely that a disease will be detected early when treatment may be cheaper and more effective. For example, uninsured cancer patients are diagnosed at later stages of the disease and die earlier than insured cancer patients.[12(p3)] Overall, studies have estimated that having health insurance could reduce mortality rates for the uninsured by 10–15%, resulting in 18,000 fewer deaths per year.[12(p3)]

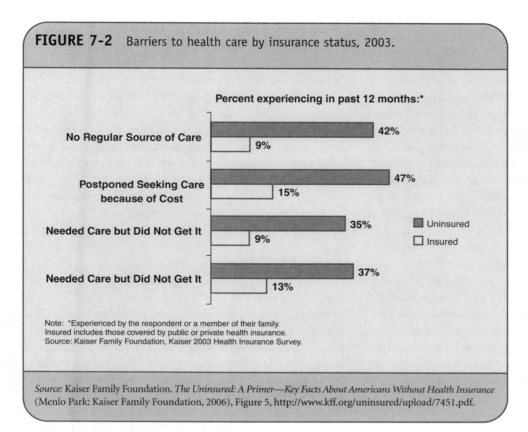

FIGURE 7-2 Barriers to health care by insurance status, 2003.

Percent experiencing in past 12 months:*

No Regular Source of Care — Uninsured 42%, Insured 9%

Postponed Seeking Care because of Cost — Uninsured 47%, Insured 15%

Needed Care but Did Not Get It — Uninsured 35%, Insured 9%

Needed Care but Did Not Get It — Uninsured 37%, Insured 13%

■ Uninsured
□ Insured

Note: *Experienced by the respondent or a member of their family.
Insured includes those covered by public or private health insurance.
Source: Kaiser Family Foundation, Kaiser 2003 Health Insurance Survey.

Source: Kaiser Family Foundation. *The Uninsured: A Primer—Key Facts About Americans Without Health Insurance* (Menlo Park: Kaiser Family Foundation, 2006), Figure 5, http://www.kff.org/uninsured/upload/7451.pdf.

WAYS TO COUNT THE COSTS OF UNINSURANCE

There are several ways to think about the costs of being uninsured. These include the health status costs to the uninsured individual, as discussed earlier; financial cost to the uninsured individual; financial cost to state and federal governments; financial cost to providers; productivity costs from lost work time due to illness; and costs to other public priorities that cannot be funded because of the resources spent on providing care to the uninsured.

The financial burden of being uninsured is significant. Although on average the uninsured spend fewer dollars on health care than the insured, those without insurance spend a greater proportion of their overall income on medical needs. Furthermore, when the uninsured receive care, it is often more expensive because the uninsured are not receiving care as part of an insurance pool with leverage to negotiate lower rates from providers. Given their lower income, relatively high health care expenses, and competing needs, the uninsured are more than twice as likely to have trouble paying their bills as the insured. Almost one-quarter of the uninsured reported that the need to pay for medical bills required them to alter their life significantly.[2(p8)]

Costs of medical care provided by health professionals but not fully reimbursed are referred to as uncompensated care costs.[b] In 2004, it was estimated that uncompensated care costs reached $41 billion in this country, with federal, state, and local spending covering 85% of the tab, mostly through "disproportionate share payments" to hospitals. Although hospitals provide about 60% of all uncompensated care services and receive significant government assistance, physicians provide about 20% of uncompensated care services, most of which is not subsidized.[13] Clinics and direct care programs account for the remaining 20% of uncompensated care dollars.[13] These providers also receive government subsidies, but to a much lesser extent than hospitals.

Providers may try to absorb uncompensated care costs into their budgets while shifting another portion of their costs from nonpaying patients to paying patients. This practice, known as cost shifting, was more common prior to the proliferation of managed care plans, which are less willing than traditional indemnity insurance plans to absorb the cost of uncompensated care. With limited opportunities to shift the cost of treating uninsured patients to insured patients, providers charge the uninsured the full cost of care, negotiate reduced rates and payment plans for patients, or provide services at little or no cost to the patient. However, if uncompensated care costs are too high, providers may turn away nonpaying patients or close their practices.

In addition, every dollar spent by providers, governments, and communities to cover uncompensated care costs is a dollar that is not spent on another public need. There are a variety of high-cost public health needs, such as battling infectious diseases like HIV/AIDS or tuberculosis, engaging in emergency preparedness planning, and promoting healthy behaviors. Public and private funds used to cover uncompensated care, especially when the care is more expensive than necessary because of the lack of preventive care or early interventions, are resources that are no longer available to meet the country's other health needs.

One additional pool of funds to cover uncompensated care costs comes from a less direct source—private insurance. As providers try to recover uncompensated care costs by charging higher rates to insurance companies, private insurers may raise their premiums to cover the additional charges.[14] One study estimated that almost $29 billion in uncompensated care to the uninsured is financed by higher premiums for privately insured patients, resulting in an 8.5% increase in the cost of private insurance.[14] However, as noted earlier, it has become more difficult to shift costs in the current era of negotiated prices and managed care plans.

One final cost associated with the uninsured is the cost of lower productivity. Productivity costs refer to the reduced productivity in the workforce due to the lower health status related to being uninsured. Productivity may be reduced when workers are absent or when they are not functioning at their highest level due to illness. In addition, several studies show that providing health insurance helps employers recruit better employees and that workers with health insurance are less likely to change jobs, reducing the costs of hiring and training new employees.[14]

SAFETY NET PROVIDERS

Whether individuals are uninsured, underinsured, or publicly insured, securing access to care can be difficult for those without comprehensive private insurance. For the uninsured, the high cost of care is often a deterrent to seeking care. For those with Medicaid or SCHIP coverage, it is often difficult to find a provider willing to accept their insurance due to the extremely low reimbursement rates and administrative burdens

Box 7-2
Discussion Questions

Given the costs just described, should it be a public priority to make sure everyone has health insurance? If so, at what point, if any, should the government step in to provide individuals with assistance to purchase insurance coverage? And should it be a federal or state responsibility? Or should everyone be part of one government-run plan or program? Should there be mandates that individuals buy health insurance, just as there are mandates that car owners buy car insurance? Should individuals be penalized financially if they do not have health insurance?

associated with participating in the program. For these patients and others, the "health care safety net" exists.[c]

The health care safety net refers to providers who serve disproportionately high numbers of uninsured and publicly insured patients. Although there is no formal designation indicating that one is a safety net provider, the Institute of Medicine defines the health care safety net as "[t]hose providers that organize and deliver a significant level of health care and other related services to uninsured, Medicaid, and other vulnerable populations."[4(p21)] According to the IOM, "core" safety net providers are those who serve vulnerable populations *and* have a policy of providing services regardless of patients' ability to pay.[4(p21)] Some safety net providers have a legal requirement to provide care to the underserved while others do so as a matter of principle.

Who are the safety net providers? It is a difficult question to answer because there is no true safety net "system." Safety net providers can be anyone or any entity providing health care to the uninsured and other vulnerable populations, whether community and teaching hospitals, private health professionals, school-based health clinics, or others. Those providers that fit the narrower definition of "core" safety net providers include some public and private hospitals, community health centers, family planning clinics, and public health agencies that have a mission to provide access to care for vulnerable populations. Safety net provider patient loads are mostly composed of people who are poor, on Medicaid, or uninsured, and are members of racial and ethnic minority groups. For example, in recent years 91% of health center patients had incomes at or below 200% FPL, 63% of public hospital patients and 76% of health center patients were on Medicaid or were uninsured, and over 60% of health center patients and 65% of public hospital patients were racial or ethnic minorities.[15–17]

Community health centers provide comprehensive primary medical care services, culturally sensitive care, and enabling services such as transportation, outreach, and translation that make it easier for patients to access services. Many health centers also provide dental, mental health, and pharmacy services. Because health centers are not focused on specialty care, public hospitals are often the sole source of specialty care for uninsured and underserved populations.[16(p4)] In addition, public hospitals provide traditional health care services, diagnostic services, outpatient pharmacies, and highly specialized trauma care, burn care, and emergency services.[16(p2)] Although not all local government health departments provide direct care, many do. Local health departments often specialize in caring for specific populations such as individuals with HIV or drug dependency, as compared to public hospitals and health centers, which provide a wider range of services.[4(pp63–65)]

Safety net providers receive funding from a variety of sources. Medicaid is the single largest funding stream for both public hospitals and health centers, accounting for over one-third of their revenue.[15(p13),16(p7)] Health centers also receive federal grants to cover the cost of caring for the uninsured; however, this grant funding has not kept pace with their cost of care. In fact, the annual cost of treating uninsured patients is $230 more per patient than health centers receive from federal grants.[18] In addition, payment from private insurance is unreliable due to the high-cost sharing plans held by many privately insured, low-income individuals. Furthermore, Medicare payments to health centers are capped under federal law at an amount that does not match the growth in health care spending. For these reasons, health centers faced over $900 million in unpaid charges in 2004, a 137% increase from 1999.[15(p13)]

Public hospitals face a similarly difficult economic picture. Even though public hospitals accept only 4.3% of all hospital admissions nationally, they provide 24% of the hospital industry's uncompensated care.[16(p8)] Additionally, many other public hospital services are not fully reimbursed because payments made by individuals or insurers do not match the cost of care. Like health centers, public hospitals receive additional funds to cover low-income patients, including Medicaid disproportionate share payments, state and local subsidies, and other revenues such as sales tax and tobacco settlement funds.[16] Even though these funds totaled almost $9 billion in 2002, many public hospitals have difficulty maintaining economic stability due to their low-income, high-uninsured patient load.[16(pp7–9)]

For all the positive work accomplished by safety net providers, they cannot solve all health care problems for the uninsured. Safety net patients may not experience continuity of care, whether because they cannot see the same provider at each visit or because they have to go to numerous sites or through various programs to receive all the care they need. Even though safety net providers serve millions of patients every year, there are not enough providers in enough places to satisfy the need for their services. And, as noted earlier, many safety net providers are under-funded and constantly struggling to meet the complex needs of their patient population. The problems facing the uninsured and the stresses to the health care safety net highlight the inadequacies of the current "system" of providing health care. Given the country's patchwork of programs and plans, decisions made in one area can significantly affect another. For example, if Medicaid reimbursement or eligibility is cut, safety net providers will have a difficult time keeping their doors open while, simultaneously, more patients will become uninsured and seek care from

Box 7-3
Discussion Questions

Safety net providers mostly serve uninsured and publicly insured low-income patients. Many of the safety net provider features you just read about are in place to assist these patients in accessing health care. If there were enough safety net providers to meet demand, would it remain important to pursue universal health insurance coverage? Are there reasons for both safety net providers and health insurance to exist? How does having insurance relate to accessing care?

safety net providers. If more people choose high-deductible private insurance plans that they cannot easily afford, individuals may go without needed services or safety net providers will end up providing an increasing amount of uncompensated care. If employers decide to cut coverage or increase employee cost sharing, previously insured people may fall into the ranks of the uninsured. Policymakers must understand how these and other pieces interact in order to develop policies that will solve existing health care problems without creating new ones.

THE DIFFICULTY OF REFORM IN THE UNITED STATES

The array of problems facing the health care system has led to numerous health reform proposals and implemented policies. The concept of health reform can have several different meanings. Given the patchwork health care system, health reform often refers to changes that seek to reduce the number of uninsured. Due to the high and increasing cost of health care services, health reform might also include changes that seek to contain costs and control utilization. The notion of health reform could also cover other features of the health care system, such as trying to reduce medical errors, strengthen patient rights, build the public health infrastructure, or confront the rising cost of medical malpractice insurance. Although all of these aspects of reform are important, this section focuses on those reforms that address the problem of the uninsured; it would be impossible to fully address all the issues raised in this chapter, and America's sizable uninsured population is arguably the most pressing health care concern of the day. We begin with a discussion about why reform is difficult to achieve in the United States and then introduce some of the reforms that have been attempted on a national or state level with varying degrees of success.

Numerous authors have addressed the main factors that deter significant social reform in this country, including health reform.[19–21] Factors that are prominently discussed include the country's culture, the nature of U.S. political institutions, the power of interest groups, and path dependency (i.e., the notion that people are generally opposed to change).

Culture

This country's culture and lack of consensus about health reform impede attempts to create universal coverage health plans. The twin concepts of entrepreneurialism and individualism have a real impact on health policy decisions: Americans generally oppose government solutions to social welfare problems.[21(p438)] Opposition is high to health reforms that rely either on a direct government-run program or public funding through tax increases.[21(p438)] For example, less than half (40%) of Americans favor a single-payer health plan.[22]

At the same time, the country also believes the government has some role to play in health reform. Large majorities favor tax credits to assist the uninsured with purchasing health insurance, expanding government programs for low-income individuals, and government mandates that employers provide insurance.[22] In addition to having different views about how to reduce the number of uninsured, there is no agreement about the overall scope of the health care problems we face.[22] Although a majority of Americans think that the current health system needs major changes, 20% thinks only minor changes are required and another 23% thinks the system needs to be rebuilt entirely.[22]

U.S. Political System

The country's federal system of government also makes it difficult to achieve universal coverage. Traditionally, social welfare programs—including the provision of health care—have been the responsibility of the states. Initially there was almost no federal involvement in the provision of health care, and when the federal government became more heavily involved in 1965, Medicaid continued to keep the locus of decision making on the state level. Of course, there are select populations, such as the elderly (Medicare) and veterans (Veterans Health Administration), who have a federalized health insurance system. However, the country appears to support a Medicaid-type expansion over a new federalized program.[22]

Although states are generally home to social welfare changes, it is very difficult to provide universal health care on a state-by-state basis. One reason is that if state health reform efforts lead the way, the country could have a patchwork of programs and policies that vary from state to state, with the potential to make health coverage even more complex and inefficient than it is currently. In addition, states must consider whether they are making policy decisions that will give employers an incentive to choose to locate in another state with fewer or less onerous requirements. If employers leave the state, it could result in loss of jobs and have downstream effects on the state's economy.

In addition, state reforming efforts are also constrained by the Employee Retirement Income Security Act of 1974 (ERISA).[d] As discussed in Chapter 9, ERISA is a federal law that regulates "welfare benefit programs," including health plans, operated by private employers. ERISA limits states' ability to reform because it broadly preempts state laws that "relate to" employer-sponsored plans and because it applies to nearly all individuals who receive health benefits through a private employer.[e] One effect of the law, for example, is that states have little regulatory control over the benefits covered in employer-sponsored health plans, because ERISA accords employers near-total discretion over the design of their benefit packages.[23(p237)]

Despite these hurdles, it is also important to recognize that a health reform strategy focusing on states has benefits as well. At its best, state-level reform can be accomplished more rapidly and with more innovation than at the federal level. State legislatures may have an easier time convincing a narrower band of constituents important to the state than Congress has in accommodating the varied needs of stakeholders nationwide. Along the same lines, states are able to target reforms to meet the particular needs of their population, instead of covering more diverse needs across the entire country. Additionally, through the use of direct democracy (referenda, ballot initiatives, etc.), citizens can more easily have an impact on decisions by state-level policymakers than by federal legislators.

Other aspects of the U.S. political system also make it difficult to institute sweeping reform. For example, although presidents have significant influence on policy agenda-setting and proposing budgets, they have very limited power to make changes without the assistance of Congress (as discussed in detail in Chapter 2). The U.S. government is often divided, with different parties holding power in the executive and legislative branches. This division often results in partisanship and policy inaction due to different policy priorities and views.

Furthermore, although members of Congress may ride the coattails of a popular president from their own party, they are not reliant on the president to keep their jobs. The issues and views their constituents care about most may not align with the president's priorities. In those cases, members of Congress have a strong incentive to adhere to the wishes of those who vote for them, instead of simply following the president's lead. Furthermore, since federal office-holders are reelected at extremely high rates—98% of incumbents successfully defended their seats in 2004[24]—those in Congress may feel confident about focusing on their district's or state's needs before those of the entire nation.

Federal legislative rules also support inaction or incremental reform over sweeping changes. In the U.S. Senate, 60 (out of 100) votes are needed to break a filibuster or to change budget rules. Thus, even the political party in the majority can have difficulty effectuating change. Also, because both the House and the Senate have to pass bills containing the same policies and language to have any chance at becoming law, a large political majority in one chamber or the other does not guarantee the ability to enact a policy. As a result, in many cases members of Congress have to work together, at least to some degree, to devise a consensus policy that satisfies enough members to pass a bill. This type of consensus requirement makes radical change unlikely.

Interest Groups

As discussed in more detail in Chapter 2, decisions by politicians are often influenced by interest groups. The role of interest groups is to represent their members' interests in policy decisions. They lobby politicians and the general public about the virtues or vices of specific proposals, work to improve proposals on the agenda, and attempt to defeat proposals they think are not in the best interest of their group. By contributing to political campaigns, interest groups gain the ear, and often the influence, of politicians who vote on issues important to the group.

In terms of health care reform, interest groups representing various providers, businesses, employer groups, insurance companies, and managed care organizations have all been opposed to comprehensive health reform.[21(pp438–439)] There are numerous points along the path from developing a policy idea to voting for or against a bill when interest groups can attempt to affect politicians' views. The more radical the policy proposal, the more interest groups are likely to become engaged in the political decision-making process, making it difficult to pass a bill that includes comprehensive reform.

In general, it is easier to oppose a proposal than develop one and pass a bill. Opponents of proposals are not required to show that they have a better alternative to whatever is on the table. Instead, they can simply point to aspects of the policy idea that are unpopular and call for the proposal to be rejected. This was the tactic used by the Health Insurance Association of America (HIAA) in their well-known "Harry and Louise" television ads that opposed the Clinton adminis-

tration's comprehensive health reform bill in 1993, the Health Security Act. In the ad, Harry and Louise, two "average" Americans, are seen discussing the health care system over breakfast. Although they both agreed that the system needed to be improved, they highlighted certain aspects of the Clinton plan that were particularly controversial, such as an overall cap on funds for health care needs and restrictions on provider choice. The punch line for the ad was "There's got to be a better way."[25] To be effective in opposing the Clinton plan, HIAA did not have to propose an alternative that was scrutinized and compared to the Clinton proposal. Simply saying "the country can do better" was enough to help create significant opposition to the plan.

Path Dependency

Finally, the concept of "path dependency" can be a hindrance to major health reform. "The notion of path dependency emphasizes the power of inertia within political institutions."[21(p439)] That is, once a certain way of doing things becomes the norm, it is hard to change course. Yet, this theory does not mean that health reform is impossible. Inertia may be overcome at "critical moments or junctures" that open a window for change.[21(p439)] For example, the passage of Medicaid and Medicare in 1965 was a radical change from the past pattern of limited federal government involvement in health care. The catalysts for this change were the growing social pressure for improving the health care system and the landslide victory of Democrat Lyndon Johnson as president and of liberal and moderate Democrats in Congress. The most recent window for national health reform was the 1992 election of Democrat Bill Clinton on a platform emphasizing broad heath reform, coupled while the Democratic majority in Congress (until 1994). Although Clinton's plan was not ultimately successful, it appeared that the American public and politicians were open to changing the course of the health care "path" that had been taken to date. The idea of path dependency suggests that inertia and fear of change make broad reform difficult to achieve, but not impossible.

Path dependency is also evident on the individual level; that is, once individuals are used to having things a certain way, it is difficult for them to accept change. Currently, about 85% of Americans have health insurance, most of them through employer-sponsored coverage. Comprehensive health reform would likely change the condition of the insured population to some degree, by changing either their source of coverage, the benefits included in coverage, the cost of coverage, or some other factor. Professor Judith Feder refers to this problem as the "crowd-out" politics of health reform.[26] "[T]he fundamental barrier to universal coverage is that our success in insuring most of the nation's population has 'crowded out' our political capacity to insure the rest."[26(p461)] In other words, many of the insured do not want a change in the health care system that will leave them worse off in order to make the uninsured better off.

According to Professor Feder, the way to solve the political crowd-out dilemma is by changing the very nature of American culture. The focus on individualism must be replaced with a concern for the community and recognition that all Americans are part of a single community. "[T]he challenge to improving or achieving universal coverage is to decide whether we are a society in which it is every man, woman or child for him/herself or one in which we are all in it together."[26(p464)] If the latter view prevails, fear of change and loss of benefits can be replaced with a desire to provide some benefits to all.

UNSUCCESSFUL ATTEMPTS TO PASS NATIONAL HEALTH INSURANCE REFORM

Since the early 1900s, when medical knowledge became advanced enough to make health care and health insurance a desirable commodity, there have been periodic attempts to implement universal coverage through national health reform. The Socialist Party was the first U.S. political party to support health insurance in 1904, but the main engine behind early efforts for national reform was the American Association for Labor Legislation (AALL), a "social progressive" group that hoped to reform capitalism, not overthrow it.[27(p243)] In 1912, Progressive Party candidate Theodore Roosevelt supported a social insurance platform modeled on the European social insurance tradition that included health insurance, worker's compensation, old-age pensions, and unemployment. With his loss to Woodrow Wilson, the national health insurance movement was without a strong national leader for three decades.

The AALL continued to support a form of health insurance after Roosevelt's defeat, and drafted a model bill in 1915. This bill followed the European model, limiting participation to working class employees and their dependents. Benefits included medical aid, sick pay, maternity benefits, and a death benefit. These costs were to be financed by employers, employees, and the state. The AALL believed that health insurance for the working population would reduce poverty and increase society's productivity and well-being through healthier workers and citizens.

Opposition to AALL's bill came from several sources.[27(pp247–249)] Although some members of the American Medical Association approved of the bill conceptually, physician support rapidly evaporated when details emerged about aspects of the plan that would negatively impact their income and autonomy. The American Federation of Labor (a labor union) opposed compulsory health insurance because it wanted workers to rely on their own economic strength, not the state, to obtain better wages and benefits. In addition, the federation was concerned that it would lose power if the government, not the union, secured benefits for workers. Employers were generally opposed to the bill, contending that supporting public health was a better way to ensure productivity and well-being. In addition, they feared that providing health insurance to employees might promote malingering instead of reducing lost work days. After experiencing the high cost associated with worker's compensation, employers also were not eager to take on an additional expensive benefit. Of course, the part of the insurance industry that had already established a profitable niche in the death benefit business was strongly opposed to a bill that included a death benefit provision. Employers, providers, and insurers have, in general, remained staunch opponents of national health reform over the years, while unions have supported national reform efforts. However, this dynamic has changed recently with more provider groups, employers, and even some insurers calling for a national solution to the problems of rising health care costs and the uninsured.

The country's entry into World War I in 1917 also changed the health reform debate. Many physicians who supported the AALL bill entered the military, shifting their focus away from the domestic health policy debate. Anti-German sentiment was high, so opponents of the bill gained traction by denouncing compulsory health insurance as anti-American. One pamphlet read: "What is Compulsory Social Health Insurance? It is a dangerous device, invented in Germany, announced by the German Emperor from the throne the same year he started plotting and preparing to conquer the world."[27(p253)]

The next time that national health insurance might have taken hold was from the mid-1930s through the early 1940s as the country was coping with the difficulties of the Depression. During this time there was a significant increase in government programs, including the creation of Social Security in 1935, which provided old-age assistance, unemployment compensation, and public assistance. Yet, the fourth prong of the social insurance package, health insurance, remained elusive. President Franklin Roosevelt heeded his staff's advice to leave health insurance out of Social Security due to the strong opposition it would create.[27(p267)]

Even so, members of Roosevelt's administration continued to push for national health insurance. The Interdepartmental Committee to Coordinate Health and Welfare Activities was created in 1935 and took on the task of studying the nation's health care needs. This job fell to its Technical Committee on Medical Care. Instead of supporting a federal program, the committee proposed subsidies to the states for operating health programs. Components of the proposal included expanding maternal and child health and public health programs under Social Security, expanding hospital construction, increasing aid for medical care for the indigent, studying a general medical care program, and creating a compensation program for those who lost wages due to disability.

Although President Roosevelt established a National Health Conference to discuss the recommendation, he never fully supported the medical care committee's proposal. With the success of conservatives in the 1938 election and the administration's concerns about fighting the powerful physician and state medical society lobbies, national health reform did not have a place on Roosevelt's priority list. Senator Robert Wagner (D-NY) introduced a bill that followed the committee's recommendations in 1939, and although it passed in the Senate, it did not garner support from the president or in the House.

World War II provided another opportunity for the opposition to label national health insurance as socialized medicine. But once the war ended, President Roosevelt finally called for an "economic bill of rights" that included medical care. President Truman picked up where Roosevelt left off, strongly advocating for national health insurance. President Truman's proposal included expanding hospitals, increasing public health and maternal and child health services, providing federal aid for medical research and education, and, for the first time, a single health insurance program for all.[27(p281)] Heeding lessons from earlier reform failures, Truman emphasized that his plan was not socialized medicine and that the delivery system for medical and hospital care would not change.

Again, there was strong opposition to the proposal. The AMA vehemently rejected the proposal and most other health care groups opposed it as well. Although the public initially approved of it, there was no consensus about how national health insurance should be structured and more people preferred modest voluntary plans over a national, compulsory, comprehensive health insurance program.[27(p282)] Additional opposition came from the American Bar Association, the Chamber of Commerce, and even some federal agencies concerned about losing control over their existing programs. In the end, only the hospital construction portion of the proposal was enacted (recall the earlier discussions about the Hill-Burton Act).

When Truman won re-election on a national health insurance platform in 1948, it appeared the tide had turned. However, the AMA continued its strong opposition and its attempts to link national health insurance to socialism. Congress considered various compromises, but never reached a consensus. The public remained uncertain about what kind of plan to favor. Employers maintained their opposition to compulsory insurance. In addition, one large group of potential supporters—veterans—were disinterested in the debate because they had already secured extensive medical coverage through the Veterans Administration. As the Korean War moved forward, Truman's focus shifted away from national health insurance and toward the war effort and other priorities.

National health insurance did not return to the national policy agenda until the 1970s. The landscape was quite different than in Truman's era. Medicaid and Medicare had been created, health care costs had begun to rise exponentially, and the economy was deteriorating. In 1969, President Nixon declared that a "massive crisis" existed in health care and that unless it was fixed immediately, the country's medical system would collapse.[27(p381)] The general public seemed to agree, with 75% of respondents in one survey concurring that the health care system was in crisis.[27(p381)] Democrats still controlled Congress by a significant margin, and Senator Edward Kennedy (D-MA) and Representative Martha Griffiths (D-MI), the first woman to serve on the powerful House Ways and Means Committee, proposed a comprehensive, federally operated health insurance system.

At the same time, a movement supporting health care and patient rights was gaining momentum. These included rights to informed consent, to refuse treatment, to due process for involuntary commitment, and to equal access to health care.[27(p389)] The public was both anxious to obtain care and willing to challenge the authority of health care providers.

The Nixon administration's first attempt at health reform focused on the need to change the financing of the health care system from one dominated by a fee-for-service system that created incentives to provide more and more expensive services, to one that promoted restraint, efficiency, and the health of the patient. The result was a "health maintenance strategy" intended to stimulate the private industry to create health maintenance organizations (HMOs) through federal planning grants and loan guarantees, with the goal of enrolling 90% of the population in an HMO by the end of the 1970s.[27(pp395–396)] Ironically, group health plans, often labeled socialized medicine, had become the centerpiece of a Republican reform strategy.

Nixon's proposal included an employer mandate to provide a minimum package of benefits under a National Health

Insurance Standards Act (NHISA), a federally administered Family Health Insurance Program for low-income families that had a less generous benefit package than the one required by NHISA, reductions in Medicare spending to help defray the costs, a call for an increase in the supply of physicians, and a change in how medical schools were subsidized. Opponents were plentiful and this plan did not come to fruition. Some felt that the plan was a gift to private insurance companies. Advocates for the poor were outraged at the second tier of benefits for low-income families. The AMA was concerned about HMOs interfering with physician practices and supported an alternative that provided tax credits for buying private insurance.

After the 1972 election, Nixon proposed a second, more comprehensive plan that covered everyone and offered more comprehensive coverage. Private insurance companies would cover the employed and a government-run program would cover the rest of the population, with both groups receiving the same benefit package. Senator Kennedy and Representative Wilbur Mills (D-AR) supported a similar plan and it appeared a compromise was close at hand. However, labor unions and liberal organizations preferred the original Kennedy plan and resisted compromising with the hope of gaining power in the 1974 post-Watergate elections. Fearing the same political shift, the insurance companies actually supported a catastrophic insurance plan proposed by Senator Russell Long (D-LA), believing it was better than any plan that would come out of a more liberal Congress after the elections. Once again, there was no majority support for any of the bills and a national health insurance plan was not enacted.

Although President Jimmy Carter gave lip service to national health reform, he never fully supported a proposal. It was not until the election of Bill Clinton in 1992 that the next, and so far last, real attempt at national health insurance was made. The Clinton administration plan, dubbed the Health Security Act, was designed to create national health insurance without spending new federal funds or shifting coverage from private to public insurance. It relied on the concept of "managed competition," which combined elements of managed care and market competition.

Under the Health Security Act, a National Health Board would have established national and regional spending limits and regulated premium increases. "Health alliances" would have included a variety of plans that were competing for the business of employees and unemployed citizens in each geographic area. All plans were to have a guaranteed scope of benefits and uniform cost sharing. Employers were required to provide coverage for their workers at a defined high level of benefits and those with 5,000 employees or fewer had to purchase plans through the health alliance. Subsidies were provided for low-income individuals and small businesses. Funding was to be provided from cost containment measures that were reinvested. Forced by the Congressional Budget Office to provide an alternative funding strategy should the cost containment not create enough funds, the plan also included the option of capping insurance premium growth and reducing provider payments.

Like the national health insurance plans before it, the Health Security Act had opponents from many directions. The health alliances were attacked as big government, employers resisted mandates and interference with their fringe benefits, some advocates feared that cost containment would lead to care rationing, the insured were concerned about losing some of their existing benefits or cost-sharing arrangements, the elderly feared losing Medicare, and academic health centers were concerned about losing funds based on new graduate medical education provisions.[26(p463)] In addition, the usually strong support from unions was missing because of an earlier disagreement with the president on trade matters. It is also generally accepted that the Clinton administration made several political mistakes that made a difficult political chore nearly impossible. The Health Security Act never made it to a vote.

Although the federal government has not been able to pass comprehensive reform, there has been some recent movement toward incremental changes in health insurance coverage. However, most of the activity on the federal level has focused on cost containment, not insurance expansion. As mentioned in Chapter 4, there is growing support for health savings accounts and high-deductible health care plans; federal pilot projects to increase the use of these plans were part of the Medicare reform bill that created the new drug benefit and of the Deficit Reduction Act of 2005 that involved numerous Medicaid changes. These incremental reforms are controversial, with advocates arguing that they promote personal responsibility and better use of the health care system and opponents contending that they will result in a larger underinsured population that will still have problems accessing and paying for their health care. At the time of this writing, Congress is also considering legislation that would make it easier for small businesses to form purchasing pools across state lines and that would expand tax deductions so individuals purchasing insurance on the private market gain the same tax benefits as those with employer-sponsored insurance. As is evident from these proposals, comprehensive health reform is not currently on the national agenda.

STATE HEALTH REFORM

With the repeated failure of comprehensive national health reform and seemingly limited federal interest in expanding insurance coverage, it is natural to look to the states as a potentially more effective avenue for change. As discussed earlier in this chapter, there are numerous reasons why it is difficult to achieve reform on the state level. Even so, states have historically had a central role in providing health care to their citizens and are often at the forefront of change in a variety of important social policy areas. When states act as policy laboratories by implementing innovative reforms, others can learn from the positive and negative consequences of the reform efforts.

States have been active in implementing a variety of health reform strategies. In addition to the Medicaid reforms discussed in Chapter 6, states have recently used a number of approaches to increase health insurance coverage for their residents. A few examples of states implementing new or expanded programs to increase insurance coverage include: [28]

- *Massachusetts*, which approved legislation that requires all residents to buy insurance or pay a penalty to cover the cost of care they will eventually need. Most employers will have to provide health coverage or pay a per-employee penalty. In addition, a new state-subsidized program will be available for residents with incomes up to 300% FPL. The state hopes to cover 90% to 95% of the state's uninsured residents over the next three years.
- *Vermont*, which established a new program that will cover about 30,000 currently uninsured residents who do not qualify for other public programs and will offer state-subsidized premiums on a sliding fee scale. The state also passed a requirement forcing employers to pay assessments if they do not offer health insurance coverage.
- *Illinois*, which passed the Covering All Kids Health Insurance Act that makes insurance coverage available to all uninsured children in the state and bases premiums on a sliding fee scale.
- *Maine*, which implemented the DirigoChoice program to provide a health insurance option to small businesses, the self-employed, and individuals without access to employer-sponsored insurance. Premium and cost-sharing discounts are available on a sliding fee scale for enrollees with income below 300% FPL.
- *New Mexico*, which implemented the State Coverage Initiative program that created a new employer-sponsored insurance program, provided through a managed care organization. This initiative is part of a larger strategy to reduce the number of uninsured in the state.

Other states have focused on increasing coverage through employer mandates with so-called "play or pay" bills that require employers to provide health insurance to their workers (play) or pay for employee health insurance (pay). Currently, Hawaii is the only state with an employer mandate,[28] and its law preceded ERISA's passage.[f] However, in 2003 the California legislature passed an employer mandate bill (although it was rejected by the voters a year later and was never implemented) and in 2005 12 other states introduced similar bills. Maryland recently passed a more tailored bill that requires employers with 10,000 or more employees to spend at least 8% of their payroll on health care. (The law is commonly referred to as the "Wal-Mart" law because Wal-Mart was the only company that did not meet its requirements at the time it was enacted.) Several other states are reportedly considering similar legislation. In addition, some states are publishing information about employers that have a large percentage of uninsured or publicly insured workers to try to sway public opinion and create pressure on those companies to increase insurance options for their employees.[28(p24)]

Other states have focused on a purchasing pool strategy. The idea is to use the state's purchasing power (or combine the purchasing power of several small groups) to enable small employers to obtain better terms for insurance coverage because through the pools they have a large group of people to insure. For example, Kansas has created the Kansas Health Care Authority, which intends to create a new insurance product for small businesses with low-income employees. Montana created a small business purchasing pool to provide tax credits and premium assistance to small employers who purchase insurance through the pool or other qualified

Box 7-4
Discussion Questions

Given the failure of national health reform, is it better to focus on state-level reforms? Or will that approach lead to a confusing and even more complex patchwork of programs? Does it matter whether the reform focuses on decreasing the number of uninsured versus another issue such as cost containment or patient rights?

As a policy advocate, what approach do you think will be the most successful in the near future? What primary policy goal guides your decision-making process?

plan.[28(p25)] West Virginia created a public/private partnership to help small businesses provide coverage to their employees. The plan allows small businesses to enjoy the purchasing power of large groups by giving participating carriers access to the West Virginia Public Employee Insurance Agency rates.[28(p25)]

In the absence of a national consensus on health reform, it is likely that reform options will continue to be implemented on the state level. States can continue to learn from the experiences of other states, and perhaps the federal government will implement some of these reforms on a national level.

CONCLUSION

The uninsurance problem has persisted over many years. Although there is general agreement about the health, financial, and social costs that are created by having an enormous group of uninsured individuals, there is little agreement about how to fix the problem or whether affirmative steps should be taken to address it. Recently, the approach to health reform has been not on expanding comprehensive health insurance coverage, but on cost containment, providing direct service through community health centers, and increasing the use of high-deductible catastrophic plans that may be combined with tax-sheltered medical savings accounts. Some people contend that universal coverage will only come when Americans consider themselves part of a whole community, with a responsibility to each other. Others believe that because the current system is unworkable, reform will succeed only when the status quo can no longer be sustained. Still others promote incremental steps, citing the failure of national health insurance plans as an indication that major health reform will not occur. And there are those who do not believe that the issue of the uninsured should be a priority item on the policy agenda. Although the future of health reform is uncertain, it promises to be an interesting and energetic policy debate.

REFERENCES

1. U.S. Bureau of the Census. *Income, Poverty, and Health Insurance Coverage in the United States: 2005.* Washington, D.C.: Economics and Statistics Administration. Bureau of the U.S. Census; 2006.
2. Kaiser Family Foundation. *The Uninsured: A Primer—Key Facts About Americans Without Health Insurance.* Menlo Park, Calif.: Kaiser Family Foundation; 2006. Available at: http://www.kff.org/uninsured/upload/7451.cfm. Accessed October 25, 2006.
3. Hoffman C, Rowland D, Carbaugh A. Holes in the health insurance system—who lacks coverage and why. *J Law Med Ethics.* 2004;32:391–396.
4. Institute of Medicine. *America's Health Care Safety Net: Intact but Endangered.* Washington, D.C.: National Academy Press; 2000.
5. Shoen C, Doty M, Collins S. et al. Insured but not protected: how many adults are underinsured? *Health Affairs.* June 2005;Web Exclusive:W5-289–W5-301: http://content.healthaffairs.org/cgi/reprint/hlthaff.w5.289v1 (Note - you can only access this if you have a subscription to health affairs). Accessed August 1, 2006.

6. Department of Health and Human Services. The 2006 HHS poverty guidelines. Available at: http://aspe.hhs.gov/poverty/06poverty.shtml. Accessed August 1, 2006.
7. Institute of Medicine. *Coverage Matters: Insurance and Health Care.* Washington, D.C.: National Academy Press; 2001.
8. Kaiser Commission on Medicaid and the Uninsured. *The Uninsured in Rural America.* Menlo Park, Calif.: Kaiser Family Foundation; 2003. Available at: http://www.kff.org/uninsured/upload/The-Uninsured-in-Rural-America-Update-PDF.pdf. Accessed August 1, 2006.
9. Institute of Medicine. *Insuring America's Health: Principles and Recommendation.* Washington, D.C.: National Academy Press; 2004.
10. Starfield B, Shi L. The medical home, access to care, and insurance: a review of evidence. *Pediatrics.* 2004;113:1493–1498.
11. Lambrew J. DeFriese G, Carey T. et al. The effects of having a regular doctor on access to primary care. *Med Care.* 1996;34:138–151.
12. Institute of Medicine. *Hidden Costs, Value Lost: Uninsurance in America.* Washington, D.C.: National Academy Press; 2003.
13. Hadley J, Holohan J. *The Cost of Care for the Uninsured: What Do We Spend, Who Pays, and What Would Full Coverage Add to Medical Spending?* Menlo Park, Calif.: Kaiser Commission on Medicaid and the Uninsured; 2004. Available at: http://www.kff.org/uninsured/upload/The-Cost-of-Care-for-the-Uninsured-What-Do-We-Spend-Who-Pays-and-What-Would-Full-Coverage-Add-to-Medical-Spending.pdf. Accessed August 1, 2006.
14. Families USA. *Paying a Premium: The Added Cost of Care for the Uninsured.* Washington, D.C.: Families USA; 2005. Available at: http://www.familiesusa.org/assets/pdfs/Paying_a_Premium_rev_July_13731e.pdf. Accessed August 1, 2006.
15. Proser M. *The Safety Net on the Edge.* Washington, D.C.: National Association of Community Health Centers; 2005. Available at: http://www.nachc.com/research/Files/SNreport2005.pdf. Accessed August 1, 2006.
16. Regenstein M, Huang J. *Stresses to the Safety Net: The Public Hospital Perspective.* Menlo Park, Calif.: Kaiser Family Foundation; 2005. Available at: http://www.kff.org/medicaid/upload/Stresses-to-the-Safety-Net.pdf. Accessed August 1, 2006.
17. National Association of Community Health Centers. *Health Center Fact Sheet—United States.* Washington, D.C.: National Association of Community Health Centers; 2004. Available at: http://www.nachc.com/research/Files/USfactsheet.pdf. Accessed August 1, 2006.
18. Taylor J. *The Fundamentals of Community Health Centers.* Washington, D.C.: The National Health Policy Forum; 2004. Available at: http://www.nhpf.org/pdfs_bp/BP_CHC_08-31-04.pdf Accessed on October 25, 2006.
19. Gordon C. *Dead on Arrival: The Politics of Health Care in Twentieth-Century America.* Princeton, N.J.: Princeton University Press; 2003.
20. Blake CH, Adolino JR. The enactment of national health insurance: a boolean analysis of twenty advanced industrial countries. *J Health Politics Policy Law.* 2001;26:670–708.
21. Jost TS. Why can't we do what they do? National health reform abroad. *J Law Med Ethics.* 2004;32:433–441.
22. National Public Radio, The Kaiser Family Foundation, and Kennedy School of Government. *National Survey on Health Care.* Menlo Park, Calif.: Kaiser Family Foundation; 2002. Available at: http://www.kff.org/kaiserpolls/loader.cfm?url=/commonspot/security/getfile.cfm&PageID=14065. Accessed August 1, 2006.
23. Weissert CS, Weissert WG. *Governing Health: The Politics of Health Policy,* 2nd ed. Baltimore: Johns Hopkins University Press; 2002.
24. Friedman J, Holden R. The gerrymandering myth. *The New Republic Online;* 2006. Available at: https://ssl.tnr.com/p/docsub.mhtml?i=w060529&s=friedmanholden060106. Accessed on October 25, 2006.
25. West DM, Heith D, Goodwin C. Harry and Louise go to Washington: political advertising and health care reform. *J Health Politics Policy Law.* 1996;21:35–68.
26. Feder J. Crowd-out and the politics of health reform. *J Law Med Ethics.* 2004;32:461–464.

27. Starr P. *The Social Transformation of American Medicine: The Rise of a Sovereign Profession and the Making of a Vast Industry.* New York: Basic Books; 1982.

28. Burton A, Campion D, Cohn D. et al. *State of the States.* Washington, D.C.: Academy Health; 2006. Available at: http://www.statecoverage.net/pdf/stateofstates2006.pdf. Accessed August 1, 2006.

ENDNOTES

a. See Chapter 6 for a full discussion of Medicaid and SCHIP eligibility.

b. Uncompensated care refers to situations when care is given but the provider does not expect to receive full payment given the patient's situation (e.g., income, insurance status). Bad debt refers to situations when care is given and the provider expects, but does not receive, full payment. It is not clear from the article whether the authors included bad debt in their calculation of uncompensated care costs.[13(pp2–3)]

c. Although we discuss the health care safety net in the context of treating uninsured and underinsured patients, safety net providers in the form of almshouses and public hospitals existed before health insurance was commonplace. For a detailed discussion of the history of hospitals in the United States, see Charles E. Rosenberg, *The Care of Strangers: The Rise of America's Hospital System* (Baltimore: Johns Hopkins University Press, 1987).

d. 88 Stat. 832.

e. ERISA § 514, 29 U.S.C. § 1144.

f. Many states consider ERISA's preemptive force to be an impediment to using employer mandates as a way to significantly reduce the uninsured rate in their state.

CHAPTER 7 ADDENDUM: Historical Contextual Timeline of Important Events in Health Policy and Law

		1800	1820	1830
Political Party in Power—Federal Government	President	Federalist (1789–1801)	Democratic–Republican (1801–1829); Democrat (1829–1841)	
		George Washington (1789–1797); John Adams (1797–1801)	Thomas Jefferson (1801–1809); James Madison (1809–1817); James Monroe (1817–1825); John Quincy Adams (1825–1829); Andrew Jackson (1829–1837); Martin Van Buren (1837–1841)	
	U.S. House of Representatives	Pro-Administration (1789–1793); Anti-Administration (1793–1795); Jeffersonian Republican (1795–1797); Federalist (1797–1801)	Jeffersonian Republican (1801–1823)	Adams-Clay Republican (1823–1825); Adams (1825–1827); Jacksons (1827–1829)	Jacksons (1829–1837); Democrat (1837–1841)
	U.S. Senate	Pro-Administration (1789–1795); Federalist (1795–1801)	Republican (1801–1823)	Jackson-Crawford Republican (1823–1825); Jacksonian (1825–1833)	Anti-Jacksonian (1833–1835; Jacksonian (1835–37); Democrat (1837–1841)
Major Social and Political Events		Industrial Revolution (~ 1790–1860) and increased urbanization	War of 1812 (1812–1814) and post-war economic growth	
Key Federal Legislative Proposals/Laws and Key Legal Decisions		1798 U.S. Public Health Service Act: Creates the **Marine Hospital Service,** predecessor to the Public Health Service, to provide medical care to merchant seamen.	*Marbury v. Madison,* 5 U.S. 137 (1803): Established the Supreme Court's power of judicial review; **1818 Office of the Surgeon General** established.	
Important Developments in Health and Medicine		State Poor Laws require communities to care for residents who are physically or mentally incapable of caring for themselves; States begin building dispensaries in the late 1700's to provide medication to the poor; Almshouses serve as primitive hospitals, providing limited care to the indigent; Public health focuses on fighting plague, cholera, and smallpox epidemics, often through quarantine.		

CHAPTER 7 ADDENDUM: Historical Contextual Timeline of Important Events in Health Policy and Law

		1840	1850	1860
Political Party in Power—Federal Government	President	Whig (1841–1845); Democrat (1845–1849); Whig (1849–1853); Democrat (1853–1861) William Henry Harrison (1841); John Tyler (1841–1845); James K. Polk (1845–1849); Zachary Taylor (1849–1850)	Millard Fillmore (1850–1853); Franklin Pierce (1853–1857); James Buchanan (1857–1861)	Republican; Democrat Abraham Lincoln (1861–1865); Andrew Johnson (1865–1869)
	U.S. House of Representatives			Republican 1859–1875
	U.S. Senate	Whig 1841–1845 (27th–28th); Democrat 1845–1861 (29th–36th)		Republican 1861–1879 (37th–45th)
Major Social and Political Events		Industrial Revolution (~ 1790–1860) and increased urbanization U.S.-Mexican War 1846–1848	Crimean War 1853–1856	U.S. Civil War (1861–1865) and postwar expansion in interstate commerce.
Key Federal Legislative Proposals/Laws and Key Legal Decisions		**1848 Import Drug Act:** Initiates drug regulation; U.S. Customs Service is required to enforce purity standards for imported medications.		**1862 Bureau of Chemistry** (forerunner of the FDA) is established as a scientific laboratory in the Department of Agriculture.
Important Developments in Health and Medicine		**1846** First publicized use of general anesthetic; use of anesthetics increases the number of surgeries performed **1847** American Medical Association is founded.	Studies by Edwin Chadwick in England, Lemuel Shattuck in Massachusetts, and others reveal that overcrowded and unsanitary conditions breed disease, and advocate establishment of local health boards; By the end of the 1800s, 40 states and several localities establish health departments.	**1861** First nursing school is founded and the role of nursing is established during the Civil War; **1860s** Louis Pasteur develops the germ theory of disease; **1865 Antiseptic surgery** is introduced by Joseph Lister, decreasing death rates from surgical operations; with the advent of licensing, the practice of medicine begins to become a more exclusive realm.

CHAPTER 7 ADDENDUM: Historical Contextual Timeline of Important Events in Health Policy and Law

		1870	1880	1890
Political Party in Power—Federal Government	President	Republican Ulysses S. Grant (1869–1877); Rutherford B. Hayes (1877–1881)	Republican (1881–1885); Democrat (1885–1889) James A. Garfield (1881); Chester A. Arthur (1881–1885); Grover Cleveland (1885–1889)	Republican (1889–1893); Democrat (1893–1897); Republican (1897–1901) Benjamin Harrison (1889–1893); Grover Cleveland (1893–1897); William McKinley (1897–1901)
	U.S. House of Representatives	Democratic 1875–1881	Republican 1881–1883; Democratic 1883–1889	Republican 1889–1891; Democratic 1891–1895; Republican 1895–1911
	U.S. Senate	Democratic 1879–1881 (46th)	Republican 1881–1893 (47th–52nd)	Democratic 1893–1895 (53rd); Republican 1895–1913 (54th–62nd)
Major Social and Political Events				
Key Federal Legislative Proposals/Laws and Key Legal Decisions		**1870s Medical Practice Acts:** Establish state regulation of physician licensing; **1870 Marine Hospital Service** is centralized as a separate bureau of the Treasury Department; **1878 National Quarantine Act:** Grants the Marine Hospital Service quarantine authority, due to its assistance with yellow fever outbreak.	**1887** National Hygienic Laboratory, predecessor lab to the National Institutes of Health, is established in Staten Island, New York, by the National Marine Health Service.	**1890 Sherman Antitrust Act:** Prohibits interstate trusts so economic power would not be concentrated in a few corporations.
Important Developments in Health and Medicine		**1877** Louis Pasteur discovers that anthrax is caused by bacteria; scientists find bacteriologic agents causing tuberculosis, diphtheria, typhoid, and yellow fever; immunizations and water purification interventions follow recent discoveries; state and local health departments create laboratories; states begin passing laws requiring disease reporting and establishing disease registries.	**1880s** First hospitals established and the importance of hospitals in the provision of medical care increases; **1882** First major employee-sponsored mutual benefit association was created by Northern Pacific Railway, includes health care benefit; Social Insurance movement results in the creation of "sickness" insurance throughout many countries in Europe; **1895** X-rays discovered.	

CHAPTER 7 ADDENDUM: Historical Contextual Timeline of Important Events in Health Policy and Law

	1900	1910
Political Party in Power—Federal Government	Republican/Progressive	Republican
President	Theodore Roosevelt (1901–1909)	William H. Taft (1909–1913)
U.S. House of Representatives	Republican 1895–1911	Democratic 1911–1919 (62nd–65th)
U.S. Senate	Republican	Republican
Major Social and Political Events	**Progressive Era** 1900–1920: Characterized by popular support for social reform, part of which included compulsory health insurance. Roosevelt campaigned on a social insurance platform in 1912.	
Key Federal Legislative Proposals/Laws and Key Legal Decisions	*Hurley v. Eddingfield*, 59 N.E. 1058 (Ind. 1901): Physicians are under no duty to treat; a physician is not liable for arbitrarily refusing to render medical assistance; **1902 Marine Health Service** renamed the **Public Health and Marine Hospital Service (PHMHS)** as its role in disease control activities expands; **1902 Biologics Control Act:** Regulates safety and effectiveness of vaccines, serums, etc.; *Jacobson v. Massachusetts*, 197 U.S. 11 (1905): State statute requiring compulsory vaccination against smallpox is a constitutional exercise of police power; **1906 Food and Drug Act** (Wiley Act): Gives regulatory power to monitor food manufacturing, labeling, and sales to FDA predecessor; **1908** Federal Employers Liability Act: Creates workers compensation program for select federal employees.	**1912 Children's Bureau of Health** established in Department of Commerce (later moved to Department of Labor); **1912 Public Health and Marine Hospital Service** is renamed the **Public Health Service** and is authorized to investigate human disease and sanitation; **1914 Clayton Antitrust Act:** Clarifies the Sherman Antitrust Act and includes additional prohibitions.
Important Developments in Health and Medicine	**1901** AMA reorganizes at local/state level and gains strength, beginning era of "organized medicine" as physicians as a group become a more cohesive and increasingly professional authority;	**1910** Flexner Report on Medical Education creates medical school standards; "Sickness" insurance established by Britain in 1911 and Russia in 1912; Socialist and Progressive parties in the United States support similar "sickness" insurance.

CHAPTER 7 ADDENDUM: Historical Contextual Timeline of Important Events in Health Policy and Law

		1910 (continued)	1920
Political Party in Power—Federal Government		Democratic	Republican
	President	Woodrow Wilson (1913–1921)	Warren G. Harding (1921–1923); Calvin Coolidge (1923–1929)
	U.S. House of Representatives	Democratic 1913–1919 (63rd–65th); Republican 1919–1933 (66th–72nd)	Republican 1919–1931 (66th–71st)
	U.S. Senate	Democratic 1913–1919 (63rd–65th); Republican 1919–1933 (66th–72nd)	Republican
Major Social and Political Events		World War I (1914–1919; U.S. enters in 1917)	
Key Federal Legislative Proposals/Laws and Key Legal Decisions		**1911:** First state workers compensation law enacted; **1918 Chamberlain-Kahn Act:** Provides first federal grants to states for public health services.	**1921 Sweet Act:** Establishes the Veterans Administration; **1922 Shepherd-Towner Act:** Provides grants for the Children's Bureau and state maternal and child health programs; it is the first direct federal funding of health services for individuals.
Important Developments in Health and Medicine		**1913 American College of Surgeons (ACS)** is founded; 1918 ACS begins accreditation of hospitals; **1918–1919 pandemic flu** kills over 600,000 people in the U.S.	**1920 AMA** passes resolution against compulsory health insurance; AMA opposition combined with entry into World War I (and the anti-German sentiments aroused), undermines support for national health reform and government insurance; **1929 Blue Cross** establishes its first hospital insurance plan at Baylor University; chronic illnesses begin to replace infectious diseases as most significant health threat; with innovations in medical care, health care costs begin to rise.

CHAPTER 7 ADDENDUM: Historical Contextual Timeline of Important Events in Health Policy and Law

	1930
Political Party in Power—Federal Government	Republican
President	Herbert Hoover (1929–1933)
U.S. House of Representatives	Democratic 1931–1947 (72nd–79th)
U.S. Senate	Democratic 1933–1947 (73rd–79th)
Major Social and Political Events	Great Depression (1929 through 1930s); New Deal 1933–1939
Key Federal Legislative Proposals/Laws and Key Legal Decisions	1930 National Institutes of Health established; 1933 Federal Emergency Relief Administration: Provides limited medical services for the medically indigent; 1935 Social Security Act: Provides federal grant-in-aid funding for states to create and maintain public health services and training, expands responsibilities for the Children's Health Bureau, and establishes Aid to Families with Dependent Children (AFDC) wefare program; 1935 Works Project Administration is created, including projects to build and improve hospitals; 1938 Food, Drug and Cosmetic Act: Expands regulatory scope of FDA to require premarket approval (in response to deaths from an untested product); 1939 Public Health Service is transferred from the Treasury Department to the new Federal Security Agency.
Important Developments in Health and Medicine	The Great Depression threatens financial security of physicians, hospitals, and individuals; commercial insurance industry rises in the absence of government-sponsored insurance plans; In the late 1930s the Blue Cross (hospital services) and Blue Shield (physician services) health insurance plan created; prepaid group health plans/medical cooperatives gain popularity with some providers and consumers, but are opposed by AMA; 1932–1972 Tuskegee syphillis study.

CHAPTER 7 ADDENDUM: Historical Contextual Timeline of Important Events in Health Policy and Law

	1940	1950
Political Party in Power—Federal Government	Democratic	Democratic
President	Franklin D. Roosevelt (1933–1945)	Harry S Truman (1945–1953)
U.S. House of Representatives	Democratic	Republican 1947–1949 (80th); Democratic 1949–1953 (81st–82nd)
U.S. Senate	Democratic	Republican 1947–1949 (80th); Democratic 1949–1953 (81st–82nd)
Major Social and Political Events	World War II (1939–1945, Pearl Harbor 1941)	Cold War ideology and McCarthyism (1950–1954); Korean War 1950–1953
Key Federal Legislative Proposals/Laws and Key Legal Decisions	1941 Manham Act: Funds wartime emergency building of hospitals; 1942 National War Labor Board rules that the provision of benefits, including health insurance, does not violate wage freeze; 1944 PublicHealth Service Act: Consolidates the laws related to the functions of the PHS; 1946 Hill-Burton Act: Funds hospital construction to improve access to hospital-based medical care; 1946 The "Communicable Disease Center" (CDC) opens as part of the Public Health Service; 1949 Truman's national health insurance proposal is defeated.	1953 Department of Health, Education, and Welfare (HEW) is created from the Federal Security Agency, and the Public Health Service is transferred to HEW.
Important Developments in Health and Medicine	1945 Nobel Prize in Medicine awarded for development of penicillin treatment for humans, which is used extensively in the war; 1945 Kaiser Permanente, a large prepaid, integrated health plan is opened to the public; 1946 the Emerson Report released proposing overall plan for public health in the U.S.; 1948 AMA opposes Truman's plan for national health insurance and sentiments against national health reform also fueled by the Cold War; employer-based health insurance grows rapidly with no national health insurance program and as employers compete for a short supply of employees due to the war and because health benefits are exempted from the wage freeze; after WWII, labor unions gained the right to bargain collectively, leading to another expansion in employee health plans; commercial insurance has taken over 40% of the market from Blue Cross.	1951 Joint Commission on Accreditation of Hospitals (JCAH) is created to provide voluntary accreditation.

CHAPTER 7 ADDENDUM: Historical Contextual Timeline of Important Events in Health Policy and Law

		1950 (continued)	1960
Political Party in Power—Federal Government		Republican	Democratic
	President	Dwight D. Eisenhower (1953–1961)	John F. Kennedy (1961–1963)
	U.S. House of Representatives	Republican 1952–1955 (83rd); Democratic 1955–1994 (84th–103rd)	Democratic
	U.S. Senate	Republican 1953–1955 (83rd); Democratic 1955–1981 (84th–96th)	Democratic
Major Social and Political Events			Economic downturn
Key Federal Legislative Proposals/Laws and Key Legal Decisions		1954 IRS declares that employers can pay health insurance premiums for their employees with pretax dollars; *Brown v. Board of Education,* 347 U.S. 483 (1954): racial segregation in public education violates the Equal Protection Clause of 14th Amendment;. 1956 Dependents Medical Care Act: Creates government medical care program for military and dependents outside VA system; 1956 Social Security Act is amended to provide Social Security Disability Insurance.	1962 Amendments to Food, Drug and Cosmetic Acts require that new drugs be "effective."
Important Developments in Health and Medicine		1953 Salk creates polio vaccine; 1954 first organ transplant is performed; continued progression in medical science and technology leads to increased costs; political focus turns to Korean War and away from medical care reform.	

CHAPTER 7 ADDENDUM: Historical Contextual Timeline of Important Events in Health Policy and Law

	1960s (continued)	1970s
Political Party in Power—Federal Government	Democratic	Republican
President	Lyndon B. Johnson (1963–1969)	Richard M. Nixon (1969–1974)
U.S. House of Representatives	Democratic	Democratic
U.S. Senate	Democratic	Democratic
Major Social and Political Events		
Key Federal Legislative Proposals/Laws and Key Legal Decisions	**1960 Kerr-Mills program** provides federal funding through vendor payments to states for medically indigent elderly; *Simkins v. Moses H. Cone Memorial Hospital,* 323 F.2d 959 (4th Cir. 1963): Racial segregation in private hospitals receiving federal Hill-Burton funds violates the Equal Protection Clause of the 14th Amendment; **1964: Civil Rights Act** passed; **1965 Medicare and Medicaid** programs created through Social Security Amendments; *Griswold v. Connecticut,* 381 U.S. 479 (1965): The Constitution protects a right to privacy; state law forbidding the use of contraceptives or provision of them to marriedcouples violates a constitutional right to marital privacy; **1966 Civilian Health and Medical Program for the Uniformed Services (CHAMPUS)** created.	President Nixon's proposed comprehensive health insurance plan fails; **1971** proposed Health Security Act from Senator Edward Kennedy (D-MA) fails. **1970** Communicable Disease Center is renamed the **Centers for Disease Control;** **1972 Social Security Amendments** extend Medicare eligibility and create Supplemental Security Income (SSI) program; *Canterbury v. Spence,* 464 F.2d 772 (D.C. Cir. 1972): Established modern law of informed consent based on a reasonable patient standard; *Roe v. Wade,* 410 U.S. 113 (1973): Constitutional right to privacy encompasses a woman's decision to terminate her pregnancy; **1973 Health Maintenance Organization Act:** Supports growth of HMOs.
Important Developments in Health and Medicine	**1965:** Medicare and Medicaid created; **1967** first human heart transplant.	Health care costs continue to rise dramatically, due to advances in medical technology, high-tech hospital care, the new pool of paying patients from Medicaid and Medicare, increased utilization of services, and increased physician specialization; 1972 computed tomography (CT) scan first used.

CHAPTER 7 ADDENDUM: Historical Contextual Timeline of Important Events in Health Policy and Law

Political Party in Power—Federal Government	1970s (continued)		1980s
President	Republican Gerald R. Ford (1974–1977)	Democratic Jimmy Carter (1977–1981)	Republican Ronald Reagan (1981–1989)
U.S. House of Representatives	Democratic	Democratic	Democratic
U.S. Senate	Democratic	Democratic	Republican 1981–1987 (97th–99th); Democratic 1987–1995 (100th–103rd)
Major Social and Political Events			1989 "New Federalism" of the Reagan administration; Berlin Wall falls
Key Federal Legislative Proposals/Laws and Key Legal Decisions	**1974 Employment Retirement Income Security Act (ERISA)** passed; **1977 Health Care Financing Administration (HCFA)** is created to administer the Medicare and Medicaid programs.	**1979** President Carter introduces a National Health Plan to Congress; **1979 Department of Health and Human Services (HHS)** is created from a reorganized HEW.	**1983** Medicare implements prospective payment system for reimbursing hospitals; **1986 Emergency Medical Treatment and Active Labor Act (EMTALA):** Ensures access to emergency services in Medicare-participating hospitals regardless of ability to pay; **1986 Health Care Quality Improvement Act:** Creates the National Practitioner Databank; **1986 Consolidated Omnibus Budget Reconciliation Act (COBRA):** Includes health benefit provisions that establish continuation of employer-sponsored group health coverage; **1989 Medicare Catastrophic Coverage Act of 1988:** Includes outpatient prescription drug benefit and other changes in Medicare (repealed 1989).
Important Developments in Health and Medicine		**1978** First baby conceived through in vitro fertilization is born.	**1981** Scientists identify AIDS; **1987** JAHC changes name to the **Joint Commission on Accreditation of Healthcare Organizations** (JCAHO); **1980** World Health Assembly declares smallpox eradicated; shift away from traditional fee-for-service insurance plans and toward managed care.

CHAPTER 7 ADDENDUM: Historical Contextual Timeline of Important Events in Health Policy and Law

	1990	
Political Party in Power—Federal Government	Republican	Democratic
President	George Bush (1989–1993)	William J. Clinton (1993–2001)
U.S. House of Representatives	Democratic	*First time since 1955 that both houses are Republican; Republican 1995–Present (104th–108th)
U.S. Senate	Democratic	Republican 1995–Present (104th–108th (Jan 3–20, 2001 and June 6, 2001–Nov 12, 2002 Democratic))
Major Social and Political Events	1990–1991 Gulf War	Foreign crises in Haiti and Bosnia; 1993 North American Free Trade Agreement (NAFTA); Whitewater investigation; 1995 Oklahoma City bombing; 1998 President Clinton impeached.
Key Federal Legislative Proposals/ Laws and Key Legal Decisions	1989 Agency for Healthcare Policy and Research created; 1990 Americans with Disabilities Act (ADA): provides protection against disability discrimination; 1990 Ryan White CARE Act: Creates federal support for AIDS-related services; *Cruzan v. Director, Missouri. Dep't of Health*, 497 U.S. 261 (1990): First "right to die" case before Supreme Court, in which the Court held that a competent person has a constitutionally-protected liberty interest in refusing medical treatment.	1993 President Clinton's proposed **Health Security Act** is defeated; 1995 PHS reorganized to report directly to the Secretary of HHS; 1996 **Health Insurance Portability & Accountability Act (HIPAA):** Includes privacy rules to protect personal health information, attempts to simplify coding for health bills, makes it difficult to exclude patients from insurance plans due to preexisting conditions; **Personal Responsibility and Work Opportunity Reconciliation Act of 996** replaces AFDC with the Temporary Assistance for Needy Families program (TANF); **1996 Mental Health Parity Act:** Requires insurance carriers that offer mental health benefits to provide the same annual and lifetime dollar limits for mental and physical health benefits; **1997 Food and Drug Administration Modernization Act:** Relaxes restrictions on direct-to-consumer advertisements of prescription drugs; **1997 Balanced Budget Act:** adds Medicare Part C, the Medicare managed care program, and creates the State Children's Health Insurance Program which allows states to extend health insurance coverage to additional low-income children; **The Ticket to Work and Work Incentives Improvement Act of 1999:** Creates a new state option to help individuals with disabilities stay enrolled in Medicaid or Medicare coverage while returning to work.
Important Developments in Health and Medicine		Enrollment in managed care doubles; greater use of outpatient services; rate of health spending is relatively stable at roughly 12% to 13% of GDP; direct-to-consumer advertising of pharmaceuticals increases dramatically and the Internet is used as a source of medical information; 1997 Ian Wilmut clones a sheep from adult human cells; 1994 Oregon Health Plan rations Medicaid services through a prioritized list of medical treatments and conditions. After the September 11 attacks, public health becomes focused on emergency preparedness.

CHAPTER 7 ADDENDUM: Historical Contextual Timeline of Important Events in Health Policy and Law

		2000
Political Party in Power—Federal Government		Republican
	President	George W. Bush (2001–)
	U.S. House of Representatives	Republican
	U.S. Senate	Republican
Major Social and Political Events		9/11/2001 terrorist attacks on World Trade Center in New York and on the Pentagon; 2001 U.S. military action in Afghanistan; Iraq War 2003 begins.
Key Federal Legislative Proposals/Laws and Key Legal Decisions		Congressional attention and spending turns to international and security concerns, little discussion of health reform; **2002 Homeland Security Act** Transfers some HHS functions, including the Strategic National Stockpile of emergency pharmaceutical supplies and the National Disaster Medical Service, to the new Department of Homeland Security; **2003 Medicare Modernization Act:** Adds a prescription drug benefit to Medicare beginning in 2006; **2004 Project BioShield Act:** Provides funding for vaccines and medications for biodefense and allows expedited FDA review of treatments in response to attacks; **2005 Deficit Reduction Act** makes significant changes to Medicaid, including state options to reduce benefits, increase cost-sharing, and impose new documentation requirements.
Important Developments in Health and Medicine		**2003** Sequencing of human genome completed; **2003 SARS** epidemic and **2004** flu vaccine shortage raises concerns about public health readiness; worldwide concern about a possible Avian flu epidemic; high level of concern in the U.S. about the rising rate of obesity.

CHAPTER 7 ADDENDUM REFERENCES

1. Mayo T. U.S. health care timelines. Available at: http://faculty.smu.edu/tmayo/health%20care%20timeline.htm. Accessed August 1, 2006.

2. Public Broadcasting Service. Healthcare crisis: who's at risk? Healthcare timeline. Available at: http://www.pbs.org/healthcarecrisis/history.htm. Accessed August 1, 2006.

3. Birn A-E. Struggles for national health reform in the United States. *Am J Pub Health.* 2003;93(1):86–94.

4. Sultz HA, Young KM. *Health Care USA: Understanding Its Organization and Delivery*, 4th ed. Sudbury, Mass.: Jones and Bartlett; 2004.

5. Shi L, Singh DA. *Delivering Health Care Services in America: A Systems Approach,* 3rd ed. Sudbury, Mass.: Jones and Bartlett; 2004.

6. National Library of Medicine. Exhibitions in the history of medicine: images from the history of the Public Health Service. http://www.nlm.nih.gov/exhibition/phs_history/contents.html. Accessed August 1, 2006.

7. Food and Drug Administration, Center for Drug Evaluation and Research. Time line: chronology of drug regulation in the United States. Available at: http://www.fda.gov/cder/about/history/time1.htm. Accessed August 1, 2006.

8. American Medical Association. Chronology of AMA history. Available at: http://www.ama-assn.org/ama/pub/category/1922.html. Accessed August 1, 2006.

9. U.S. Senate. People. Party leadership. Available at: http://www.senate.gov/pagelayout/history/one_item_and_teasers/partydiv.htm. Accessed August 1, 2006.

10. U.S. House of Representatives. Historical highlights. Party divisions. Available at: http://clerk.house.gov/histHigh/Congressional_History/partyDiv.html. Accessed August 1, 2006.

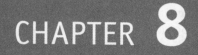

CHAPTER 8

Individual Rights in Health Care and Public Health

LEARNING OBJECTIVES

By the end of this chapter you will be able to:

- Describe the meaning and importance of the "no-duty" principle
- Explain generally how the U.S. approach to health rights differs from that of other high-income countries
- Describe the types and limitations of individual legal rights associated with health care
- Describe the balancing approach taken when weighing individual rights against the public's health

INTRODUCTION

The real-life scenarios in the vignette touch upon the key issues you will confront in this chapter, namely, the ways in which the law creates, protects, and restricts individual rights in the contexts of health care and public health. As described in Chapter 3, individuals in society are deeply impacted by law on a daily basis, and this fact is no less true when individuals navigate the health care system, or when an individual's actions are measured against the broader interests of the public's health. Over many decades, legal principles have been rejected, developed, and refined as the law continually struggles to define the appropriate relationship between individuals and the physicians, hospitals, managed care companies, and

VIGNETTE

At the turn of the 20th century, an Indiana physician named George Eddingfield repeatedly refused to come to the aid of Charlotte Burk, who was in labor, even though he was Mrs. Burk's family physician. Dr. Eddingfield conceded at trial that he made this decision for no particular reason, and despite the facts that he had been offered monetary compensation in advance of his performing any medical services and that he was aware that no other physician was available to provide care to Mrs. Burk. Unattended by any medical providers, Mrs. Burk eventually fell gravely ill, and both she and her unborn child died. After a trial and subsequent appeals, Dr. Eddingfield was found to not have wrongfully caused either death.

Around the same time as the scenario just described, the Cambridge, Massachusetts, Board of Health ordered everyone within city limits to be vaccinated against the smallpox disease under a state law granting local boards of health the power, under certain circumstances, to require the vaccination of individuals. After refusing to abide by the Cambridge Board's order, Henning Jacobson was convicted by a state trial court and sentenced to pay a $5 fine. Remarkably, Mr. Jacobson's case not only made its way to the United States Supreme Court, it resulted in one of the Court's most important public health rulings and a sweeping statement about limitations to fundamental individual rights in the face of threats to the public's health.

others they encounter in the health care delivery system, and between individuals and governmental actors charged with protecting public health and welfare. These balancing acts are made all the more difficult as the legal system bumps up against the quick pace of technological advancements in medicine and against amorphous, potentially deadly risks to the public's health, such as bioterrorism and fast-spreading influenzas.

After a background section, this chapter considers individual legal rights in health care, beginning with a brief overview of health rights under international and foreign law. This sets up a much lengthier discussion of health care rights in the United States, which for purposes of this chapter are classified according to an important distinction: legal rights *to* health care, and rights that individuals can claim only *within* the context of the health care system, that is, only once they have found a way to access needed care.[a] Examples of the latter type of rights include the right to refuse unwanted treatment, the right to autonomy in making personal health care decisions, and the right to be free from wrongful discrimination when receiving care. Finally, the chapter turns to a discussion of individual rights in the context of government-initiated public health efforts. This topic is dominated by the role and scope of government "police powers," which permit governments, when acting to promote or protect public health, to curtail individual freedoms and liberties.

BACKGROUND

Lurking behind any discussion of individual rights in a health context is one of the most basic principles in U.S. health law: Generally speaking, individuals have no legal right to health care services (or to public health insurance) and, correspondingly, there exists on the part of health care providers no general legal duty to provide care. This is referred to as the "no-duty" principle, which is aptly described by the Indiana Supreme Court in the well-known case of *Hurley v. Eddingfield*,[b] the facts of which we referred to in the first vignette at the opening of this chapter.[c] In its decision, the court wrote that the state law permitting the granting of a medical license

> provides for . . . standards of qualification . . . and penalties for practicing without a license. The [state licensing] act is preventive, not a compulsive, measure. In obtaining the state's license (permission) to practice medicine, the state does not require, and the licensee does not engage, that he will practice at all or on other terms than he may choose to accept.[d]

In other words, obtaining a license to practice medicine does not obligate an individual to actually practice, or to prac-

tice in a particular fashion or with a particular clientele; the licensure requirement exists instead to filter out individuals who may not have the requisite knowledge or skills to practice medicine. The same can be said for obtaining a law license, or even a driver's license: The former does not obligate a lawyer to practice, or to choose certain types of clients or cases; the latter does not require that a person actually drive, or drive a certain make of car. As with a medical license, the point of a law or driver's license is to guarantee that should the licensee *choose* to practice law or operate a motor vehicle, she is qualified to do so.

As you begin to think through the significance and implications of the no-duty principle, however, it is important to understand that there are many other legal principles and health laws that, in the language of the discussion from Chapter 3 concerning the scope of legal rights, define the relationship between an individual and another health system stakeholder (e.g., a physician, hospital, or government program). In fact, there are several federal and state laws that narrow the scope of the no-duty principle. For example, a federal law called the Examination and Treatment for Emergency Medical Conditions and Women in Labor Act enables all individuals to access needed hospital care in medical emergencies, irrespective of the individual's ability to pay for that care or a hospital's willingness to treat the individual. Also, both federal and state laws that generally prohibit certain forms of discrimination (say, based on race or disability) apply with equal force in the context of health care, and might require an accessibility to health services that otherwise would not exist. Furthermore, some public health insurance programs—Medicaid and Medicare, most prominently—create entitlements (a legal concept denoting a legal claim to something) to services for individuals who meet the programs' eligibility criteria,[1] and some health insurance products obligate physicians participating in the plan's networks to extend care to plan members. Finally, some states have implemented universal health care coverage programs, such as Maine's 2003 Dirigo Health Reform Act, which is designed to provide access to health coverage to every person in Maine by the year 2009.

When thinking about the law's no-duty principle, you must also take into account the role of medical ethics, which might require more of a health care professional than does the law. For example, no law mandates that licensed physicians aid a stranger in medical distress, but many believe an ethical obligation exists in this instance. And although legally the no-duty principle would dictate otherwise, most health care providers undoubtedly consider themselves ethically obligated to furnish at least some level of care to those who cannot pay for it. In short, although in reality there is no universal legal right to health care in the United States, certain situations give rise to health care rights, and specific populations may be entitled to health care or receive it purely through the magnanimity of ethics-conscious providers.

Perhaps because of the federal and state laws that chip away at the no-duty-to-treat principle, many students new to the study of health law erroneously assume that the principle is a legal anomaly, borne solely of the incredible historical power and autonomy of the medical profession and without modern precedent. In this sense, it is instructive to place the principle in a broader "welfare rights" context. During the 1960s, public interest lawyers, social reform activists, and others pressed for an interpretation of the federal Constitution that would have created an individual right to welfare. Under this view, government must provide individuals with minimally adequate levels of education, food, housing, health care, and so on.[2] But in a series of cases, the Supreme Court rejected the notion of a constitutional right to welfare.

Consider the right to education. Even though every state provides free public schools and makes education for minors compulsory, there is no national, generalized legal right to education. In the case of *San Antonio Independent School District v. Rodriguez*,[e] the Supreme Court ruled that education is not a fundamental right under the federal Constitution's Equal Protection Clause. The plaintiffs in the *Rodriguez* case were Mexican-American parents whose children attended elementary and secondary schools in an urban San Antonio school district. They had attacked as unconstitutional Texas's system of financing public education and filed the suit on behalf of schoolchildren throughout the state who were members of minority groups or who resided in relatively poor school districts. But the Court turned the plaintiffs' argument away, noting that although education is one of the most important services states perform, it

> is not among the rights afforded explicit protection under our Federal Constitution. Nor do we find any basis for saying it is implicitly so protected. . . . [T]he undisputed importance of education will not alone cause this Court to depart from the usual standard for reviewing a State's social and economic legislation.[f]

In the wake of the *Rodriguez* decision, several states interpreted their own constitutions as prohibiting inequitable methods of financing public education, thereby recognizing on some level a right to a minimally "meaningful" education. Subsequently, lawyers and social activists seeking to promote equal access to all manner of critical services seized on these state determinations, arguing that an egalitarian approach to

constitutional interpretation should not be limited to education.[3] Note, for example, how easily one author's writings about the right to education could just as well have been written with respect to health care:

> Requiring an adequate education will help to fulfill our nation's promise, articulated in *Brown* [*v. Board of Education*], that an individual be free to achieve her full potential. Ensuring educational adequacy will promote children's emotional and intellectual development, their career path and earning potential and thus their success throughout life. A meaningful education offers the hope that children can escape the degradation of poverty and its lack of opportunity, and attain pride, participation in this country's economic and political life, and financial and emotional success.[4(p825)]

However, efforts around ensuring adequate education have not been emulated in other social policy areas, such as health care. In fact, health care is treated not as a right, but as a commodity (like televisions or vacuum cleaners) subject to private market forces and socioeconomic status. During the public debate in 1993 over President Bill Clinton's failed attempt at national health reform, U.S. Representative Dick Armey (R-TX) stated that "health care is just a commodity, just like bread, and just like housing and everything else."[5(p102)] But why should this be the case, particularly when the private health insurance market has presumably found equilibrium at a point that continually leaves tens of millions of Americans uninsured, and particularly because health care (like education) is different from vacuum cleaners and other everyday goods in that it has "a fundamental bearing on the range of one's opportunities to realize one's life plans"?[3(p80)]

There is no single answer to the question of why health care is generally treated in this country as something less than an individual legal right. Many factors beyond the scope of this chapter are implicated: the nature and interpretation of the federal Constitution, politics, a weak labor movement, powerful interest groups, the nation's free market philosophies, the public's often negative view of the government, and more.[1,68] In this chapter, we limit the discussion to describing the kinds of health rights that do exist, how they operate in the context of the health care delivery system, and when considered against government-initiated public health efforts. Before we explore in depth the scope of individual health-related rights under U.S. law, however, we briefly describe these same types of rights under international law and under the law of other countries. Through this examination we provide a backdrop for understanding this country's approach to legal rights in the context of health.

INDIVIDUAL RIGHTS AND HEALTH CARE: A GLOBAL PERSPECTIVE

Despite being the world leader in terms of the development of medical technologies and the quantity of medical services, the United States is one of the only high-income nations that does not guarantee health care as a fundamental right, and it is the only developed nation that has not implemented a system for insuring at least all but the wealthiest segment of its population against health care costs.[1(p3)] In essence, other high-income nations with social democracies treat the provision of health care as a social good[g] (i.e., something that could be supported through private enterprise but is instead supported by the government and financed from public funds). And it is worth noting that nations that provide universal health care entitlements have not been bankrupted as a result. In fact, according to Professor Timothy Jost, "All of the other developed nations spend less on health care than does the U.S., in terms of both dollars per capita and proportion of gross domestic product."[1(p3)]

A foreign nation's universal health care rights—whether an unlimited right to health, a right to medical care generally or to a basic package of services, a right to health care insurance, or something else—exist under international human rights principles or under its national constitution. When recognized by governments, human rights accrue to all individuals because the rights are based upon the dignity and worth of the human being; so technically, a human right exists regardless of whether positive law (a constitution, a statute) has given it expression.[9] Examples of positive expressions of health as a human right include Article 25 of the 1948 Universal Declaration of Human Rights, which states that "[e]veryone has the right to a standard of living adequate for the health and well-being of himself and of his family, including . . . medical care . . . and the right to security in the event of . . . sickness, disability . . .", and the Constitution of the World Health Organization, which says that "The enjoyment of the highest attainable standard of health is one of the fundamental rights of every human being without distinction of race, religion, political belief, economic or social condition."

In terms of national constitutions, a 2004 survey reported that some two-thirds of constitutions world-wide address health or health care, and that almost all of these do so in universal terms, rather than being limited to certain populations.[10] For example, consider the health-related constitutional aspects of four politically and culturally diverse countries—Italy, the Netherlands, South Africa, and Poland—that have some type of

"right to health": Italy's Constitution guarantees a right to health; under the Dutch Constitution, the government is mandated "to promote the health of the population"; the Constitution of South Africa imposes on government the obligation to provide access to health services; and under Polish constitutional law, citizens are guaranteed "the right to health protection" and access to publicly financed health care services.[11]

Of course, including language respecting health rights in a legal document—even one as profound as a national constitution—does not guarantee that the right will be recognized or enforced. As in the U.S., multiple factors might lead a foreign court or other tribunal to construe rights-creating language narrowly, or to refuse to force implementation of what is properly considered a right. Examples of these factors include the relative strength of a country's judicial branch vis-à-vis other branches in its national governance structure, and a foreign court's view of its country's ability to provide services and benefits inherent in the health right.

INDIVIDUAL RIGHTS AND THE HEALTH CARE SYSTEM

The "global perspective" you just read was brief for two reasons. First, a full treatment of international and foreign health rights is well beyond the scope of this chapter. Second, historically speaking, international law has played a limited role in influencing this nation's domestic legal principles. As one author commented, "Historically the United States has been uniquely averse to accepting international human rights standards and conforming national laws to meet them."[12(p1156)] This fact is no less true in the area of health rights than in any other major area of law. As described earlier in this chapter, universal rights to health care are virtually nonexistent in the U.S., even though this stance renders it almost solitary among industrialized nations of the world.

This is not to say that this country has not contemplated health care as a universal, basic right. For instance, in 1952, a presidential commission stated that "access to the means for attainment and preservation of health is a basic human right."[13(p4)] Medicaid and Medicare—the importance of which you read about in Chapter 6—were the fruits of a nationwide debate about universal health care coverage. And during the 1960s and 1970s, the claim that health care was not a matter of privilege, but rather of right, was "so widely acknowledged as almost to be uncontroversial."[14(p389)] Nor is it to say that certain populations do not enjoy health care rights beyond those of the general public. Prisoners and others under the control of state governments have a right to minimal health care,[15] some state constitutions expressly recognize a right to health or health care benefits (for example, Montana includes an affirmative right to health in its constitution's section on inalienable rights), and individuals covered by Medicaid have unique legal entitlements. Finally, it would be inaccurate in describing health care rights to only cover rights to obtain health care in the first instance, because many important health care rights attach to individuals once they manage to gain access to needed health care services.

The remainder of this section describes more fully the various types of individual rights associated with the health care system. We categorize these rights as follows:

1. Rights related to receiving services explicitly provided under health care or health financing laws; for example, the Examination and Treatment for Emergency Medical Conditions and Women in Labor Act, and Medicaid, respectively;

2. Rights concerning freedom of choice and freedom from government interference when making health care decisions; for example, choosing to have an abortion;

3. The right to be free from unlawful discrimination when accessing or receiving health care; for example, Title VI of the federal Civil Rights Act of 1964, which prohibits discrimination on the basis of race, color, or national origin by entities that receive federal funding.[9(p12),16]

Rights Under Health Care and Health Financing Laws

We begin this discussion of rights-creating health laws with the Examination and Treatment for Emergency Medical Conditions and Women in Labor Act (also referred to as EMTALA, which is the acronym for the law's original name—the Emergency Medical Treatment and Active Labor Act—or, for reasons soon to become clear, the "patient anti-dumping statute"). We then briefly discuss the federal Medicaid program in a rights-creating context.

Rights Under Health Care Laws: EMTALA

Because EMTALA represents the only truly universal legal right to health care in this country—the right to access emergency hospital services—it is often described as one of the building blocks of health rights. EMTALA was enacted by Congress in 1986 to prevent the practice of "patient dumping," that is, the turning away of poor or uninsured persons in need of hospital care. Patient dumping was a common strategy among private hospitals aiming to shield themselves from the potentially uncompensated costs associated with treating poor and/or uninsured patients. By refusing to treat these individuals and instead "dumping" them on public hospitals, private institutions were effectively limiting their patients to those whose treatment costs would likely be covered out-of-pocket or by insurers. Note that the no-duty principle made this type of strategy possible.

EMTALA was a conscious effort on the part of elected federal officials to chip away at the no-duty principle: By creating legally enforceable rights to emergency hospital care for all individuals regardless of their income or health insurance status, Congress created a corresponding legal *duty* of care on the part of hospitals. At its core, EMTALA includes two related duties.[h] The first requires covered hospitals to provide an "appropriate" screening examination to all individuals who present at a hospital's emergency department seeking care for an "emergency medical condition." Under the law, an appropriate medical screening is one that is nondiscriminatory—remember, indigency or health insurance status are irrelevant for purposes of EMTALA's mandates—and that adheres to a hospital's established emergency care guidelines. EMTALA defines an emergency medical condition as a

> medical condition manifesting itself by acute symptoms of sufficient severity (including severe pain) such that the absence of immediate medical attention could reasonably be expected to result in (i) placing the health of the individual (or, with respect to a pregnant woman, the health of the woman or her unborn child) in serious jeopardy, (ii) serious impairment to bodily functions, or (iii) serious dysfunction of any bodily organ or part; or with respect to a pregnant woman who is having contractions, that there is inadequate time to effect a safe transfer to another hospital before delivery, or that transfer may pose a threat to the health or safety of the woman or the unborn child.[i]

The second key duty required of hospitals under EMTALA is to either stabilize any condition that meets the above definition or, in the case of a hospital without the capability to treat the emergency condition, undertake to transfer the patient to another facility in a medically appropriate fashion. A proper transfer is effectuated when, among other things, the transferring hospital minimizes the risks to the patient's health by providing as much treatment as is within its capability, when a receiving medical facility has agreed to accept the transferred patient, and when the transferring hospital provides the receiving facility all relevant medical records.

The legal rights established under EMTALA are accompanied by heavy penalties for their violation. The federal government, individual patients, and "dumped on" hospitals can all initiate actions against a hospital alleged to have violated EMTALA, and the federal government can also file a claim for civil money penalties against individual physicians who negligently violate an EMTALA requirement.

Rights Under Health Care Financing Laws: Medicaid

Many laws fund programs that aim to expand access to health care, such as state laws authorizing the establishment of public hospitals or health agencies, and the federal law establishing the vast network of community health clinics that serve medically underserved communities and populations. However, the legal obligations created by these financing laws are generally enforceable only by public agencies, not by individuals.

The Medicaid program is different in this respect. (Because Medicaid is discussed at length in Chapter 6, we do not cover it in depth here; however, because of its importance in the area of individual health care rights, we mention it also in this context.) Although most certainly a law concerning health care financing, Medicaid is unlike most other health financing laws in that it confers the right to individually enforce program obligations through the courts.[17(pp419–424)] This right of individual enforcement is one of the reasons why Medicaid, more than 40 years after its creation, remains a hotly debated public program. This is because the legal entitlements to benefits under Medicaid are viewed as a key contributor to the program's high cost. Yet whether Medicaid's legal entitlements are any more of a factor in the program's overall costs than, say, the generally high cost of health care is not clearly established.

Rights Related to Freedom of Choice and Freedom from Government Interference

EMTALA and Medicaid are remarkable in terms of the rights *to* health care that they each provide, though as mentioned earlier in this chapter, individual rights that attach *within* the context of health care provision can be equally important. Important individual rights within health care include the right to make informed health care decisions and the right to personal privacy and autonomy.[j]

The Right to Make Informed Health Care Decisions

One of the most important health care rights is the right of individual patients to make informed decisions about the scope and course of their own care. This includes the right to *refuse* treatment, regardless of its nature or urgency: The right to refuse treatment exists whether the patient is considering whether to ingest prescribed medication for minor pain, to undergo a minimally invasive test or procedure, or to consent to a major, potentially life-sustaining operation like the removal of a brain tumor. However, the right pertaining to informed decision making does not come without qualifiers and exceptions, as described below.

Modern notions of informed consent have their roots in the Nuremberg Code, which derived from the Nuremberg trials in the late 1940s of German physicians who performed horrendous experiments on prisoners in Nazi concentration camps during the Second World War. The code spells out principles of research ethics, including the need to secure in advance the voluntary consent of the research subject. These principles have been codified and expanded in American federal statutory and regulatory law concerning federally funded biomedical research.[k] But if the Nuremberg Code can be thought of as the roots of U.S. informed consent law, then the decision in *Canterbury v. Spence*[l] can be thought of as the trunk.

In 1959, Jerry Canterbury was a 19-year-old suffering from severe back pain. His neurosurgeon, Dr. William Spence, informed him that he would need a laminectomy—a surgical procedure where the roof of spinal vertebrae are removed or trimmed to relieve pressure on the spinal cord—to correct what the doctor believed was a herniated disc. However, Dr. Spence did not inform Canterbury of any risks associated with the surgery. The day after the operation, while appearing to recuperate normally, Canterbury fell from his hospital bed while no attendant was on hand and a few hours later began suffering from paralysis from the waist down. This led to a second spinal surgery, but Canterbury never fully recovered; years later, he needed crutches to walk and he suffered from paralysis of the bowels.

Canterbury sued Dr. Spence, alleging negligence in both the performance of the laminectomy and the doctor's failure to disclose risks inherent in the operation. The federal trial judge ruled in Dr. Spence's favor and Canterbury appealed, setting the stage for the now-famous decision in 1972 by the

Individual Rights and the Health Care System

federal Court of Appeals for the D.C. Circuit (considered second in national importance to the Supreme Court).[m] The decision includes two important determinations pertinent to this chapter. The first is that "as a part of the physician's overall obligation to the patient, [there exists a] duty of reasonable disclosure of the choices with respect to proposed therapy and the dangers inherently and potentially involved."[n] The court viewed this duty as a logical and modest extension of a physician's existing general duty to his patients. Importantly, the court discarded the notion that "the patient should ask for information before the physician is required to disclose."[o] In other words, the duty to disclose requires more than just answering patient questions; it demands voluntary disclosure on the part of the physician of pertinent medical information.

The *Canterbury* court's second key determination concerns the actual scope of the disclosure required—in other words, once the physician's duty to disclose is triggered, what information satisfies the legal requirement? On this matter the court made several observations: that the patient's right of "self-decision" is paramount, that the right to consent can be properly exercised only if the patient has sufficient information to make an "intelligent choice," that the sufficiency test is met when all information "material to the decision" is disclosed, and that the disclosure's legality should be measured objectively, not subjectively from the perspective of a particular physician or patient. From these observations, the court settled on three required pieces of disclosed information: a proposed treatment's inherent and potential risks, any alternatives to a proposed treatment, and the likely outcome of not being treated at all. Applying these criteria, the court ruled that Dr. Spence's failure to disclose even the tiniest risk of paralysis resulting from the laminectomy entitled Canterbury to a new trial.

As mentioned earlier, the right to make informed health care decisions is not boundless. For example, the court in *Canterbury* wrote that where disclosure of a treatment's risks would pose a threat of harm to the patient (for example, because it would severely complicate treatment or psychologically damage the patient) as to become "unfeasible or contraindicated from a medical point of view," the physician's duty to disclose could be set aside. Furthermore, a patient's competency from a legal vantage point plays a major role in her ability to consent to treatment.

The *Canterbury* decision, and subsequent decisions based on it, have over the years been interpreted expansively, and today the right to make informed health care decisions has many facets beyond a clear explanation of proposed treatments, potential risks and complications, and the like. For example, patients have the right to know whether outside factors,

Box 8-2
Discussion Questions

Go back to the first legal principle drawn from the *Canterbury* decision, namely, that physicians have a duty of reasonable disclosure to include therapy options and the dangers potentially involved with each. Do you agree with the court that this duty is both a logical and modest extension of physicians' "traditional" obligation to their patients? Why or why not? And depending on your answer, are you surprised to learn that some states have opted not to follow the *Canterbury* court's patient-oriented standard of informed consent, relying instead on the more conventional approach of measuring the legality of physician disclosure based on what a reasonable physician would have disclosed?

like research interests or financial considerations, are coloring a physician's thinking about a proposed course of treatment; patients whose first language is not English have the right to an interpreter; and patients have the right to designate in advance their treatment wishes, whether through written advance directives or another individual.

The Right to Personal Privacy

Another right related to freedom of choice/freedom from government interference is the constitutional right to personal privacy. Although the federal Constitution makes no explicit mention of the right to privacy, the Supreme Court has recognized some form of it since the 1890s.[p] The Court has taken a more or less two-pronged approach to the right. The first defines the protected personal interest as "informational privacy," meaning the limiting of others' access to and use of an individual's private information.[q] The second approach is concerned with individual autonomy and freedom from governmental interference in making basic personal decisions, and is the type of privacy right focused on in this section. This right is one of the most debated in law, both because of its implicit nature (constitutionally speaking) and because it has served as the legal underpinning of several divisive social issues, including abortion, intimate associations, and the decisions as to whether, when, and how to end one's life.

The right to privacy achieved prominence beginning with the Supreme Court's landmark 1965 decision in *Griswold v. Connecticut*,[r] in which the Court considered the constitutionality of a state law criminalizing the provision of contraception to married couples. In the early 1960s, Estelle Griswold, the Executive Director of the Planned Parenthood League of

Connecticut, and one of her colleagues were convicted of aiding and abetting "the use of a drug, medicinal article, or instrument for the purpose of preventing conception" by providing contraceptives to a married couple in violation of Connecticut law. The Court determined that although the Constitution does not explicitly protect a general right to privacy, certain provisions in the Bill of Rights create "penumbras," or zones, of guaranteed privacy, and that Connecticut's law constituted an undue intrusion into one of these zones (i.e., marriage).[s]

After the *Griswold* decision, advocates of the constitutional right to privacy flooded the federal courts with cases designed to expand the scope of the right. Quickly, laws banning interracial marriage were struck down,[t] as were laws prohibiting unmarried individuals from using contraception.[u] At the same time, federal courts were confronted with cases asking them to determine how the right to privacy applied in the context of abortion. The remainder of this section analyzes the courts' response to this particular issue. We selected the constitutional right to abortion as the focal point of the right to privacy discussion because it is not only one of the most contested rights in a health context, but also one of the most contested areas of public policy generally.

THE ROE V. WADE DECISION.   Few judicial decisions have affected this country's legal, political, and social landscape as much as *Roe v. Wade*.[v] In 1970, an unmarried pregnant woman filed a lawsuit under the pseudonym "Roe" challenging the constitutionality of a Texas criminal law that prohibited procuring or attempting an abortion at any stage of pregnancy, except for the purpose of saving the pregnant woman's life. Roe was joined in the lawsuit by a doctor who performed abortions in violation of the law. They argued that the constitutional right to privacy articulated in *Griswold* and its progeny included a woman's right to choose to obtain an abortion. Texas, through district attorney Henry Wade, claimed that the law was permissible because the state had a compelling interest in protecting women from an unsafe medical procedure and in protecting prenatal life. The federal trial court agreed with Roe and declared the law unconstitutional, and Texas immediately appealed to the U.S. Supreme Court, which agreed to hear the case.[w]

At the Supreme Court, the work of drafting the majority opinion in *Roe v. Wade* fell to Justice Harry Blackmun, who earlier in his legal career had been counsel to a well-known and highly regarded medical clinic. By a 7–2 margin, the Court ruled that the constitutional right to privacy, which in its view most strongly emanates from the Fourteenth Amendment's due process protections, is broad enough to encompass a woman's decision to terminate her pregnancy.

Once the Court established that a woman has a constitutional right to obtain an abortion, it went on to discuss the limits of that right. Roe had argued that the right to obtain an abortion is absolute, and that no state or federal law abridging the right could be enacted. The Court did not agree. Justice Blackmun wrote that states have both an interest in protecting the welfare of its citizens and a duty to protect them, and that the duty extends to the unborn. According to the Court, "a State may properly assert important interests in safeguarding health, in maintaining medical standards, and in protecting potential life. At some point in pregnancy, these respective interests become sufficiently compelling to sustain regulation of the factors that govern the abortion decision."[x] The Court then linked both a woman's "right to choose" and states' interest in protecting potential life to the viability of the fetus, setting forth the following "trimester framework" that enhances state power to regulate the abortion decision and restricts a pregnant woman's right as the fetus grows older:

> (a) For the stage prior to approximately the end of the first trimester, the abortion decision and its effectuation must be left to the medical judgment of the pregnant woman's attending physician.
>
> (b) For the stage subsequent to approximately the end of the first trimester, the State, in promoting its interest in the health of the mother, may, if it chooses, regulate the abortion procedure in ways that are reasonably related to maternal health.
>
> (c) For the stage subsequent to viability, the State, in promoting its interest in the potentiality of human life may, if it chooses, regulate, and even proscribe, abortion except where it is necessary, in appropriate medical judgment, for the preservation of the life or health of the mother.[y]

As a matter of both policy and law, the *Roe* decision has been vigorously criticized.[19–22] For example, detractors claim that the Court improperly made social policy by "finding" an expansive constitutional right to privacy (one broad enough to include the right to terminate a pregnancy) where one did not expressly exist. As a legal matter, many have argued that the decision relied too heavily on medical concepts that would be rendered obsolete as medical technology advanced and that would in turn result in a narrowing of the constitutional right advanced in the decision.[z]

Regardless of these and other criticisms, the *Roe* decision was monumental beyond its legal implications. It galvanized political forces opposed to abortion and prompted a movement to create ways to discourage the practice through state policies designed to regulate the factors involved in the abortion decision. For example, as described next, Pennsylvania enacted a law that imposed a series of requirements on women seeking abortion services, and it was this law that nearly 20 years after *Roe* set the stage for another battle at the Supreme Court over abortion and the right to privacy.

THE PLANNED PARENTHOOD OF SOUTHEASTERN PENNSYLVANIA V. CASEY DECISION.

At issue in the 1992 case of *Planned Parenthood of Southeastern Pennsylvania v. Casey*[aa] were several amendments to Pennsylvania's Abortion Control Act that made it more difficult for a pregnant woman to obtain an abortion: one provision required that a woman seeking an abortion be provided with certain information at least 24 hours in advance of the abortion; a second stated that a minor seeking an abortion had to secure the informed consent of one of her parents, but included a "judicial bypass" option if the minor did not wish to or could not obtain parental consent; a third amendment required that a married woman seeking an abortion had to submit a signed statement indicating that she had notified her husband of her intent to have an abortion, though certain exceptions were included; and a final provision imposed new reporting requirements on facilities that offered abortion services. The revised law exempted compliance with these requirements in the event of a "medical emergency."

Before any of the new provisions took effect, they were challenged by five Pennsylvania abortion clinics and a group of physicians who performed abortions. The federal trial court struck down all of the provisions as unconstitutional violations under *Roe*. On appeal, the Third Circuit Court of Appeals reversed and upheld all of the provisions, except for the husband notification requirement, as constitutional. The plaintiffs appealed to the Supreme Court, which agreed to hear the case.

The Court's 5–4 decision in favor of the plaintiffs in *Casey* expressly acknowledged the widespread confusion over the meaning and reach of *Roe*, and it used its opinion in *Casey* to provide better guidance to legislatures seeking to regulate abortion as a constitutionally protected right. Specifically, the Court in *Casey* sought to define more precisely both the constitutional rights of pregnant women and the legitimate authority of states to regulate some aspects of the abortion decision. The deeply divided Court wrote:

> It must be stated at the outset and with clarity that *Roe*'s essential holding, the holding we reaffirm, has three parts. First is a recognition of the right of the woman to choose to have an abortion before viability and to obtain it without undue interference from the State. Before viability, the State's interests are not strong enough to support a prohibition of abortion or the imposition of a substantial obstacle to the woman's

effective right to elect the procedure. Second is a confirmation of the State's power to restrict abortions after fetal viability, if the law contains exceptions for pregnancies which endanger the woman's life or health. And third is the principle that the State has legitimate interests from the outset of the pregnancy in protecting the health of the woman and the life of the fetus that may become a child. These principles do not contradict one another; and we adhere to each.[bb]

Notice how in interpreting *Roe* the Court in *Casey* makes some remarkable alterations to the contours of the right to choose to have an abortion. First, trimesters were replaced by fetal viability as the regulatory touchstone. Second, the pregnant woman, not her attending physician, effectuates the abortion decision. Third, a state's interest in protecting pregnant women and fetuses now attaches "from the outset of the pregnancy," not at the beginning of the second trimester. Fourth, and perhaps most important, the Court's invalidation of the trimester framework enabled the establishment of a new "undue burden" standard for assessing the constitutionality of state abortion regulations. Under this new standard, a state may not prohibit abortion prior to fetal viability, but it may promulgate abortion regulations as long as they do not pose a "substantial obstacle" to a woman seeking to terminate a pregnancy. The Court did not, however, alter its decision in *Roe* that post-viability, a state may proscribe abortion except when pregnancies endanger a woman's life or health. Taken together, these alterations both maintain a pregnant woman's basic constitutional right to obtain an abortion pre-viability, and enhance state interest in protecting the potentiality for human life.

Once the Court established the undue burden standard for assessing the constitutionality of state abortion regulations, it applied the standard to each constitutionally questionable amendment to Pennsylvania's Abortion Control Act. In the end, only the spousal notification provision was struck down as an unconstitutional burden; the Court determined that some pregnant women may have sound reasons for not wishing to inform their husbands of their decision to obtain an abortion, including fear of abuse, threats of future violence, and withdrawal of financial support. As a result, the Court equated the spousal notification requirement to a substantial obstacle because it was likely to prevent women from obtaining abortions.

The Court majority in *Casey* provided a new template for lower courts to use in deciding the constitutionality of state abortion regulations. Likewise, the opinion offered guidance to state legislatures as to what kinds of abortion restrictions were likely to withstand a constitutional attack. Nonetheless, some state legislatures have tested the boundaries of *Casey* by enacting bans on a procedure known as "partial birth" abortion,[cc] an issue to which we now turn.

The Stenberg v. Carhart Decision. The undue burden standard articulated in *Casey* for assessing the constitutionality of abortion regulations was put to the test in *Stenberg v. Carhart*.[dd] At issue in the case was a Nebraska criminal law banning "an abortion procedure in which the person performing the abortion partially delivers vaginally a living unborn child before killing the unborn child and completing the delivery."[ee] It further defined "partially delivers vaginally a living unborn child before killing the unborn child" to mean "deliberately and intentionally delivering into the vagina a living unborn child, or a substantial portion thereof, for the purpose of performing a procedure that the person performing such procedure knows will kill the unborn child and does kill the unborn child."[ff] The Nebraska law penalized physicians who performed a banned abortion procedure with a prison term of up to 20 years, a fine of up to $25,000, and the automatic revocation of the doctor's license to practice medicine in Nebraska.

Dr. Leroy Carhart, a Nebraska physician who performed abortions, filed a lawsuit seeking a declaration that the Nebraska law violated the constitutional principles set forth in *Roe* and *Casey*. After a lengthy trial, a federal district court agreed with Dr. Carhart and declared the Nebraska law unconstitutional. The Court of Appeals for the Eighth Circuit agreed, concluding that Nebraska's statute violated the Constitution as interpreted by the Supreme Court in *Casey*. The Supreme Court then granted review.

The Court was unequivocal in its opinion in *Stenberg* that the case was not a forum for a discussion on the propriety of *Roe* and *Casey*, but rather an application of the rules stated in those cases. In applying the undue burden standard to pre-viability abortions, the Court considered trial court testimony from expert witnesses regarding several different abortion procedures then-current in medical practice to flesh out the procedures' technical distinctions and to determine whether the procedures fell within Nebraska's definition of "partial birth" abortion. The Court determined that two distinct abortion procedures were relevant—dilation and evacuation (D&E), and dilation and extraction (D&X)—and that the Nebraska law's vague definition of "partial birth" abortion effectively banned both procedures.

Again by a 5–4 majority, the Supreme Court struck down the Nebraska law as unconstitutional on two separate grounds. First, the Court concluded that the statute created an undue burden on women seeking pre-viability abortions.

The Court reasoned that banning the most commonly used method for pre-viability second trimester abortions—the D&E procedure—unconstitutionally burdened a woman's ability to choose to have an abortion. Second, the Court invalidated the state law because it lacked an exception for the preservation of the health of the pregnant woman. The Court rejected Nebraska's claim that the banned procedures were never necessary to maintain the health of the pregnant woman and held that "significant medical authority" indicated that the D&X procedure is in some cases the safest abortion procedure available.[gg]

At the time *Stenberg* was decided, nearly 30 states had laws restricting D&E- and D&X-type abortions in some manner. Attempts to enact bans on these abortion procedures, however, have not been made only by state legislatures. Congress has tried numerous times to promulgate a federal ban, and after *Stenberg* was handed down, congressional opponents to abortion vowed to craft a ban that would pass constitutional muster. This effort culminated in the Partial Birth Abortion Ban Act of 2003 (PBABA).

Partial Birth Abortion Ban Act of 2003. PBABA represents Congress's third attempt since 1996 to ban "partial birth" abortions. Previous bills were vetoed by President Bill Clinton in 1996 and 1997, but in late 2003 PBABA easily passed both houses of Congress and was signed into law by President George W. Bush. Immediately, the constitutionality of PBABA was challenged, and the law's ultimate fate will be decided by the Supreme Court, which in February 2006 agreed to review the law.

PBABA establishes criminal penalties for "[a]ny physician who . . . knowingly performs a partial birth abortion and thereby kills a human fetus. . . ."[hh] Attempting to avoid the definitional vagueness that affected the Nebraska law's constitutionality, the drafters of the federal law used more precise language in an effort to ban only D&X procedures, although PBABA does not specifically refer to any medical procedure by name. Instead, the law defines a "partial birth" abortion as:

> An abortion in which the person performing the abortion deliberately and intentionally vaginally delivers a living fetus until, in the case of a head-first presentation, the entire fetal head is outside the body of the mother, or, in the case of a breech presentation, any part of the fetal trunk past the navel is outside the body of the mother, for the purpose of performing an overt act that the person knows will kill the partially delivered living fetus.[ii]

Furthermore, PBABA contains an exception allowing for these otherwise illegal abortions when necessary to protect a pregnant woman's life, but not health. The law's authors claim that the banned procedure is never necessary to protect the health of a pregnant woman and thus that an exception is not required.

Separate lawsuits challenging PBABA were filed in federal courts in California, Nebraska, and New York. All three federal trial courts concluded that the lack of a health exception necessarily rendered the law unconstitutional under Supreme Court precedent. With enforcement of PBABA halted, the federal government appealed all three cases. The appellate courts that examined PBABA all found that substantial medical authority exists supporting the necessity of the banned procedure and declared PBABA unconstitutional because of its lack of a health exception. As noted, the fate of PBABA now rests with the Supreme Court.

The Right to Be Free from Wrongful Discrimination

We now transition to the final topic in the discussion of individual legal rights to and within health care, namely, the topic of health care discrimination.[jj] Like discrimination generally, health care discrimination has a lurid and lengthy history in this country. Prior to the *Brown v. Board of Education* decision in 1954 and the Civil Rights Movement of the 1960s, health care injustice and exclusion based on race and other factors were commonplace, dating to slavery times and plantation-based racially segregated health care. After the end of the First Reconstruction, states passed so-called Jim Crow laws, cementing in place legally segregated health care. As a result, hospitals, physician practices, medical/nursing/dental schools, and professional medical societies were all separated based on race. In places where Jim Crow laws had not been passed, corporate bylaws and contracts between private parties often had the same discriminatory effect, and these "Jim Crow substitutes" were generally honored and enforced by the courts that interpreted them.

Federal law also played a role in perpetuating racially segregated health care. For example, the Hospital Survey and Construction Act of 1946 (more commonly known as the Hill-Burton Act, after the key sponsors of the measure) provided federal money to states to build and refurbish hospitals after World War II, but explicitly sanctioned the construction of segregated facilities:

> A hospital will be made available to all persons residing in [its] territorial area . . . , without discrimination on account of race, creed, or color, but an exception shall be made in cases where

separate hospital facilities are provided for separate population groups, if the plan makes equitable provision on the basis of need for facilities and services of like quality for each such group.[kk]

This provision was not ruled unconstitutional until the 1963 case of *Simkins v. Moses H. Cone Memorial Hospital*, which has been referred to as the "*Brown v. Board of Education* of health care."[23] *Simkins* also helped fuel the passage of the Civil Rights Act of 1964, this country's most important civil rights legislation of the 20th century. For purposes of health care, Title VI of the 1964 Act was of specific importance. Title VI is discussed in more depth later in this chapter; in sum, this portion of the Civil Rights Act makes it illegal for programs and activities that receive federal funding to discriminate on the basis of race, color, or national origin.

Notwithstanding the health care rewards brought about by the civil rights movement—Title VI, the passage of Medicaid and Medicare, the establishment of federally financed community health centers—the focus on health care civil rights was waning as early as 1968. Several factors led to this decline, but what is most striking is that compared to the progress made by public and private civil rights efforts over the past 40 years in education, employment, and housing, civil rights enforcement in the health care field has been anything but sustained.

Of course, even an enduring and well-funded enforcement effort is no guarantee of wiping out discrimination, regardless of its social context. There are, unfortunately, vestiges of discrimination in many important aspects of American society, including the health care system. Moreover, although historically health care discrimination on the basis of race and ethnicity has received the most attention, the existence of discrimination in health care on the basis of socioeconomic status, disability, age, and gender also raise troubling questions. The remainder of this section touches briefly on each of these areas, describing laws (where applicable) or legal theories used to combat the particular health care discrimination at issue.

Race/Ethnicity Discrimination

The fact that health care discrimination premised on race or ethnicity has dominated the health care civil rights landscape should not be surprising, because racist beliefs and customs have infected health care no less so than other areas of life, such as education, employment, and housing. This fact is chronicled to a staggering degree by W. Michael Byrd and Linda A. Clayton,[24,25] two physician-researchers at the Harvard School of Public Health. Byrd and Clayton paint a complex and disturbing picture of a health care system that itself perpetuates racism in health care in three distinct ways: by not destroying the myth that minority Americans should be expected to experience poorer health relative to Caucasians; by organizing itself as a private, for-profit system that marginalizes the indigent and minorities; and by refusing to acknowledge the historical and ongoing problem of racial exclusion in health care.

One key problem that in part results from the design of the health care system is that of racial and ethnic health disparities—differences in health care access, treatment, and outcomes between populations of color and Caucasians. In 2003, the Institute of Medicine (IOM) released an influential report that included overwhelming evidence of racial and ethnic health disparities and documented that these disparities could not be explained solely by the relative amount of health care needed by populations of color and nonminority populations.[26] For example, the report concluded that African Americans are relatively less likely to receive treatment for early-stage lung cancer, publicly insured Latinos and African Americans do not receive coronary artery bypass surgery at rates comparable to publicly insured nonminorities, and Latino and African-American children on Medicaid experience relatively higher rates of hospitalization.

Furthermore, the IOM study revealed that even when relevant patient characteristics are controlled for, racial and ethnic differences arise not only in terms of accessing care initially, but also after individuals have entered the health care system, a finding that supports the notion that the system itself and physician practice style contribute to disparities. This notion is, of course, quite controversial, because it suggests that physician decision making and clinical practice can increase the likelihood of racially disparate outcomes.

The key law used to combat race and ethnicity discrimination in health care is Title VI of the 1964 Civil Rights Act,[ll] which states that "[n]o person in the United States shall, on the ground of race, color, or national origin, be excluded from participation in, be denied the benefits of, or be subjected to discrimination under any program or activity receiving federal financial assistance."[mm] Because it only attaches to recipients of federal funding, Title VI does not reach, for example, health professionals who do not directly participate in government-sponsored health programs (nor does it reach physicians whose only participation in federal assistance programs is under Medicare Part B; the basis for this exemption is purely historical [and political], and the exemption is not codified in Title VI statutory or regulatory law[23(pp115–128)]). Nonetheless, Title VI has long had the potential to greatly impact the field of health care, because an enormous amount of federal funding has been poured into the health care enterprise over the past 40-plus years.

The concept of "discrimination" under Title VI applies both to *intentional* acts and to actions or policies that unintentionally have the *effect* of discriminating against racial and ethnic minorities. This is so because federal regulations implementing the Title VI statute (which explicitly only prohibits intentional discrimination) reach actions that, even if neutral on their face, have a disproportionate adverse impact (or effect) on members of minority groups. In the case of health care access and delivery, you can imagine several types of conduct that might potentially violate the Title VI disproportionate impact regulations. For example, were a hospital to segregate patients by source of payment—say, by maintaining a ward or floor that only treated patients covered under Medicaid—this might have the effect of adversely impacting racial and ethnic minorities, given the overall makeup of the Medicaid population. Similarly, the Title VI regulations could be violated if a managed care organization enrolled both privately and publicly insured persons, but allowed participating providers to refuse to accept as patients those individuals covered by Medicaid.

The disproportionate impact regulations are critically important to realizing Title VI's full force, because much of the racism in post-1954 America does not take the form of overt, intentional acts. However, as a result of the 2001 Supreme Court decision in *Alexander v. Sandoval*,[nn] these regulations were severely undercut. Under *Sandoval*, private individuals were barred from bringing a lawsuit under the disparate impact regulations, leaving the federal government as the sole enforcer when racial or ethnic minorities allege a violation of the regulations.[oo]

Physical and Mental Disability Discrimination

Like discrimination based on race or ethnicity, health care discrimination premised on disability has a long, sad history in this country and, as with race, the health system itself is partly to blame for its perpetuation. For instance, historically persons with mental disabilities were viewed from a medical standpoint as having little to offer to society, and they were as a matter of practice shipped to mental asylums isolated from communities. But those with physical disabilities were not spared discriminatory practices; because individuals with Down syndrome were viewed by medical practitioners as "Mongoloid idiots," and children with cerebral palsy or other serious physical limitations were regularly viewed as unable to contribute to society, they were all simply institutionalized. These historical practices and perspectives resonate even in the modern health care system, in which treatment opportunities for the disabled are skewed toward institutional, rather than community, settings, and disease-specific limitations in health insurance are commonplace.

However, passage of the Americans with Disabilities Act (ADA)[pp] in 1990 alleviated at least some of the problems associated with disability discrimination in health care. Like Title VI, the ADA is not specifically a "health law"—its intent is to extend to the disabled the maximum opportunity for community integration in many sectors of society, including employment, public services, public accommodations (i.e., privately owned entities open to the public), telecommunications, and more. For this reason, it prohibits discrimination generally against disabled individuals who satisfy the essential requirements of a particular job, or who meet the qualification standards for a program, service, or benefit.

But the ADA's impact on health care for disabled individuals is notable, in large part because the law defines "places of public accommodation" to include private hospitals and other private health care providers. So, for example, a dentist in private practice who does not receive any federal funds for his services is nonetheless prohibited from discriminating against a person who is HIV-positive, as the well-known case of *Bragdon v. Abbott*[qq] makes clear. This represents an important expansion of federal disability law, because prior to the ADA only recipients of federal funds were proscribed from discriminating on the basis of disability. Note also how this expanded concept of public accommodations differs from Title VI of the Civil Rights Act, which still requires the receipt of federal money on the part of the offending entity to trigger protections for racial and ethnic minorities.

Although the ADA has dramatically altered the disability law landscape, it is not without limitations. For example, the regulations implementing the ADA's statutory text only require entities that implement public programs and services to make "reasonable modifications"—but not "fundamental alterations"—to those programs and services. Under the ADA, a fundamental alteration is one that would change the essential nature of a public program or service. Whether a requested change to a public program or service by a disabled individual amounts to a "reasonable" or "fundamental" one is po-

tentially determinative to the outcome of the request. Why? Because if a court determines that the request would alter the essential nature of the program or service at issue, it is powerless under the ADA to order the change. Another way of understanding this reasonable modification/fundamental alteration dichotomy is to recognize that fundamental alterations to public services—alterations that might actually be necessary to achieve at least the spirit of the ADA's loftiest goals and meet the expectations of a modern, enlightened society—could only be made by the political branches of government, not by the courts.

Another important limitation of the ADA (at least as it has been interpreted by most courts) is that it does not prohibit arbitrary insurance coverage limits attached to certain medical conditions. A stark example of this is found in the case of *Doe v. Mutual of Omaha Insurance Company*,[rr] in which a federal appellate court ruled that a lifetime benefit limitation in a health insurance policy of $25,000 for AIDS or AIDS-related conditions did not violate the ADA, even though the very same policy set a $1 million lifetime limit for other conditions.

Socioeconomic Status Discrimination

Compared to race or disability discrimination in health care access and treatment, health care discrimination based on class gains little attention—even though socioeconomic status is independently associated with health status, and the negative effects of poverty on health and health care access are incontrovertible. Class-related health care discrimination can take many forms. For example, health care providers might refuse to accept as patients individuals who are covered under Medicaid. Or low-income individuals might fall victim to the practice of redlining, which refers to discrimination based on geographic location when companies offer goods and services to consumers.[ss] Another example stems from the fact that health care providers (physician and dental practices, hospitals, etc.) sometimes elect to not operate in relatively poor communities, leaving residents of these communities at heightened risk for experiencing a shortage of adequate health care resources.

Gender Discrimination

Gender discrimination against women is also a problem in health care. This bias appears to be of particular concern in the area of coronary heart disease,[28] where delayed or disparate care could have severe consequences. At least in theory, gender discrimination in health care could be remedied under the Equal Protection Clause of the federal Constitution. However, Equal Protection claims are difficult to win, because they require proof of both state action (a sufficient government connection to the discriminatory acts) and proximate causation (a cause-and-effect link between the discrimination and the harm suffered). And consider the fact that health care practitioners who receive federal funds cannot face suit under Title VI for even obvious gender discrimination, because Title VI's prohibitions relate only to race, color, and national origin discrimination.

Age Discrimination

Finally, the medical care system also seems to be biased against the elderly. Just one of several disturbing facts on the treatment front is that the elderly sometimes do not receive needed surgical care because health professionals wrongfully assume that the chances of recovery are not good.[29] Another concern pertains to insurance coverage, in that many employers are attempting to rescind lifetime health coverage benefits to retired workers, even where the benefits had been promised as part of negotiated labor contracts. At first blush, this may not seem like a critical issue, because many retirees are at or beyond the age required for Medicare eligibility. But some retirees are of course not yet 65 years old, a retiree's employer-sponsored benefits might provide more or different coverage than Medicare, and employer benefits might cover a retiree's dependents, which Medicare does not do.

INDIVIDUAL RIGHTS IN A PUBLIC HEALTH CONTEXT

The discussion thus far has focused on health care legal rights that individuals can claim in the context of access, receipt of services, freedom of choice, and anti-discrimination. In each of these areas, however, the right claimed is not absolute. For example, EMTALA does not make illegal all transfers of indigent patients from private hospitals to public ones; rather, it requires that patients be medically stabilized before a transfer can occur. Even eminent civil rights laws do not provide blanket protections, because they might only be triggered where federal funding is present, or where the assistance requested would not fundamentally alter a government health program.

In this section, we consider restrictions on individual rights and liberties of a different sort. These derive not from the limitations of specific laws, but rather from governmental police powers used to protect the general public's health and welfare. One simple way to think about individual rights in a public health context is to use a balancing approach—what might the appropriate legal trade-offs be between private rights and public welfare? Public discussion of this trade-off intensified after the tragic terrorist attacks of September 11, 2001, because many government actions taken in their wake—the passage of new laws, the tightening of existing regulations, the detainment of alleged terrorists—starkly raised the question of where to draw the line between individual autonomy and government authority to restrain that autonomy in the name of public welfare and national security. The attacks raised new public health law–related questions as well, including whether the potential for a bioterrorist attack utilizing smallpox should compel the federal government to vaccinate individuals against the virus—even against their will—in order to protect the public at large in the event of an attack.

Overview of Police Powers

Police powers represent state and local government authority to require individual conformance with established standards of conduct. These standards are designed to promote and protect the public's health, safety, and welfare, and to permit government control of personal, corporate, and other private interests. The government's police powers are broad and take many forms. Health care professionals are required to obtain licenses from government agencies. Health care facilities face accreditation standards. Food establishments are heavily regulated. Employers are bound by numerous occupational health and safety rules. Businesses are constrained by pollution control measures. Tobacco products can only be marketed in certain ways. The purchase of guns is controlled, buildings have to abide by certain codes, motorcyclists must wear helmets. The list goes on and on.

The government's police powers are oftentimes invasive, a result that stems in part from the fact that the American colonies were battling multiple communicable diseases during the time of the writing of the Constitution, and its drafters were thus well aware of the need for pervasive governmental public health powers. At the same time, the government may not overreach when restricting private autonomy in the name of public health promotion and protection. For example, police powers cannot be used as a form of punishment, they cannot be used arbitrarily and capriciously, and they cannot be used for purposes unrelated to public health and welfare.

A key principle inherent to the use of police powers is that of coercion.[30] This is so because, in a country founded upon the twin ideals of individualism and a limited government, many individuals and businesses do not respond kindly to being told to conform with public health regulations that limit their actions. For example, sometimes a public health concern (e.g., pollution) requires a response (enhanced governmental regulation) that may not be in the best economic interests of an implicated party (a refinery). This is not to say that individuals and businesses do not voluntarily assume responsibilities and measures that are in the public's interest. For instance, one effect of poor exercise habits—obesity—has enormous implications for the public's health and for national health care costs. As a result, the government would prefer that all individuals exercise for a minimum amount of time each week, but there is of course no law requiring this; rather, voluntarism is the guiding principle when it comes to personal exercise. Nonetheless, personal coercion and industrial regulation have long been adopted (and accepted) practices of public health officials, and all of the major communicable disease outbreaks have been combated with some combination of compulsory screening, examination, treatment, isolation, and quarantine programs.

The Jacobson v. Massachusetts Decision

The fact that government coercion can be justified by important public health goals does not answer the question of where to draw the line between personal/economic freedom on the one hand, and the public welfare on the other. This question was taken up by the Supreme Court in *Jacobson v. Massachusetts*,[tt] perhaps the most famous public health law decision in the Court's history.[uu]

The facts in *Jacobson* are straightforward enough. At the turn of the 20th century, the state of Massachusetts enacted a law granting local health boards the power to require vaccination when necessary to protect the public's health or safety. In 1902 the Cambridge Board of Health, in the throes of attempting to contain a smallpox outbreak, took the state up on its offer, and issued an order requiring all adults in the city to be vaccinated against the disease. Henning Jacobson refused vaccination on the ground that he previously suffered negative reactions to vaccinations. Jacobson was fined $5 for his refusal, a penalty upheld by the state's highest court. Jacobson appealed to the U.S. Supreme Court, setting the stage for a decision that more than 100 years later remains both controversial and at least symbolically forceful.[31,32]

Like the enduring private interest/public welfare tension underpinning public health law generally, the *Jacobson* decision amounts to "a classic case of reconciling individual interests in bodily integrity with collective interests in health and safety."[31(p577)] The 7–2 decision went the state's way, with the Supreme Court recognizing that police powers were generally broad enough to encompass forced vaccination. Responding to Jacobson's argument that the Massachusetts law impermissibly infringed on his constitutional right to liberty, the Court wrote:

> [T]he liberty secured by the Constitution of the United States to every person within its jurisdiction does not import an absolute right in each person to be, at all times and in all circumstances, wholly freed from restraint. There are manifold

restraints to which every person is necessarily subject for the common good. On any other basis organized society could not exist with safety to its members. Society based on the rule that each one is a law unto himself would soon be confronted with disorder and anarchy.[vv]

Due to this and other language used by the Court in the decision, *Jacobson* is often described as sweepingly deferential to public health officials and their use of police powers. And without question, social compact theory (the idea that citizens have duties to one another and to society as a whole) animates the Court's decision. However, the *Jacobson* decision also recognizes the individual liberties protected by the Constitution, and in fact requires a deliberative governmental process to safeguard these interests.

According to the *Jacobson* Court, public health powers must be exercised in conformity with four standards in order to pass constitutional muster:

- The first standard, that of "public health necessity," requires that government use its police powers only in the face of a demonstrable public health threat.
- The second standard, termed "reasonable means," dictates that the methods used when exercising police powers must be designed in such a way as to prevent or ameliorate the public health threat found to exist under the first standard.
- "Proportionality" is the third *Jacobson* standard; it is violated when a particular public health measure imposes a burden on individuals totally disproportionate to the benefit to be expected from the measure.

Box 8-4
Discussion Question

Jacobson v. Massachusetts is a product of the early 20th century, and the public health law principles supporting it are vestiges of an even earlier time. This, coupled with a century of subsequent civil liberties jurisprudence and societal advancement, has led some commentators to question whether *Jacobson* should continue to retain its paradigmatic role in terms of the scope of government police powers. At the same time, other public health law experts call for *Jacobson's* continued vitality, arguing that it is settled doctrine and a still-appropriate answer to the private interest/collective good question. What do you think?

• Finally, and axiomatically, the public health regulation itself should not pose a significant health risk to individuals subject to it. This is the standard of "harm avoidance."

These standards have never been explicitly overturned, but it can be argued that they have at the very least been implicitly replaced, given that in the hundred years since *Jacobson* was decided, the Supreme Court has developed a much more complex approach to applying constitutional provisions to cases implicating individual autonomy and liberty.

The "Negative Constitution"

The discussion of police powers up to this point might reasonably lead you to believe that the Constitution *obligates* the government to protect the public's health and welfare through affirmative use of its powers. This view, however, has never been adopted by the Supreme Court. Instead, the prevailing view is that the Constitution *empowers* government to act in the name of public health but does not require it to do so. This interpretation of the Constitution refers to what is known as the "negative constitution," that is, the idea that the Constitution does not require government to provide any services, public health or otherwise. This approach to constitutional law derives from the fact that the Constitution is phrased mainly in negative terms (e.g., the First Amendment prohibits government abridgment of free speech). Professor Wendy Parmet describes the "negative constitution" this way:

> In the century that has witnessed Auschwitz and Chernobyl, it is easy to see the dangers posed by state power. This recognition tempers enthusiasm for public authority and leads us to use law as a limiting device. In our legal tradition, this view of law is integral to constitutional structure, with its emphasis on separation of powers, checks and balances, procedural protections, and individual rights. We rely on the Constitution to limit the power of the government to restrain our freedoms and cause us harm. In this sense, law is a negative force that prevents the state from intruding upon the individual. This negative conception of law, which sees legal rights as a restraint upon the state, has played a dominant role in the formulation of contemporary American public health law. It explains the central pillars of constitutional public health law: the search for limits on governmental authority to restrain individual freedoms in the name of public health, and the concomitant assumption

that government has no obligation to promote public health.[33(pp267,271)]

In two important decisions, *DeShaney v. Winnebago County Department of Social Services*[ww] and *Town of Castle Rock, Colorado v. Gonzales*,[xx] the Supreme Court has advanced this view of the negative constitution. In the former case, one-year-old Joshua DeShaney was placed in his father's custody after his parents divorced. Two years later, the father's second wife complained to county officials in Wisconsin that the father had been abusing Joshua physically. Social service workers opened a file on the case and interviewed Joshua's father, but the county did not pursue the matter further after the father denied the charges. One year after that, an emergency room physician treating Joshua alerted social services of his suspicion that Joshua's injuries were the result of abuse. The county again investigated but decided that insufficient evidence of child abuse existed to remove Joshua from his father's custody. This emergency room scenario played out two additional times over the next several months, but Joshua's caseworkers still believed that they had no basis on which to place Joshua in court custody. Some months later, when Joshua was four years old, he suffered a beating so severe that he fell into a life-threatening coma. He survived but was left with permanent, severe brain damage, and he was expected to live his life in an institution for the profoundly mentally retarded. Joshua's father was subsequently convicted of child abuse.

Joshua's mother filed a civil rights claim on Joshua's behalf against the county officials who failed to take the boy into their custody. The lawsuit was based on the Due Process Clause of the federal Constitution, which prohibits states from depriving any person of property without due process of law. However, the Supreme Court in *DeShaney* concluded that the "substantive" component of the Due Process Clause—which focuses on challenges to government conduct—could not be read to provide Joshua with a property interest in having state child welfare officials protect him from beatings by his father. For a 6–3 majority, Chief Justice Rehnquist held that state officials had no affirmative constitutional duty to protect Joshua:

> [N]othing in the language of the Due Process Clause itself requires the State to protect the life, liberty, and property of its citizens against invasion by private actors. The Clause is phrased as a limitation on the State's power to act, not as a guarantee of certain minimal levels of safety and security. It forbids the State itself to deprive individuals of life, liberty, or property without "due process of law," but its language cannot fairly be

extended to impose an affirmative obligation on the State to ensure that those interests do not come to harm through other means.[yy]

The majority further rejected the argument that the state's knowledge of the danger Joshua faced, and its expression of willingness to protect him against that danger, established a "special relationship" that gave rise to an affirmative constitutional duty to protect.

In dissent, three justices in *DeShaney* argued that through the establishment of its child protection program, the state of Wisconsin undertook a vital duty and effectively intervened in Joshua's life, and its failure to live up to its child protection duty amounted to a constitutional violation. According to the dissenters, the majority opinion "construes the Due Process Clause to permit a State to displace private sources of protection and then, at the critical moment, to shrug its shoulders and turn away from the harm that it has promised to try to prevent."[zz]

Sixteen years after *DeShaney*, the Supreme Court in *Castle Rock v. Gonzales* had an opportunity to again consider whether the government has a duty to affirmatively protect its citizens. This time, however, the Court was concerned not with substantive due process, but rather with procedural due process, which mandates that when a state establishes a benefit or right for its citizens, it is not entitled to deny individuals the benefit or right in an arbitrary or unfair way.

Unfortunately, the facts in *Gonzales* are as tragic as those in *DeShaney*. In May 1999, Jessica Gonzales received a court order protecting her and her three young daughters from her husband, who was also the girls' father. On June 22nd, all three girls disappeared in the late afternoon from in front of the Gonzales home, and Jessica suspected that her husband had taken them, in violation of the restraining order. This suspicion was confirmed in a phone conversation she had with her husband. In two initial phone conversations with the Castle Rock Police Department, she was told there was nothing the police could do and to wait until 10:00 p.m. to see if her husband brought the girls home.

Shortly after 10:00 Jessica called the police to report that her children were still missing, but this time she was told to wait until midnight to see what transpired. She called the police again at midnight, reported that her children were still missing, and left her home to go to her husband's apartment. Finding nobody there, she called the police again at 12:10 a.m. and was told to wait for an officer to arrive. Thirty minutes later, after no officer showed up, she went to the police station to submit a report. According to the Supreme Court decision, the officer who wrote up the report "made no reasonable effort to enforce the [restraining order] or locate the three children.

Instead, he went to dinner." A couple hours later, Jessica's husband pulled his truck up to, and began shooting at, the Castle Rock Police Department. After he was killed by police during the gunfight, the three Gonzales daughters were found dead in the back of the truck; they had been murdered by their father hours earlier.

Jessica sued the police department, claiming that her constitutional right to procedural due process was violated by the department's inaction. She argued that the restraining order she received was her "property" under the Constitution's Due Process Clause and that it was effectively "taken" from her without due process. Overturning the federal appellate court that ruled in her favor, the Supreme Court decided by a 7–2 margin that Jessica did not have a property interest in police enforcement of the restraining order against her husband.

The Court said it was not clear that *even if* it had found an individual entitlement to enforcement of a restraining order under a Colorado state statute requiring officers to use every reasonable means to enforce restraining orders, that this entitlement would constitute a protected "property" interest that triggers due process protections under the federal Constitution. Justice Antonin Scalia wrote that the Due Process Clause does not protect all government "benefits," including those things that government officials have discretion to grant or deny. Applying this standard, the Court ruled that Colorado's protection order law did not create an individual entitlement to police enforcement of restraining orders, explaining that police have discretion to act or not act under many circumstances, including when to enforce a restraining order (e.g., police officers have discretion to consider whether a violation of a protection order is too "technical" or minor to justify enforcement). Furthermore, the Court noted that if the Colorado legislature included statutory language making police enforcement of a restraining order "mandatory," even that would not necessarily mean that Mrs. Gonzales had a personal entitlement to its enforcement, given that the statute makes no mention of an individual's power to demand—or even request—enforcement.

In dissent, two justices in *Gonzales* argued that restraining orders amount to a personal, enforceable property interest. They asserted that the majority opinion wrongly ruled that a citizen's interest in government-provided police protection does not resemble a "traditional conception" of property. Looking to the legislative history and text of Colorado's own protection order law and to the purpose of the state's domestic violence legislation, the dissent concluded that a particular class of individuals were indeed entitled beneficiaries of domestic restraining orders.

Box 8-5
Discussion Questions

The "negative constitution" is a concept over which reasonable people can easily disagree. Notwithstanding the "defensive" manner of some of the Constitution's key provisions, there are several arguments in support of more affirmative action on the part of government health and welfare officials than current Supreme Court jurisprudence requires. For example, the dissent in *DeShaney* argues persuasively that Wisconsin's implementation of a child protection program effectively created a constitutional duty to actually protect children from seemingly obvious danger. As one leading scholar put it, "If an agency represents itself to the public as a defender of health, and citizens justifiably rely on that protection, is government 'responsible' when it knows that a substantial risk exists, fails to inform citizens so they might initiate action, and passively avoids a state response to that risk?"[30(p34)] What do you think of this argument? And can you think of others that call into question the soundness of the negative theory of constitutional law?

CONCLUSION

This chapter offered a snapshot of the current state of health-related legal rights. But as alluded to early on in the chapter, there were times in its relatively short history that this country was closer to recognizing broader individual health care rights than is currently the case, just as there have been times (as the aftermath of September 11, 2001, proved) when concerns for the public's health and safety have eclipsed the nation's more natural inclinations toward individualism and a deregulated marketplace. That this is so is of no surprise: Legal rights are, by nature, subject to shifts in the political terrain. For example, the Aid for Families with Dependent Children program (commonly known as AFDC), the federal welfare entitlement program for low-income populations, was dismantled in 1996 after more than 60 years in existence. Originally enacted under a slightly different name as part of the New Deal in 1935, AFDC was replaced with the Temporary Assistance for Needy Families (TANF) program by a moderate Democrat (President Bill Clinton) and a conservative, Republican-controlled Congress. Compared to AFDC, TANF dramatically limited the receipt of individual benefits and focused much more heavily on creating work opportunities for needy families. Like legal rights generally, health-related legal rights are similarly

subject to changing political currents. For example, at the time of this writing, several state legislatures are considering bills that protect health professionals from providing care that conflicts with their personal beliefs, reflecting the current political power of social conservatives.[aaa]

Of course, changes to legal rights are not always represented by restrictions of those rights. The enactment of Medicaid and Medicare, which created new health-related rights, is an obvious example. Other major examples include EMTALA and expanded state consumer rights for persons in managed care. On a less noticed scale, legal rights for persons with HIV/AIDS have expanded since the 1980s,[35] and federal courts now review the constitutionality of the treatment provided in, and conditions of, psychiatric hospitals.[bbb] These are just a few of many examples.

Nonetheless, vast challenges remain. After all, many scholars, politicians, and consumers point to the 45 million uninsured Americans as just one example of not only a failing health care financing and delivery system, but also a failing of the legal system. To fix—or even significantly reduce—a problem as profound and seemingly intractable as this nation's huge uninsured population takes not just political will but also an enormous undertaking to change the law. A "rights revolution" in a health context, like other major legal upheavals, requires something else, too: a substantial amount of general economic and social unrest.[36] As historian Brooks Adams once noted, "Law is merely the expression of the will of the strongest for the time being, and therefore laws have no fixity, but shift from generation to generation."[37(p197)]

REFERENCES

1. Jost TS. *Disentitlement? The Threats Facing Our Public Health-Care Programs and a Rights-Based Response.* New York: Oxford University Press; 2003.

2. Davis MF. *Brutal Need: Lawyers and the Welfare Rights Movement, 1960–1973.* New Haven, Conn.: Yale University Press; 1993.

3. Stacy T. The courts, the constitution, and a just distribution of health care. *Kans J Law Public Policy.* 1993/1994;3:77-94.

4. Smith PS. Addressing the plight of inner-city schools: the federal right to education after *Kadrmas v. Dickinson Public Schools. Whittier Law Rev.* 1997;18:825.

5. Reinhardt U. The debate that wasn't: the public and the Clinton health care plan. In Aaron H., ed. *The Problem That Won't Go Away: Reforming U.S. Health Care Financing.* Washington, D.C.: Brookings Institution; 1996: 70-109.

6. Vladeck B. Universal health insurance in the United States: reflections on the past, the present, and the future [editorial]. *Am J Pub Health.* 2003;93:16.

7. Blum JD, Talib N, Carstens P, et al. Rights of patients: comparative perspectives from five countries. *Med Law.* 2003;22:451.

8. Rich RF. Health policy, health insurance and the social contract. *Comp Labor Law Policy J.* 2000;21:397.

9. Barnes A, McChrystal M. The various human rights in health care. *Human Rights.* 1998;25:12.

10. Kinney ED, Clark BA. Provisions for health and health care in the constitutions of the countries of the world. *Cornell Int Law J.* 2004;37:2.

11. Littell A. Can a constitutional right to health guarantee universal health care coverage or improved health outcomes?: A survey of selected states. *Conn Law Rev.* 2002;35:289.

12. Yamin AE. The right to health under international law and its relevance to the United States. *Am J Public Health.* 2005;95(7):1156.

13. President's Commission for the Study of Ethical Problems in Medicine and Biomedical and Behavioral Research. *Securing Access to Health Care: A Report on the Ethical Implications of Differences in the Availability of Health Services.* Washington, D.C.: The National Academies Press; 1983.

14. Starr P. *The Social Transformation of American Medicine: The Rise of a Sovereign Profession and the Making of a Vast Industry.* New York: Basic Books; 1982.

15. Wing KR. The right to health care in the United States. *Ann Health Law.* 1993;2:163.

16. Annas GJ. *The Rights of Patients,* 3rd ed. Carbondale: Southern Illinois University Press; 2004.

17. Rosenblatt RE, Law SA, Rosenbaum S. *Law and the American Health Care System.* New York: The Foundation Press; 1997.

18. Warren SD, Brandeis LD. The right to privacy. *Harvard Law Rev.* 1890;4:193.

19. Barzelay DE, Heymann PB. The forest and the trees: Roe v. Wade and its critics. *Boston Univ Law Rev.* 1973;53:765.

20. Ely JH. The wages of crying wolf: a comment on Roe v. Wade. *Yale Law J.* 1973;82:920.

21. Regan DH. Rewriting Roe v. Wade. *Mich Law Rev.* 1979;77:269.

22. Bopp J, Coleson R. The right to abortion: anomalous, absolute, and ripe for reversal. *Brigham Young Univ J Public Law.* 1989;3:181.

23. Smith DB. *Health Care Divided: Race and Healing a Nation.* Ann Arbor: The University of Michigan Press; 1999.

24. Byrd WM, Clayton LA. *An American Health Dilemma: A Medical History of African Americans and the Problem of Race, Beginnings to 1900.* New York: Routledge; 2000.

25. Byrd WM, Clayton LA. *An American Health Dilemma: Race, Medicine, and Health Care in the United States, 1900–2000.* New York: Routledge; 2002.

26. Smedley BD, Stith AY, Nelson AR, eds. *Unequal Treatment: Confronting Racial and Ethnic Disparities in Health Care.* Washington, D.C.: The National Academies Press; 2003.

27. Perez TE. The civil rights dimension of racial and ethnic disparities in health status. In: Smedley BD, Stith AY, Nelson AR , eds. *Unequal Treatment: Confronting Racial and Ethnic Disparities in Health Care.* Washington, D.C.: The National Academies Press; 2003; 626-663.

28. Bess CJ. Gender bias in health care: a life or death issue for women with coronary heart disease. *Hastings Women's Law J.* 1995;6:41.

29. Smith GP, II. Our hearts were once young and gay: health care rationing and the elderly. *Univ Fla J Law Public Policy.* 1996;8:1.

30. Gostin LO. *Public Health Law: Power, Duty, Restraint.* Berkeley: University of California Press/New York: The Milbank Memorial Fund; 2000.

31. Gostin LO. Jacobson v. Massachusetts at 100 years: police powers and civil liberties in tension. *Am J Public Health.* 2005;95(4):576.

32. Mariner WK, Annas GJ, Glantz LH. *Jacobson v. Massachusetts*: it's not your great-great-grandfather's public health law. *Am J Public Health.* 2005;95(4):581.

33. Parmet W. Health care and the constitution: public health and the role of the state in the framing era. *Hastings Constitutional Law Q.* 1992;20:267, 271.

34. Stein R. Health workers' choice debated: proposals back right not to treat. *Washington Post.* January 30, 2006:A01

35. Halpern SA. Medical authority and the culture of rights. *J Health Politics Policy Law.* 2004;29(4–5):835.

36. Friedman LM. The idea of right as a social and legal concept. *J Social Issues.* 1971;27(2):189-198.

37. Nash B, Zullo A, eds. *Lawyer's Wit and Wisdom: Quotations on the Legal Profession, In Brief.* Philadelphia: Running Press; 1995.

ENDNOTES

a. These competing concepts were given life in Paul Starr's influential book, *The Social Transformation of American Medicine: The Rise of a Sovereign Profession and the Making of a Vast Industry* (New York: Basic Books, Inc., 1982). Incidentally, *The Social Transformation of American Medicine* should be read by all students with an interest in the history of medicine; the book's significance across a range of disciplines is hard to overstate. See "Special Issue: Transforming American Medicine: A Twenty-Year Retrospective on *The Social Transformation of American Medicine,*" *Journal of Health Politics, Policy, and Law* 29, nos. 4-5 (August-October 2004).

b. 59 N.E. 1058 (Ind. 1901).

c. Recall from those facts that Dr. Eddingfield was already Mrs. Burk's family physician. However, the general legal rule is that past treatment is not tantamount to an *existing* physician–patient relationship; rather, that type of relationship is specific to a "spell of illness" and must be established (or renewed) accordingly.

d. 59 N.E. 1058 (Ind. 1901).

e. 411 U.S. 1 (1973).

f. Ibid., 35.

g. For an interesting article describing the importance of political structures in determining the level of equalities/inequalities in a society, including the level of government-provided health care coverage, see Vicente Navarro and Leiyu Shi, "The Political Context of Social Inequalities and Health," in *Health and Social Justice: Politics, Ideology, and Inequity in the Distribution of Disease,* ed. Richard Hofrichter (San Francisco: Jossey-Bass, 2003).

h. Under EMTALA, only hospitals that participate in the Medicare program are bound by the emergency care duties. However, nearly all hospitals participate in Medicare.

i. 42 U.S.C. § 1395dd(e)(1).

j. One other right that falls in this category—the patient's right to an advocate who is not the patient's physician—is authoritatively described in Annas, *The Rights of Patients.*[16](28–43)

k. 45 C.F.R. Part 46.

l. 464 F.2d 772 (D.C. Cir. 1972).

m. Incidentally, the *Canterbury* decision was authored by Spottswood Robinson, III who, prior to becoming a highly regarded federal judge, was instrumental in the fight for civil rights, in part as one of the National Association for the Advancement of Colored People (NAACP) lawyers who initially brought suit in one of the cases that eventually morphed into *Brown v. Board of Education.*

n. 464 F.2d, 782.

o. Ibid., 783 fn. 36.

p. A now-famous 1890 article is often credited with introducing the constitutional "right to be let alone."[18]

q. In a health context, this type of privacy is embodied by the Health Insurance Portability and Accountability Act (HIPAA), found in large part in 29 U.S.C. §§ 1181 - 1187, 42 U.S.C. §§ 300gg *et seq.* and 42 U.S.C. §§ 1320a *et seq.*, which creates a federal right to maintain the confidentiality of one's personal health information.

r. 381 U.S. 479 (1965).

s. Ibid., 484–486.

t. *Loving v. Virginia,* 388 U.S. 1 (1967).

u. *Eisenstadt v. Baird,* 405 U.S. 438 (1972).

v. 410 U.S. 113 (1973). For a compelling look at what the case has meant to society, see David J. Garrow, *Liberty and Sexuality: The Right to Privacy and the Making of Roe v. Wade* (California: University of California Press, 1994).

w. In rare circumstances, the Supreme Court will hear a case without an intermediate appellate court ruling.

x. 410 U.S., 154.

y. Ibid., 164–165.

z. For example, notice how the Supreme Court linked states' power to ban abortions (with certain exceptions) to fetal viability, even though the progression of medical knowledge and technology could push back the point of viability earlier into pregnancy. Also, who appears to hold the power, under "(a)" above, to decide whether an abortion should occur? The *physician*, a fact often overlooked by those who hail *Roe* as a seminal women's rights case and one that calls into question how the pregnant woman's constitutional right to privacy could be effectuated by her treating physician.

aa. 505 U.S. 833 (1992).

bb. Ibid., 847.

cc. Furthermore, in February 2006, South Dakota enacted the South Dakota Women's Health and Human Life Protection Act, which makes it a felony for doctors to perform any abortions in South Dakota except to save the life of a pregnant woman. Naturally, this law is being challenged by Planned Parenthood and is not being enforced until its constitutionality is determined.

dd. 530 U.S. 914 (2000).

ee. Ibid., § 28-326 (9).

ff. Ibid.

gg. Ibid., 932.

hh. 18 U.S.C.A. § 1531 (a) (2004).

ii. Ibid., (b).

jj. This section was adapted from Joel B. Teitelbaum, "Health Care and Civil Rights: An Introduction," *Ethnicity and Disease* 15, no. 2, Supp. 2, (2005): 27–30.

kk. 42 U.S.C. § 291e(f).

ll. 42 U.S.C. §§ 2000a *et seq*.

mm. 42 U.S.C. § 2000d.

nn. 532 U.S. 275 (2001).

oo. For a discussion of the implications of the *Sandoval* decision in a health care context, see Sara Rosenbaum and Joel Teitelbaum, "Civil Rights Enforcement in the Modern Healthcare System: Reinvigorating the Role of the Federal Government in the Aftermath of *Alexander v. Sandoval*," *Yale Journal of Health Policy, Law, and Ethics* III:2 (2003): 1.

pp. 42 U.S.C. §§ 12101 *et seq*.

qq. 524 U.S. 624 (1998).

rr. 179 F.3d 557 (7th Cir.1999), cert. denied, 528 U.S. 1106 (2000).

ss. Although insufficient data exist to know the extent of redlining in health care–related goods and services, several industries (home health care, pharmaceutical, and managed care) have come under particular scrutiny.[27]

tt. 197 U.S. 11 (1905).

uu. Incidentally, it was the *Jacobson* case to which we alluded in the second factual scenario at the opening of this chapter.

vv. 197 U.S. at 26.

ww. 489 U.S. 189 (1989).

xx. 125 S.Ct. 2796 (2005).

yy. 489 U.S. at 195.

zz. Ibid., 212.

aaa. These bills represent a "surge of legislation that reflects the intensifying tension between asserting individual religious values and defending patients' rights. . . . The flurry of political activity is being welcomed by conservative groups that consider it crucial to prevent health workers from being coerced into participating in care they find morally repugnant—protecting their 'right of conscience' or 'right of refusal.'. . . The swell of propositions is raising alarm among advocates for abortion rights, family planning, AIDS prevention, the right to die, gays and lesbians, and others who see the push as the latest manifestation of the growing political power of social conservatives."[34(pA01)]

bbb. See *Wyatt v. Stickney*, 344 F. Supp. 373 (M.D. Ala. 1972).

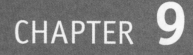

CHAPTER 9

Health Care Quality Policy and Law

LEARNING OBJECTIVES

By the end of this chapter you will be able to:

*   Describe the scope and causes of medical errors
*   Describe the meaning and evolution of the medical professional standard of care
*   Identify and explain certain state-level legal theories under which health care professionals and entities can be held liable for medical negligence
*   Explain how federal employee benefits law often preempts medical negligence lawsuits against insurers and managed care organizations

INTRODUCTION

This chapter steps away from the broad topics of health care access and coverage to focus on health care quality. As with access and coverage, health care quality has various dimensions—defining, measuring, and improving quality are all topics appropriately addressed as part of the study of health care—and the topic of health care quality has increasingly been a focal point of researchers, analysts, health professionals, and consumers. For instance, in the last several years alone, the influential Institute of Medicine of the National Academies of Science has released two major reports pertaining to health care quality: *To Err Is Human: Building a Safer Health System*,[1] which focused on the specific quality concern of patient safety, and *Crossing the Quality Chasm: A New Health System for the*

VIGNETTE

Michelina Bauman was born on May 16, 1995, in New Jersey. The managed care organization (MCO) through which her parents received health care coverage had precertified coverage for one day in the hospital post-birth, and both Michelina and her mother were discharged from the hospital 24 hours after Michelina was born. The day after the discharge, Michelina became ill. Her parents telephoned the MCO, but they were neither advised to take Michelina back to the hospital nor provided an in-home visit by a pediatric nurse as promised under the MCO's "L'il Appleseed" infant care program. Michelina died that same day from meningitis stemming from an undiagnosed strep infection.

21st Century,[2,a] which described how the health care delivery system should be overhauled to improve care.

Also like health care access and coverage issues, health care quality is a key concern in health policy and law. For example, long-standing problems related to the administration of health care—like racial and ethnic health disparities, and the geographic variation in the amount or type of care provided to patients—have drawn responses from policymakers and the legal system. Furthermore, policy and legal responses are often needed as health care quality is affected by changes in the marketplace or by advances in medical technology. For instance, as described in Chapter 4, institutional payers for health care services—traditional insurers, employers, and managed care companies—are more involved in health care practice now than was the case historically,[3(p26)] a fact that has spurred policymakers and courts to reconsider traditional notions of health care quality and liability.

The role of law as a monitor of the quality of health care was on display in the previous chapter, in the context of the no-duty-to-treat principle and the case of *Hurley v. Eddingfield*.[b] Recall from that discussion how Indiana's physician licensure law was described as a filter to weed out individuals without the requisite skills to safely and adequately practice medicine. Licensure performs a second health care quality function, as well—it allows state regulators to monitor the conduct of medical practitioners even after they have been licensed.

Holding health care professionals and entities liable for substandard care is another (and perhaps the most well-known) legal tool used to promote quality in health care. As described in Chapter 8, physicians have no legal duty to accept a patient into their practice or to provide care upon request, except in limited circumstances. However, a doctor's decision to treat a patient establishes a legally significant physician–patient relationship, under which the physician owes the patient a reasonable duty of care. Failure to meet what is termed the *professional standard of care*—the legal standard used in medical negligence cases to determine whether health professionals and entities have adequately discharged their responsibility to provide reasonable care to their patients—can result in legal liability for reasonably foreseeable injuries.[c]

As you will soon discover, the laws and legal principles that define the circumstances under which aggrieved individuals can successfully sue a managed care organization for substandard care or coverage determinations are complex. This complexity stems from multiple facts. First, the legal framework applied to medical negligence cases was developed long before the advent of managed care. Second, the hybrid nature of managed care (combining as it does the financing and delivery of care) defies easy categorization and makes application of the legal framework challenging. And third, a federal law (the Employee Retirement Income Security Act, or ERISA) pertaining to employee benefit plans preempts (i.e., precludes) many typical state-level legal claims against MCOs.

The next section of this chapter provides an overview of errors in health care. Although medical errors are only one component of the broad subject of health care quality, they are commonly included in the quality discussion and serve as a jumping off point for a discussion of health care liability. The chapter then turns to a full discussion of the professional standard of care and its evolution, followed by a description of some of the state legal theories under which hospitals, traditional insurers, and MCOs can be held liable for substandard medical professional conduct. Finally, the chapter explores the complex area of ERISA preemption of lawsuits premised on these same legal theories.

MEDICAL ERRORS AS A PUBLIC HEALTH CONCERN

Health care providers and public health professionals have in recent years committed increased attention to the problem of medical errors. Although medical errors are obviously not a new problem, framing the issue as a public health problem is a relatively new phenomenon.

The extent to which medical errors both occur at all and ultimately result in adverse health outcomes and mortalities indicates that the problem is not confined to one ethnic or racial population, socioeconomic group, or geographic area. A study conducted in Colorado and Utah suggests that 44,000 Americans die each year as a result of hospital-related medical error,[1(p1)] while a similar study in New York estimates the number to be as high as 98,000.[1(p1)] Another study suggested that every year approximately 1.5 million adverse medical events in hospitals seriously and permanently disable approximately 150,000 patients.[4(pp840–841)] Overall, more people die each year from medical errors than from motor vehicle accidents, breast cancer, or AIDS.[1(p1)] The negative effects of medical errors on individual patients and on society as a whole—including associated reductions in work productivity, lost income, and the costs associated with correcting injuries resulting from errors—support the conclusion that medical errors are properly classified as a public health problem requiring a strong response from, among others, policymakers and the legal system.

There are various causes of medical errors. They can be caused by actions that are, relatively speaking, concrete—such as failing to complete an intended medical course of action, implementing the wrong course of action, using faulty equipment or products in effectuating a course of action, failing to stay abreast of one's field of medical practice, or health professional inattentiveness.[d] There are more abstract causes of medical errors, as well. For example, they can result from the fact that "[m]uch of medical treatment is still primitive: the etiologies and optimal treatments for many illnesses are not known [and] many treatment techniques, such as cancer chemotherapy, create substantial side effects."[3(p30)] Also, many people argue that the culture of medicine—including its history of elitism, its focus on memorization in both diagnosing and treating illness, and its dedication to secrecy when adverse medical outcomes occur—helps to explain the extent of medical errors.

Just as there are multiple causes of medical errors, so are there various strategies—some broad and systemic, others more incremental—for preventing and reducing their occurrence. For instance, hospitals usually employ two vehicles to minimize medical errors and assure quality care for patients: risk management programs and peer review processes. Risk management programs monitor risks associated with non-physician personnel and with facilities under the direct control of hospital administrators; peer review processes entail a secretive evaluation of hospital-based physician practices by physicians themselves. Most physicians encounter the peer review process when they apply for "staff privileges" at a hospital, which grant doctors the ability to use the hospital for their own private practice, including the ability to admit patients and use the hospital's resources in treating patients. Once a doctor is granted such privileges he or she is subject to ongoing peer review. Many analysts maintain that the secretive manner in which the peer review process is conducted stifles meaningful improvements to patient safety, and that it is too reactive, responding to errors only after they have occurred.

Recently, public and private policymakers have begun shifting their attention to medical error reforms that are less reactive and more centered on error prevention and patient safety improvements. There are two primary objectives of these reforms: to redesign health care delivery methods and structures to limit the likelihood of human error, and to prepare in advance for the inevitable errors that will occur in health care delivery regardless of the amount and types of precautions taken. Medical error reform could entail various approaches, including more standardization of medical procedures, mandatory reporting of medical errors, reducing reliance on memory in medical care, increasing and improving medical information technology systems, encouraging patients to be more participatory in their own medical care, and establishing a national focus on the topic of patient safety.[3(pp43–64)] For example, the federal Patient Safety and Quality Improvement Act (PSQIA)[e] was signed into law in 2005 in response to the IOM's *To Err Is Human* report. PSQIA created a system for use by health care providers to anonymously report medical error data for systematic analysis. The hope is that by aggregating,

Box 9-1
Discussion Questions

What do you think of the term *medical error* as a descriptor of adverse medical outcomes? After all, there are many medical procedures (e.g., invasive surgeries) and treatments (e.g., chemotherapy) that not only are inherently risky, but also cause painful and dangerous (and often unpreventable) side effects (i.e., that lead to "adverse" medical results). Given this fact, is it conceivable that the health care delivery system could ever operate free of "error"? Can you think of other terms that better (or more fairly) convey the range of adverse outcomes attending health care practice?

analyzing, and disseminating the data analyses to health care providers nationwide, health care professionals and entities will increase their knowledge about what leads to adverse medical outcomes and alter their practice methods accordingly. Similarly, U.S. Senators Hilary Rodham Clinton and Barack Obama have proposed the National Medical Error Disclosure and Compensation (MEDiC) bill, which would go farther than PSQIA by creating an Office of Patient Safety and Health Care Quality within the federal Department of Health and Human Services aimed, in part, at reducing preventable error rates.[7]

PROMOTING HEALTH CARE QUALITY THROUGH THE STANDARD OF CARE

Not all medical errors rise to the level of being contrary to law. This section details the measure used by the legal system to determine which errors trigger legal protections: the professional standard of care. The standard of care is key both to the provision of high-quality health care and to legal claims that a health professional's, hospital's, or managed care organization's negligence in rendering medical care resulted in injury or death. This type of liability falls under the law of *torts*, a term that derives from the Latin word for "twisted," and which applies to situations where the actions of an individual or entity "twists away" from being reasonable and results in harm to others. Proving tort liability is not easy generally, and this is no less true in the specific context of medical care. A patient seeking to hold a health professional or entity responsible for substandard care or treatment must demonstrate the appropriate standard of care, a breach of that standard by the defendant, measurable damages (for example, physical pain or emotional suffering), and a causal link between the defendant's breach and the patient's injury.[f]

The Origins of the Standard of Care

The professional standard of care has its origins in 18th-century English common law. Courts in England had established that a patient looking to hold a physician legally accountable for substandard care had to prove that the doctor violated the *customs of his own profession*, as determined by *other professionals within the profession*. In other words, no objective standard was utilized by courts to measure the adequacy of physician practice.[g] Furthermore, courts were not in the habit of making searching analyses of whether the customs and standards proffered by the profession as defensible were at all reasonable. As noted above and in Chapter 1, this type of physician deference was incorporated into America's legal fabric, as policymakers and courts delegated key decisions about medical practice—including determinations as to whether a specific practice undertaken in the treatment of a particular patient was acceptable or negligent—to the medical profession itself.

The law's reliance on health professionals to determine the appropriate standard of medical care was not without its problems. In effect, this *laissez-faire* approach made it virtually impossible for an injured patient to successfully recover monetary damages from a negligent doctor, because the patient was required to find another health professional willing to testify that the doctor's treatment violated the customary standard of care. (This type of testimony was certainly uncommon, as health professionals rarely openly questioned the practices of other members of the profession.) Moreover, using professional custom as the touchstone for determining legal liability had the effect of thwarting the modernization of medical care, because practicing physicians knew they would be judged, in essence, based on how other physicians customarily practiced.

Furthermore, establishing a violation of professional custom was not the only hurdle injured patients had to clear in their effort to hold their physicians legally accountable for substandard care. English courts also developed what became known as the "locality rule," which held that testimony provided on behalf of a patient as to whether a physician's actions met the standard of care could only come from physicians who practiced *within the same or similar locality* as the physician on trial. Thus, not only did aggrieved patients need to find a physician willing to testify that a fellow member of the profession violated customary practice, they needed to find this expert witness within the (or a similar) locality in which the defendant-doctor actually practiced.[4(p844),h] As they did with the professional custom rule, U.S. courts gradually adopted the English locality rule. For example, the Supreme Judicial Court of Massachusetts ruled that a small-town physician was

> bound to possess that skill only which physicians and surgeons of ordinary ability and skill, prac-

ticing in similar localities, with opportunities for no larger experience, ordinarily possess; and he was not bound to possess that high degree of art and skill possessed by eminent surgeons practicing in larger cities and making a specialty of the practice of surgery.[i]

Courts' application of the locality rule severely limited patients' ability to bring medical malpractice actions against their physicians. Indeed, some injured patients were prevented from even initially mounting a case, because they were unable to convince a "geographic colleague" of their own physician to serve as an expert witness. (This problem was particularly acute in rural communities where there were fewer doctors to begin with, and where collegiality was the norm.) Furthermore, the locality rule likely resulted in at least a few local medical standards that were set by doctors who were less than completely skilled. The rule had another effect, as well: It led to a gulf among localities and cities in the standard of medical care practiced, and thus to different standards of care for similarly situated patients. Imagine, for example (notwithstanding the fact that the professional custom rule generally discouraged advancements in the standard of medical care), that physicians in a large town or city upgraded their practice techniques to reflect new medical technologies. Small-town practitioners had little incentive to model their big-city colleagues in the improvement of their own practice techniques, because the locality rule limited testimony as to the reasonableness of a physician's care to practitioners in the same or similar locality as the doctor on trial and their own actions would never be measured against the elevated techniques of their big-city counterparts.

By the 1950s or so, policymakers and the legal system grew wary of a health care system effectively in charge of policing itself; not surprisingly, this view was reflective of society more broadly, which during the civil rights era adopted a set of values heavily influenced by social justice and circumspect of concentrated institutional power. It also reflected the fact that no matter how chilling the effects of the professional custom and locality rules were, the practice of medicine—particularly the dissemination of medical research findings—had obviously evolved from the 1800s. These facts both vastly altered the law's approach to measuring physician care and promoted higher quality health care.[4(pp844–845)]

The Evolution of the Standard of Care

Under the law's modernized approach to the standard of care, both legal pillars of the physician autonomy era—the professional custom rule and the locality rule—were more or less razed.[j]

The Professional Custom Rule

Courts no longer defer to professional custom as solely determinative of whether a physician's actions reached the accepted standard of care. Instead, courts now analyze whether the custom itself is reasonable in light of existing medical knowledge and technology.[k] Although evidence of professional custom remains probative in determining whether the standard of care has been met, courts consider a range of other relevant evidence as well. Thus, the benchmark courts employ today to determine whether a health professional's treatment of a particular patient rose to the standard of care is whether it was *reasonable given the "totality of circumstances."*

Furthermore, it is no longer the case that evidence as to what is and is not customary medical practice is limited to what medical professionals themselves testify. Although evidence as to medical custom may still be introduced by medical professionals, objective clinical and scientific evidence—such as scientific research and clinical trial results—are now considered relevant in determining medical negligence. For example, the well-known case of *Helling v. Carey*[l] shows how advances in medical knowledge can obliterate long-standing medical customs and replace them with new requirements. In *Helling*, a 32-year-old woman sought treatment from a series of ophthalmologists for glaucoma-type symptoms. The ophthalmologists, however, refrained from screening the patient for glaucoma, on the ground that professional custom only called for the screen in patients beyond the age of 40 because the incidence of glaucoma in younger people was low. The State of Washington's Supreme Court ruled that notwithstanding the fact that the ophthalmologists had properly adhered to accepted custom, the *custom itself* was outdated based on current medical knowledge and was therefore unreasonable. The court effectively determined that a new treatment standard was required of the ophthalmology profession, and held that the defendant-physicians were liable for the patient's blindness.

The key legal principle at work in *Helling* is that courts can (and do, in rare circumstances) determine for an entire industry (medical or otherwise) what is legally required of them, despite long-standing industry practices. This principle is premised on the famous case of *The T.J. Hooper*,[m] in which the U.S. Second Circuit Court of Appeals held that a tugboat company was liable for damages to cargo it was shipping, because the company failed to maintain radio receiving equipment that could have warned the boats of a storm that battered the boat. The company argued that it should not be liable for the damage because at the time it was not typical practice in the tugboat industry to carry radio equipment. In response, the court wrote:

There are, no doubt, cases where courts seem to make the general practice of the calling the standard of proper diligence. . . . Indeed in most cases reasonable prudence is in fact common prudence; but strictly it is never its measure; *a whole calling may have unduly lagged in the adoption of new and available devices.* It never may set its own tests, however persuasive be its usages. *Courts must in the end say what is required*; there are precautions so imperative that even their universal disregard will not excuse their omission.[n]

Essentially, the court determined that the tugboat company was not acting reasonably under the circumstances, but was instead hewing too closely (and foolishly) to what should have been considered an outmoded industry practice. This same view appeared to drive the court in *Helling v. Carey*, as well. Indeed, the idea that the quality of health care provided by a health professional should be measured by an objective standard based on reasonableness under the circumstances—rather than by other professionals cloaked in the protections of outright autonomy—is today considered the norm. Furthermore, this view extends to big cities and small towns alike, and to both well-off and indigent patients.

The Locality Rule

Just as professional custom was transformed by the courts from being conclusive evidence of proper medical practice to being merely one piece of the evidentiary puzzle, so too was the locality rule undone (in most states) by more modern judicial thinking. Based in part on the fact that medical education and hospital-based care were becoming increasingly standardized under national accreditation efforts, courts stopped restricting evidence regarding the appropriate standard of care to the locality in which a physician practiced. Instead, most states have adopted what could be termed the "reasonably competent physician" standard, described as

that degree of care and skill which is expected of a reasonably competent practitioner in the same class to which he belongs, acting in the same or similar circumstances. Under this standard, advances in the profession, availability of facilities, specialization or general practice, proximity of specialists and special facilities, together with all relevant considerations, are to be taken into account.[o]

Under this revised standard, the practice of medicine nationally is key, because for purposes of determining medical liability a physician's actions are now measured objectively against those of a reasonably prudent and competent practitioner under similar circumstances, not against the actions of physicians who practice within a particular defendant's locality. Thus, in the eyes of the law, local medical practice customs have properly given way to higher expectations where health quality is concerned. Together, the revamped legal rules pertaining to medical custom and local practice were combined to create what is called the *national standard of care*.[4(pp844–845)]

TORT LIABILITY OF HOSPITALS, INSURERS, AND MANAGED CARE ORGANIZATIONS

Just as physicians are now held to a national standard of care in cases challenging the quality of their care and treatment, so too have courts moved to apply this same standard to hospitals, traditional health insurers, and managed care organizations. The following sections consider each of these in turn.

Hospital Liability

By the early 1900s, the health care industry began to rely much more heavily on hospitals (as opposed to physicians' offices or patients' homes) as a locus of patient care than had been the case previously. As with all health care settings, hospital-based medical practice created circumstances that led patients to challenge the quality of care provided. Out of necessity, the legal system (specifically, state-level courts) responded to these challenges by applying theories of liability—premised on the national standard of care—meant to hold hospitals accountable for negligence that occurred within their walls. Two theories—one premised on hospitals' relationship with doctors and one based on the actions and decisions of hospitals themselves—dominate the field of hospital liability. The former theory is called vicarious liability; the latter is termed corporate liability. We discuss each in turn.

Vicarious Liability

The concept of vicarious liability, which maintains that one party can be held legally accountable for the actions of another party based solely on the type of relationship existing between the two parties, is premised on the long-standing principles of "agency" law. Under this field of law, where one party to a relationship effectively serves (or is held out to society) as an agent of another party, a court can assign legal responsibility to the other party where the agent's actions negligently result in injury to a person or damage to property. For example, vicarious liability allows a hospital to be held responsible in some situations for the negligent acts of the doctors that practice medicine under its roof—not because the hospital itself somehow acted negligently, but rather because the doctor is (or is viewed as by the law) an agent of the hospital.

One relatively easy way for a plaintiff to win a lawsuit premised on vicarious liability is to establish through evidence that the two parties at issue are engaged in an employer–employee relationship, and that the employee (i.e., the agent) was acting within the normal scope of her professional duties when the act of negligence occurred. In these instances, courts frequently look to the employer to adequately supervise the employee while on the job and hold the employer responsible when an employee's negligent acts occur within the parameters of the employee's job responsibilities.

However, many "agents" of the companies they are hired to work for are not formal employees; rather, they are hired as independent contractors. Indeed, this is true of most hospital–physician relationships. Historically, agency law respected hiring entities' decisions to hire individuals as independent contractors rather than as employees, and the general legal rule is that employers are not accountable for the illegal actions of these contractors. Nonetheless, there are exceptions to this rule, and courts have developed theories of vicarious liability—such as *actual agency*, *apparent agency*, and *nondelegable duty*—that are more concerned with the scope of an employer–independent contractor relationship than with the formal characterization of the relationship as determined by the parties themselves. In other words, employers cannot avoid legal liability simply by labeling a hired worker as an independent contractor, because courts will analyze evidence of an employer–independent contractor relationship to determine the specifics of the relationship.

Actual agency exists—and the negligence of an independent contractor can be imputed to his employer—when the employer exercises *de facto* supervision and control over the contractor. Thus, for example, agency can be shown to exist between a health care corporation and a health professional when the particular facts pertaining to the relationship reveal that the corporation actually exercises control over the professional, even though the professional is not technically an employee. Similarly, the doctrine of apparent agency (also called ostensible agency) is another exception to the general rule that employers should not be legally exposed for the negligence of their independent contractors. In the context of health care, this type of agency exists, for example, when a patient seeks care from a hospital emergency department (rather than from any particular physician working in that department) and the hospital leads patients to believe that physicians are employees of the hospital (for example, via a billboard extolling the skills of the physicians who practice in its emergency department).[p] Finally, courts have also associated the doctrine of vicarious liability with certain duties considered so important to society as to be legally "nondelegable." For example, the importance of a hospital's obligation to maintain control over the care provided in its emergency department led one court to rule that it would be improper for the hospital to claim immunity from vicarious liability when its independent contractor furnished substandard medical care.[q]

Corporate Liability

In the context of the quality of hospital care, the concept of corporate liability has been just as important as that of vicarious liability. However, as opposed to vicarious hospital liability, which is predicated on the negligence of individual health professionals, corporate liability holds hospitals accountable for their own "institutional" acts or omissions. In other words, a hospital can be held liable when its own negligent acts as a corporation cause or contribute to a patient's injury. Several general areas give rise to litigation around hospitals' direct quality of care duties to patients: failure to screen out incompetent providers (i.e., negligence in the hiring of clinicians), failure to maintain high quality practice standards, failure to take adequate action against clinicians whose practices fall below accepted standards, and failure to maintain proper equipment and supplies.[4(p927)]

The most famous hospital corporate liability case is *Darling v. Charleston Community Memorial Hospital*.[r] In *Darling*, the Illinois Supreme Court found Memorial Hospital liable for negligent treatment provided to plaintiff Dorrence Darling, an 18-year-old who suffered a broken leg while playing in a college football game. The poor treatment Darling received by the hospital's emergency room staff—his leg cast was not properly constructed and its application cut off blood circulation—ultimately resulted in amputation of Darling's leg below the knee. The court held the hospital liable not for the actions of the emergency room staff, but for *its own* negligence: According to the court, Memorial Hospital did not maintain a sufficient number of qualified nurses for poste-

mergency room bedside care (when Darling's leg became gangrenous), and it neither reviewed the care provided by the treating physician nor required the physician to consult with other members of the hospital staff.

Insurer Liability

Like hospitals, conventional (i.e., indemnity) health insurers historically were not susceptible to being sued under tort principles; rather, they were subject mainly to breach of contract lawsuits when they failed to reimburse medical claims for services covered under beneficiaries' health insurance policies. This stemmed from two related facts: First, normative insurer practice was to leave medical judgments and treatment decisions in the hands of doctors, meaning that it was rare for an insurer-related action to lead to the type of injury covered by tort law; second, to the extent that an insurer did deny a beneficiary's claim for insurance coverage, it did so retrospectively—in other words, *after* the beneficiary received needed diagnostic tests, treatments, medications, and so on. This effectively meant that when beneficiaries sued their health insurer, they did so not because they had been physically or emotionally injured by the insurer's decision to deny an insurance claim, but because there was a dispute as to whether the insurer was going to pay for the already-received medical care.[s] Thus, although coverage denials had potentially enormous economic implications for affected beneficiaries, they did not tend to raise health care access or quality issues.

In the years following the *Darling* decision, however, courts began to apply tort liability principles to traditional indemnity insurers when their coverage decisions were at least partially responsible for an individual's injury or death,[t] which had the effect of opening insurers to a fuller range of potential damages (e.g., pain and suffering) than had been the case previously (when under breach of contract principles insurers were only liable for the actual cost of care they had initially declined to cover). This increased exposure to liability grew out of the fact that insurers were becoming more aggressive in their use of *prospective* coverage decisions, and courts were aware of how these types of coverage determinations could impact access to and the quality of health care. The advent of managed care as the primary mechanism for delivering and financing health care only magnified this concern (given managed care's use of techniques such as utilization review), and opened the door to one of the most contentious aspects of health services quality today—the extent to which patients can sue managed care organizations for negligent coverage or treatment decisions.

Managed Care Liability

Just as state courts were important in the extension of tort principles to health professionals, hospitals, and insurers, so too did they inaugurate application of these principles to managed care organizations.[4] As described in Chapter 4, modern managed care organizations are complex structures that heavily regulate the practices of their network physicians. Indeed, perhaps the most defining aspect of managed care is its oversight of physician medical judgment through various mechanisms—utilization review, practice guidelines, physician payment incentives, and so on.

A function of managed care's oversight of physician practice is that there is no longer any doubt that application of the professional standard of care for the purpose of determining negligence extends beyond the literal quality of health care delivered and reaches the very *coverage* of that care. This is because managed care has so altered coverage decision-making practices to focus on prospective decisions; where this type of coverage determination used to be the exception, it is now the rule. Instead of coverage denials leading to disputes over who was going to pay for an already-received medical service, prospective managed care coverage decisions more or less determine whether an individual receives treatment at all.[8]

Needless to say, prospective coverage decisions' negative impact on individuals' ability to access necessary, high quality care is no small policy matter. At the same time, in one critical legal sense it does not particularly matter whether a dispute between an MCO and one of its beneficiaries is framed as one of negligence in health care *quality* or health care *coverage*—either way, the key issue is whether the medical judgment exercised by the MCO met the professional standard of care. In applying this standard, courts have had little trouble finding MCOs liable under state law both for the negligence of their network physicians and for their own direct negligence. (However, as discussed in the next section, these court decisions presume the nonapplicability of ERISA, a federal law that often precludes individuals from suing their managed care company under state tort laws.)

There have been a number of cases in which courts have determined that MCOs can be held vicariously liable for the negligent actions of their network physicians where a patient can prove an agency relationship under one of the theories (actual agency, apparent agency, or nondelegable duty) described above. In these cases, courts perform an exhaustive examination of the facts to determine the specific relationship between the treating physician and the MCO or the ways in which the MCO portrays and obligates itself to its beneficiaries. For example, in the leading case of *Boyd v. Albert Einstein Medical Center*,[u] a Pennsylvania court closely analyzed a health maintenance organization's (HMO's) literature for any contractual relationship to its beneficiaries to determine whether it could be held vicariously liable under a theory of apparent agency for the treatment of a woman who

died after physicians negligently treated her for a lump in her breast. Among other things, the court noted that the HMO's contract with its beneficiaries agreed to "provide health care services and benefits to members in order to protect and promote their health," and that the patients' contractual relationship was with the HMO, not with any individual physician in the HMO's network. In the end, the court determined that because the patient "looked to" the HMO itself for care and the HMO held itself out as providing care through its network physicians, the HMO was vicariously liable for the patient's negligent treatment.

Similarly, courts have applied the doctrine of corporate liability to managed care organizations. Courts have given various reasons for subjecting MCOs to this type of liability: At least in their role as arrangers or providers of health care, MCOs are much like hospitals; MCOs have the resources to monitor and improve the quality of health care delivery; and MCOs maintain tremendous authority over the make-up of their physician networks. The case of *Jones v. Chicago HMO Ltd. of Illinois*[v] is a good example of the application of corporate liability principles to managed care. In *Jones*, the plaintiff called her MCO-appointed physician (Dr. Jordan) after her three-month-old daughter (Shawndale) fell ill with constipation, fever, and other problems. Both an assistant to Dr. Jordan and, eventually, Dr. Jordan himself, explained that Shawndale should not be brought to the physician's office but should instead be treated at home with castor oil. A day later Shawndale was still sick and her mother took her to a hospital emergency room, where she was diagnosed with bacterial meningitis, secondary to an ear infection. Shawndale was permanently disabled as a result of the meningitis. It emerged through pretrial testimony that the defendant MCO had assigned 4,500-6,000 patients to Dr. Jordan, far more than its own medical director deemed acceptable under the professional standard of care. The Illinois Supreme Court agreed, ruling that MCOs breach a legal duty as a corporate entity by assigning an excessive number of patients to any single network physician, because doing so can affect the quality of care provided to beneficiaries.

Box 9-3
Discussion Questions

What do you think about the role and success of tort law in promoting high-quality health care? Does it help to deter errors? If not, why?

This section reviewed generally the application of the professional standard of care to hospitals, insurers, and managed care organizations and described certain state-level theories of liability that are implicated when patients claim that the care they received fell short of this standard. However, as alluded to earlier, the federal Employee Retirement Income Security Act often preempts (i.e., supersedes) these kinds of state law liability claims against insurers and managed care organizations. This chapter now turns to a discussion of ERISA and its preemptive force.

FEDERAL PREEMPTION OF STATE LIABILITY LAWS UNDER THE EMPLOYEE RETIREMENT INCOME SECURITY ACT (ERISA)

Generally speaking, ERISA prohibits individuals from recovering damages for death and injuries caused by substandard medical professional conduct to the extent that the individual receives her health coverage through a *private employer-sponsored* benefit plan. (Among others, individuals who work for federal, state, and local *public* employers are not covered by ERISA's rules.) Because approximately 150 million workers and their families in the United States receive this type of health coverage, and because managed care represents the dominant structure of health care delivery, the issue of whether individuals with private employer-sponsored managed care coverage can recover damages for substandard medical professional conduct is paramount.

Overview of ERISA

One of the most complex areas of federal civil law, the Employee Retirement Income Security Act[w] was established in 1974 mainly to protect the employee pension system from employer fraud. However, the law was drafted in such a way as to extend to all benefits offered by ERISA-covered employers, including health benefits. Because ERISA does not distinguish among employers based on size, essentially all employees in this country who receive health and other benefits through a private employer can be said to work for an "ERISA-covered" employer.

ERISA employs two main devices to protect employee pensions and other benefits. First, it imposes "fiduciary" responsibilities on those individuals or entities that administer various types of employer-sponsored benefit plans (in the case of health benefits, these are often conventional insurers or MCOs, or the employers themselves). A person or entity with fiduciary responsibilities is analogous to a trustee, who is expected to act primarily for another's benefit in carrying out his or her duties. Put differently, a fiduciary is one who manages money or property (like a pension fund or health care benefit) for another person and who is expected

to act in good faith in that management. One critical fiduciary responsibility is to act with an eye toward the best interests of the person who has placed his or her trust in the fiduciary, rather than seeking personal enrichment through trustee activities.

The second tool used by Congress in ERISA to regulate employee benefits is a set of uniform, nationwide rules for the administration of employee benefits. However, although ERISA closely regulates the structure and operation of pension plans, the law includes few substantive standards governing the design or administration of health (or other) employee benefits. This stems mainly from the fact that Congress's main purpose in passing ERISA was to confront the employer fraud and underfunding evident in the pension system in the early 1970s (after all, the title of the law hints that its purpose is to specifically protect employee *retirement income*), not to regulate all employee benefit plans. However, the language used by ERISA's drafters is both broad and ambiguous, and courts have interpreted the statute as applying well beyond the field of pensions.[4(pp173–177)] As a result of the dearth of substantive standards pertaining to employee health benefits, employers enjoy discretion under ERISA to decide whether to offer health benefits at all and, if they do, to offer a benefit package of their choosing. This discretion allows the employer to design the benefit plan itself or buy an "off the shelf" insurance policy from a health insurer. If the employer chooses the latter, it also must decide whether to use a conventional insurer or a managed care company; if using a managed care company, it must decide whether to include physician incentive schemes in its benefit plan.

ERISA's lack of substantive health benefit regulations is compounded by the fact that the law contains few avenues for employees to remedy negligent benefit plan administration, including substandard conduct in the administration of health plan benefits. As mentioned, ERISA precludes the recovery of monetary damages under state law theories of liability when employer-sponsored benefits are improperly denied; Congress was of the opinion in fashioning ERISA that payment of these types of damages would drain employer benefit plans of needed resources. However, one might assume that when Congress broadly displaces state laws aimed at remedying negligence (as it did with ERISA), it would put in place meaningful enforcement provisions in the federal law. Yet the remedies available under ERISA are dramatically more limited than those available under state law. Under ERISA, employees and their beneficiaries are effectively limited to suing to prospectively force a plan administrator to grant a covered benefit, to recover payment retrospectively when a covered benefit was improperly denied, and to enforce a plan administrator's fiduciary responsibilities.[x] The upshot of these rights is that they allow an employee injured by an action or decision of his benefit plan to recover *nothing beyond the actual cost of the benefit due in any event.*

Furthermore, in *Pilot Life Insurance Co. v. Dedeaux*,[y] the U.S. Supreme Court held that ERISA's enforcement provision constituted not merely *a* remedy for negligent administration of an employee benefit plan, but rather the *exclusive* remedy. This means that all other state remedies generally available to individuals to remedy corporate negligence are preempted (and thus not available) to employees whose health benefits are provided through an ERISA-covered plan. We turn now to a full discussion of ERISA preemption.

ERISA Preemption

In order to ensure the uniform regulation and administration of employee pension plans (and, as it turned out, other employee benefits) across the nation, Congress included in ERISA one of the most sweeping preemption provisions ever enacted under federal law. The uniqueness of the scope of ERISA's preemptive force is underscored by the fact that, as you read in Chapter 3, the states in America's governmental structure maintain broad authority to regulate many fields (including the fields of health care and health insurance) as they see fit, and federal law generally supplements, but does not replace, state law.

Furthermore, ERISA actually implicates two different types of preemption. The first, known as "conflict preemption," occurs when specific provisions of state law clearly conflict with federal law, in which case the state law is superceded. The second form of preemption triggered by ERISA is "field preemption," which the courts employ when they interpret federal law to occupy an entire field of law (e.g., employee benefit law), irrespective of whether there are any conflicting state law provisions (this is the type of preemption at work in ERISA's remedial provisions, described earlier). The practical import of this second type of preemption is that a wide range of state laws are preempted by ERISA even though they do not directly conflict with it. All in all, it is little wonder that ERISA is considered to function as a "regulatory vacuum."[4(p177)]

The length of ERISA's conflict preemption provision belies its preemptive scope, and its wording belies the enormous amount of litigation it has engendered. The substantive entirety of the preemption clause reads: "[ERISA] shall supersede any and all State laws insofar as they may now or hereafter relate to any employee benefit plan."[z] Courts have grappled with the meaning of this language for decades. For example, the term "relate to" has been interpreted by the U.S. Supreme Court to include any state law that has "a connection with or reference to" an employee benefit plan,[aa] but not those that only have a "remote and tenuous" relationship to benefit plans.[bb]

Thus, the former types of state laws are preempted, while the latter are not. The Supreme Court has also weighed in on the meaning of "employee benefit plan."[cc]

In addition to the preemption clause itself, however, there are two additional pieces to the ERISA conflict preemption puzzle that only add to the law's complexity. The second piece is referred to as the "insurance savings" clause, which says that the preemption clause shall not "be construed to exempt or relieve any person from any law of any State which regulates insurance...."[dd] This essentially means that even where a state law relates to an employee benefit plan, it is saved from preemption if it regulates insurance.[ee] The Supreme Court has interpreted this provision to mean a state law is saved from preemption if it is specifically directed toward entities engaged in insurance and substantially affects the risk pooling arrangement between an insurer and its beneficiaries.[ff] The practical effect of the savings clause, then, is to narrow the reach of the preemption clause, because state laws that meet the "regulates insurance" test fall outside the scope of ERISA preemption.

The final element of ERISA conflict preemption is the "deemer" clause, which addresses the distinction between fully insured and self-insured employee health benefit plans.[gg] ERISA's deemer clause reads in pertinent part: "[A]n employee benefit plan shall [not] be deemed to be an insurance company or other insurer, ... or to be engaged in the business of insurance ... for purposes of any law of any State purporting to regulate insurance companies."[hh] The purpose of this clause is to prohibit states from deeming employee benefit plans as the functional equivalent of health insurers, and its practical effect is critical for the tens of millions of employees who receive their health benefits under self-insured plans: The deemer clause prevents state laws that meet the "regulates insurance" test from applying to self-insured employee health benefit plans.[ii] In other words, even state laws "saved" from preemption do not apply to self-insured plans because under ERISA these types of plans are "deemed" not to be insurance companies. The ultimate result of the deemer clause's application is to *exempt completely* self-funded employee benefit plans from state insurance law. This allows sponsors of self-funded plans enormous discretion to design the plans as they choose.

The Intersection of ERISA Preemption and Managed Care Professional Medical Liability

The final matter to discuss in the context of ERISA preemption has been one of the most unstable over the past several years: the extent to which ERISA preempts state tort law claims by individuals against managed care companies for negligent coverage decisions and substandard provision of care. This issue has played out over a series of federal court decisions attempting to define with some precision ERISA's application in the context of employer-sponsored managed care plans.

In the 1992 case of *Corcoran v. United HealthCare, Inc.*,[jj] the Fifth Circuit Court of Appeals ruled that Florence Corcoran's state law claim against United HealthCare for the wrongful death of her fetus had to be dismissed under ERISA, regardless of any medical negligence on the part of the MCO. The court held that even if the company improperly denied coverage of pre-term labor management services for Mrs. Corcoran, her state lawsuit seeking damages for a negligent coverage decision was preempted because the company's determination was, in the language of ERISA, sufficiently "related to" Mrs. Corcoran's employee benefit plan.

Three years later, the Third Circuit Court of Appeals ruled in *Dukes v. U.S. Healthcare, Inc.*[kk] that although individuals in ERISA-covered health benefit plans may not be able to sue under state law for an MCO's negligent coverage denial (i.e., for a company's decision as to the *quantity* of care covered under the plan), they can seek state law damages where a managed care company's negligence is connected to the *quality* of care actually provided. The Third Circuit essentially ruled that Congress did not intend in passing ERISA to supersede state laws aimed at the regulation of health care quality, historically a subject area under the states' purview. Instead, according to the court, federal policymakers enacted ERISA to alleviate national companies' concerns over abiding by many different state pension and employee benefit laws and to instead subject them to a uniform set of funding and administration rules. Whatever Congress meant by a "state law that relates to an employee benefit plan," the *Dukes* court did not interpret ERISA's preemption provision to sweep in laws pertaining to the quality of medical care provided to beneficiaries of employer-sponsored health benefit plans.

In the five years after *Dukes* was decided, federal court decisions applying ERISA to managed care plans more or less subscribed to this quantity/quality distinction. However, the Supreme Court stepped into the fray in 2000 in the case of *Pegram v. Herdrich*,[ll] seemingly altering the approach lower courts had been taking when analyzing ERISA preemption of state law negligence claims against MCOs. The main issue in *Pegram* was whether physician incentive arrangements were violative of the fiduciary responsibility rules contained in ERISA (incidentally, the Court ruled they were not). However, the Court included several paragraphs in its decision about the role of the treating physician in the case, who also happened to be one of the owners of the managed care company being sued for negligently failing to order a diagnostic test. In so doing, the Court described two different kinds of decisions made by MCOs:

What we will call pure "eligibility decisions" turn on the plan's coverage of a particular condition or medical procedure for its treatment. "Treatment decisions," by contrast, are choices about how to go about diagnosing and treating a patient's condition: given a patient's constellation of symptoms, what is the appropriate medical response? *These decisions are often practically inextricable from one another.* . . . This is so not merely because . . . treatment and eligibility decisions are made by the same person, the treating physician. It is so because a great many *and possibly most* coverage questions are not simple yes-or-no questions, like whether appendicitis is a covered condition (when there is no dispute that a patient has appendicitis), or whether acupuncture is a covered procedure for pain relief (when the claim of pain is unchallenged). The more common coverage question is a when-and-how question. Although coverage for many conditions will be clear and various treatment options will be indisputably compensable, physicians still must decide what to do in particular cases. . . . In practical terms, these eligibility decisions cannot be untangled from physicians' judgments about reasonable medical treatment.[mm]

Importantly, the Court went on to suggest that these intertwined decisions fall beyond ERISA's reach and that state laws implicated when these decisions are negligently made are not preempted, though the Court provided no clear guidance as to when managed care decisions tipped sufficiently toward coverage or care to pull them out of the realm of being "mixed." Following the decision, many federal courts faced with ERISA's application to claims by managed care beneficiaries adopted *Pegram*'s approach over the one developed in *Dukes*. Courts favored *Pegram*'s approach because it opened the door to state law remedies for individuals (like Florence Corcoran) who were injured as a result of managed care negligence but who otherwise had no way to recover for their loss.

In the 2004 case of *Aetna Health, Inc. v. Davila*,[nn] however, the Supreme Court appeared to close the door it appeared to open in *Pegram*, suggesting that lawsuits premised on the intertwined or "mixed" decisions made daily by MCOs escape ERISA's preemptive force only when the decisions include actual treatment by an MCO medical employee. The *Davila* decision actually represented a pair of cases (the other one originally called *Cigna v. Calad*) consolidated by the Court due to the similarity of the respective plaintiffs' claims. Both Juan Davila and Ruby Calad were members of ERISA-covered employee health benefit plans. Davila was injured when Aetna chose to substitute a less expensive medication for the one he normally took to control his arthritis pain; Calad suffered complications after being prematurely discharged from the hospital subsequent to Cigna's decision to cover just one day of hospitalization post-surgery. Rather than filing appeals directly with their insurance companies, Davila and Calad sued under a state law called the Texas Health Care Liability Act. They argued that their respective insurer's decision breached a duty under the Texas law to exercise reasonable care in health care decision making, and that the breach caused their injuries.

In rejecting both plaintiffs' claims, the Supreme Court ruled that ERISA preempts lawsuits for damages against ERISA-covered plans for negligent health care coverage decisions, even when the coverage decision was predicated on flawed medical judgment. Thus, *Davila* makes clear that when an individual covered by an ERISA plan complains only of negligent coverage decision making (including the wrongful denial of a benefit) on the part of an MCO, ERISA shields the MCO from liability beyond the actual value of the benefit itself.[oo] However, the Supreme Court in *Davila* also explained that notwithstanding ERISA, MCOs remain liable under state tort laws for negligence when acting in their capacity as providers or arrangers of health care. Although this ruling sustains the general distinction made by the federal court of appeals in the *Dukes* decision, its effect on the legal remedies available to injured patients is likely to be limited, given that policymakers and courts still view coverage decision making, rather than the provision of health care, as the primary aim of MCOs.

Box 9-4
Discussion Questions

The critical intersection between health care and health insurance as exemplified by the *Davila* decision leads to an important question: Is it reasonable to treat a health care coverage decision as having nothing to do with health care itself? Put another way, given the expense of health care today, do you believe that individuals and families can afford necessary health care if there is no third party responsible for covering at least some of the cost?

CONCLUSION

This chapter introduced the concept of health care quality generally, described the specific quality concern of medical errors, and detailed the topic of legal liability for substandard health care provision and decision making, including the preemptive role played by ERISA. Of course, holding health professionals and entities legally accountable for negligence in health care is just one method used to promote high quality care. Policymakers, health services researchers, the health professions themselves, and others have proposed or implemented several additional strategies (e.g., related to the health care system's organizational structure, or to evidence-based medicine, or to information technology) aimed at remedying existing quality concerns and improving the quality of care going forward. Many of these strategies have yet to take hold on a national scale, however, and finding effective ways to mesh them with existing legal rules—and navigating the legal system's responses to them—are issues the country will grapple with in future years.

REFERENCES

1. Kohn LT, Corrigan JM, Donaldson MS, eds. *To Err Is Human: Building a Safer Health System.* Washington, D.C.: National Academy Press; 2000.

2. Committee on Quality of Health Care in America. *Crossing the Quality Chasm: A New Health System for the 21st Century.* Washington, D.C.: National Academy Press; 2001.

3. Furrow BR, Greaney TL, Johnson SH, Jost TS, Schwartz RL. *Health Law: Cases, Materials and Problems.* St. Paul, Minn.: West Group; 2001.

4. Rosenblatt RE, Law SA, Rosenbaum S. *Law and the American Health Care System.* Westbury, Conn.: The Foundation Press; 1997.

5. Kaufman M. Medication errors harming millions, report says. *Washington Post,* July 21, 2006:A08.

6. Nordenberg T. Make no mistake: medical errors can be deadly serious. Available at: http://www.fda.gov/fdac/features/2000/500_err.html. Accessed August 1, 2006.

7. Clinton HR, Obama B. Making patient safety the centerpiece of medical liability reform. *New Engl J Med.* 2006;354(21):2205.

8. Rosenbaum S, Frankford D, Moore B, Borzi P. Who should determine when health care is medically necessary? *New Engl J Med.* 1999;340(3):229–233.

ENDNOTES

a. Among many important contributions to the discussion of how best to improve health care quality, *Crossing the Quality Chasm* delineated six elements of quality health care: safety, effectiveness, patient-centeredness, timeliness, efficiency, and equity.

b. 59 N.E. 1058 (Ind. 1901).

c. For example, in the lawsuit stemming from the facts described at the outset of this chapter, the parents of the infant who died alleged that their MCO's decision to precertify only 24 hours of hospital care coverage did not meet the requisite standard of care in several health care quality respects: it was not medically appropriate and was motivated by financial profit, not Michelina's health and well-being; it forced Michelina's premature discharge from the hospital; it was made despite the MCO's knowledge that newborns are particularly at risk for developing illnesses; and it discouraged physicians participating in the MCO's provider network from re-admitting infants to the hospital when problems arose after discharge.

d. By way of example, according to the Institute of Medicine (IOM), errors in the prescribing, administering, and dispensing of medications result in at least 1.5 million injuries or deaths annually in the United States.[5(pA08)] Furthermore, "mistakes in giving drugs are so prevalent in hospitals that, on average, a patient will be subjected to a medication error each day he or she occupies a hospital bed."[5(pA08)] Yet according to the IOM, "at least a quarter of the injuries caused by drug errors are clearly preventable,"[5(pA08)] and some of the errors are spawned by something as simple as name confusion among pharmaceuticals. For example, it is easy to see how physicians, nurses, and pharmacists could easily confuse the arthritis drug Celebrex, the anticonvulsant drug Cerebyx, and the antidepressant drug Celexa when prescribing, administering, and filling medications.[6]

e. P.L. 109-41 (July 29, 2005).

f. Because the law's evolving view of the standard of care closely mirrors its view of the medical profession more generally, it is worth pausing for a moment to reflect on Chapter 1's discussion of the health policy and law conceptual framework that is focused on historical, social, political, and economic views. This framework includes three perspectives: professional autonomy, social contract, and free market. The first perspective, dominant from about 1880–1960, argues that physicians' scientific and medical expertise leaves them in the best position to determine whether care rendered to patients is of adequate quality, and thus that legal oversight of the medical profession should be driven by the profession itself. The second perspective guided policymaking and legal principles for roughly 20 years beginning around 1960, and maintains that health care delivery and financing should be governed by enforcement of a "social contract" that generally elevates patient rights and societal values over physician autonomy and control. The free market perspective—dominant since the 1990s—contends that health care services are most efficiently delivered in a deregulated marketplace controlled by commercial competition. Bear in mind the first two perspectives specifically as you read this section.

g. One of the most commonly cited English cases for this rule is *Slater v. Baker and Stapleton*, in which the court ruled that the appropriate legal standard for determining a surgeon's liability was "the usage and law of surgeons . . . the rule of the profession" as testified to by practicing surgeons. 95 Eng. Rep. 860, 862 (King's Bench 1767).

h. Naturally, permitting a "similar" locality to be used as the benchmark for allowing standard of care testimony gave rise to litigation around what was, and was not, "similar" to the locality in which a defendant-doctor practiced.

i. *Small v. Howard*, 128 Mass. 131, 132 (1880).

j. However, some states still retain the locality rule as the appropriate standard for the admissibility of medical evidence, and some states utilize a modified rule that takes into account local resources and other factors in determining whether a defendant-doctor was able to meet the standard of care. For an example of the latter point, see *Hall v. Hilbun*, 466 So.2d 856 (Miss. 1985), in which the Mississippi Supreme Court determined that the locality rule still had relevance to the extent that a physician's imperfect care resulted not from his substandard medical knowledge and skills, but from the fact that he did not have access to needed resources and equipment. In this type of situation, the court reasoned, health professionals who genuinely attempt to meet the requisite standard of care should not be held legally responsible when factors outside their control prevent them from doing so. The court in *Hall* went on to explain that under these circumstances, a physician is required to be aware of extant limitations and to actively demonstrate an effort to assist patients as best he can by, for example, referring them to doctors and facilities better able to care for them.

For purposes of determining legal liability for substandard treatment, the notion of distinguishing between medical knowledge and skills on the one hand and medical resources and other factors on the other has particular relevance when the treatment involves an indigent patient whose care implicates broad contextual problems, such as poor living conditions or insufficient access to providers. Here, again, many courts look to see whether the treating physician's actions demonstrate an understanding of the proper level of care and a sincere effort to reach that level. However, do not confuse the fact that the law does not generally hold physicians liable for the consequences of re-

source problems attending the health care system, or of poverty, with the idea that different standards of care exist for the well-off and for the poor. As far as the law is concerned, there is a unitary standard of care to be applied regardless of a patient's socioeconomic status, and physicians can certainly be held legally responsible for mistreating an indigent patient.

k. An example of this shift can be seen in the case of *Canterbury v. Spence*, 464 F.2d 772 (D.C. Cir. 1972), which was discussed at length in the preceding chapter in the context of a patient's right to make informed health care decisions. The *Canterbury* court ruled that a professional-oriented standard for measuring the legality of a physician's disclosure of information to a patient should be replaced by an objective standard predicated on what a reasonable patient would need to be told to effectuate the aforementioned right.

l. 519 P.2d 981 (Wash. 1974).

m. 60 F.2d 737 (2d Cir. 1932).

n. Ibid., 740 (italics added).

o. *Shilkret v. Annapolis Emergency Hospital Association*, 349 A. 2d 245, 253 (Md. 1975).

p. *Mehlman v. Powell*, 378 A. 2d 1121 (Md. 1977).

q. *Jackson v. Power*, 743 P. 2d 1376 (Alaska, 1987).

r. 211 N.E.2d 253 (Ill. 1965).

s. For example, see *Van Vector v. Blue Cross Association*, 365 N.E. 2d 638 (Ill. App. Ct., 1977).

t. For example, see *Gruenberg v. Aetna Insurance Co.*, 510 P. 2d 1032 (Cal., 1973).

u. 547 A. 2d 1229 (Pa. Super., 1988).

v. 730 N.E. 2d 1119 (2000). Interestingly, this important corporate health care decision was handed down by the Illinois Supreme Court, which also decided the landmark *Darling v. Charleston Community Memorial Hospital* case.

w. Even citations to ERISA are complicated, because the law's section numbers in the U.S. Code (where much of ERISA can be found under Title 29) do not always correspond to the section numbering in the original act as written by Congress. For a helpful Website effectively decoding where ERISA provisions are located in the U.S. Code, go to http://benefitslink.com/erisa/crossreference.html.

x. 29 U.S.C. § 1132.

y. 481 U.S. 41 (1987).

z. 29 U.S.C. §1144(a).

aa. *Shaw v. Delta Air Lines, Inc.*, 463 U.S. 85 (1983).

bb. *New York State Conference of Blue Cross & Blue Shield Plans v. Travelers Insurance Co.*, 514 U.S. 645 (1995).

cc. *Fort Halifax Packing Co. v. Coyne*, 482 U.S. 1 (1987).

dd. 29 U.S.C. § 1144(b)(2)(A).

ee. *Metropolitan Life Insurance Co. v Massachusetts*, 471 U.S. 724 (1985).

ff. *Kentucky Association of Health Plans, Inc. v. Miller*, 538 U.S. 329 (2003).

gg. A fully insured health plan (sometimes referred to simply as an insured plan) is one in which an employer purchases health insurance coverage (i.e., pays premiums) to a conventional insurance company or MCO, and in return the insurance company or MCO accepts the financial risk of paying claims for covered benefits. A self-insured health plan (also called a self-funded plan) exists when an employer retains some or all of the financial risk for its employees' claims for covered benefits. Nearly half of all U.S. employers self-insure their health benefit plans.

hh. 29 U.S.C. § 1144(b)(2)(B).

ii. *Metropolitan Life Insurance Co. v Massachusetts*, 471 U.S. 724 (1985).

jj. 965 F.2d 1321 (5th Cir. 1992).

kk. 57 F. 3d 350 (3d Cir. 1995).

ll. 530 U.S. 211 (2000).

mm. Ibid., 228-29 (italics added).

nn. 542 U.S. 200 (2004).

oo. Note how this outcome can reasonably be viewed as incentivizing ERISA plans to arbitrarily deny patients' claims for health care coverage, because even in the event that plans are found to have acted negligently, they are only responsible for paying the cost of the denied benefit, but nothing more.

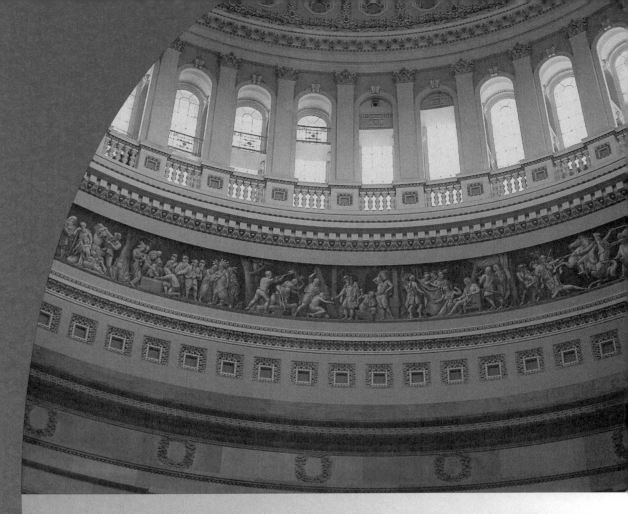

PART III

Basic Skills in Health Policy Analysis

Parts I and II covered fundamental concepts of health policy and law and engaged in a substantive discussion of essential issues in health policy. Part III examines the concept of policy analysis and spells out how to write a health policy analysis, one of the most important skills in health policy.

CHAPTER 10

The Art of Structuring and Writing a Health Policy Analysis

INTRODUCTION

Imagine you work for the governor of a state that recently received a large sum of federal money for anti-bioterrorism efforts and your boss asks you how it should be spent. How are you going to respond? Or, assume you are an assistant to the director of a state nutrition program for low-income children and the program's budget was slashed by the legislature. The program's director needs to reduce costs and turns to you for help; how will you approach this problem? Finally, pretend you work in the White House as a domestic policy advisor and the president is considering revising the administration's national stem cell research guidelines. What guidance will you offer? The prior chapters guided you through the substance of health policy and law. This chapter teaches you what policy analysis is and how to address complex health policy questions through a written policy analysis that thoroughly analyzes the question with which you are grappling.

POLICY ANALYSIS OVERVIEW

In this section we define policy analysis and review the purposes for developing one. In the following section, we provide a step-by-step process detailing how to create a written health policy analysis.

Defining Policy Analysis

We use the following definition to describe a policy analysis: *An analysis that provides informed advice to a client that relates to a public policy decision, includes a recommended course of action/inaction, and is framed by the client's powers and values.* We briefly review each element of this definition below.

Client-Oriented Advice

The "client" is the particular stakeholder that requests the policy analysis, and the analysis must be developed to suit the needs of the client. (The client could be a policymaker who hires you, a fictional policymaker in an exercise developed by your professor, an employer who asks you to analyze a problem, etc.) In general, a stakeholder refers to an individual or a group that has an interest in the issue at hand. There may be many stakeholders related to a particular policy issue. Of course, the client requesting an analysis is also a stakeholder because that person or entity has an interest in the issue. However, to avoid confusion we refer to the person or group that requests the analysis as the client, and the other interested parties as stakeholders.

Informed Advice

Providing informed advice means the analysis is based on thorough and well-rounded information. The information included in the analysis must convey all sides of an issue, not just the facts and theories supporting a particular perspective. If a decision maker is only presented with evidence supporting one course of action or one side of a debate, it will be impossible for the client to make a well-informed decision. In addition, to be effective in persuading others to favor the recommended policy, your client must be able to understand and, when necessary, refute alternative solutions to the problem.

Public Policy Decision

As discussed in detail in Chapter 2, policy analyses involve public policy decisions. A public policy problem goes beyond the individual sphere and affects the greater community.

Providing Options and a Recommendation

A key component of any policy analysis is providing the client with several options to consider, analyzing those options, and settling on one recommendation. In other words, a policy analysis is not simply a background report that identifies a variety of issues relating to a particular problem; instead, it gives the client ideas about what steps to take to address the problem and concludes by recommending a specific course of action.

Your Client's Power and Values

Finally, the analysis should be framed by the client's power and values. The first requirement is fairly straightforward and uncontroversial: The options presented and the recommendation made must be within the power of the client to accomplish. On the other hand, the notion of framing an analysis according to the client's values is more controversial. In most conceptualizations of policy analysis, including the one discussed later in this chapter, the process is roughly the same: Define the problem and provide information about it, analyze a set of alternatives to solve the problem, and implement the best solution based on the analysis.[1(p3)] As new information is uncovered or the problem is reformulated, analysts may move back and forth among these steps in an iterative process.[2(p47)] However, although there is general agreement that politics and values play a role in policy analysis, there is disagreement over at which stage of the analysis they come into play.

To understand this controversy it is necessary to discuss two models of policy analysis—the rational model and the political model. The rational model was developed in an attempt to base policy decisions on reason and science, rather than the vagaries of politics.[2(p7)] In the traditional rational model, the analyst does not consider politics and values. Instead, she should recommend the "rational, logical, and technically desirable policy."[2(p51)] According to the rational model, the *decision maker* infuses the analysis with politics and values once the analyst's work is complete.

Professor John Kingdon and others have moved away from the rational model and toward a political model. Kingdon suggests that policy analysis occurs through the development of three streams: problems, policies, and politics.[3,a] The problem stream is where problems are defined and noticed by de-cision makers. The policy stream is where solutions are proposed. These proposals may be solutions to identified problems, but they are often favored projects of policymakers or advocates that exist separate from specific problems that have garnered attention. Finally, the political stream refers to the ever-changing political mood. As a general matter these streams develop separately, only coming together at critical junctures when the problem reaches the top of the agenda, the solutions to that problem are viable, and the political atmosphere makes the time right for change.[3(p87)]

Kingdon's approach discusses occurrences the rational model does not, such as why some problems are addressed and others are not, why some solutions are favored even if they are not technically the best approach, and why action is taken at some junctures but not at others.[3] In addition, the rational model only refers to one cycle of problems. As Kingdon and others have noted, solutions to one problem often lead to unintended consequences that create other problems to be addressed, resulting in an ongoing policy analysis cycle instead of an event with a start and a finish.[5(p260)]

Professor Deborah Stone also focuses on the role of politics and values in analysis.[2(pp1-14)] She argues that the idea of the rational policy analysis model misses the point because "analysis itself is a creature of politics."[2(p8)] According to Stone, everything from defining a problem, to selecting analytic criteria, to choosing which options to evaluate, to making a recommendation is a political and value-laden choice. "[R]ational policy analysis can begin only after the relevant values have been identified and . . . these values change over time as a result of the policymaking process."[2(p32)] She contends that policy analysis should do the very things that the rational model does not permit—allow for changing objectives, permit contradictory goals, and turn apparent losses into political gains.[2(p9)] The goal of the rational model founders—to divorce analysis from the vagaries of politics—is simply not possible in Stone's view.

Having differentiated these models, we now return to our definition of policy analysis: *An analysis that provides informed advice to a client that relates to a public policy decision, includes a recommended course of action/inaction, and is framed by the client's powers and values.* You can see that this definition follows Stone's political model of policy analysis, requiring the analysis to be developed with a particular client's values in mind. After reviewing the numerous examples provided in the following section, it will be evident that client values permeate all aspects of a policy analysis. Only after you take into account your client's values, combine it with the information you have gathered, place it in the prevailing political context, and understand your client's powers, can you make an appropriate policy recommendation.

Multiple Purposes

The ultimate product of a policy analysis is a recommendation to a specific client about how to address a problem. However, a policy analysis has several other purposes as well. It provides general information necessary to understand the problem at hand and may be an important tool to inform stakeholders about a policy problem. In addition, the analysis may be a vehicle for widespread dissemination of ideas and arguments. Although your analysis is targeted to the client requesting advisement, it may also be used to inform and persuade other supporters, opponents, the media, the general public, and others. Finally, it will help you, the policy analyst, learn how to think through problems and develop solutions in an organized, concise, and useful way.

Policy analyses can take many forms—a memorandum, an oral briefing, a report, and so on—and, correspondingly, have varying degrees of formality. This chapter explains how to construct a *short, written* analysis because it is a commonly used, highly effective, and often practical way to provide a policy analysis to your client. Whether you are aiding a governor, the director of a state program, the CEO of a private business, or any other decision maker, you often will not have the opportunity to discuss issues in person or for a significant length of time. Furthermore, given time pressures, the demands on high-level policymakers, the need for rapid decision making, and the variety of issues most policymakers deal with, many clients will not read a lengthy analysis. That is why it is essential for anyone who wants to influence policy to be able to craft a clear and concise written analysis.

STRUCTURING A POLICY ANALYSIS

We now turn to a five-step method for writing a thorough yet concise policy analysis. Regardless of the subject matter, you can use this structure to analyze the question your client is considering. As you review each part of the analysis, notice the various disciplines and tools that may be part of writing an effective policy analysis. Analysts draw from a variety of disciplines—law, economics, political science, sociology, history, and others—and use a number of quantitative and qualitative tools when explaining issues, analyzing options, and making recommendations.

Although policy analyses come in various formats and use different terminology, they will all contain these essential elements:

- *Problem statement:* Defines the problem addressed in the analysis
- *Background:* Provides factual information needed to understand the problem
- *Landscape:* Reviews the various stakeholders and their concerns
- *Options:* Describes and analyzes several options to address the problem
- *Recommendation:* Offers one option as the best action to pursue

The following sections discuss each of these elements in detail.

The Problem Statement

The first step in writing a policy analysis is to clearly define the problem you are analyzing. A problem statement should be succinct and written in the form of a question that identifies the problem addressed in the analysis. It usually consists of a single sentence, though it may be two sentences if you are analyzing a particularly complex issue. Although a problem statement is simple to define, it is often one of the most difficult parts of the analysis to do well. It is also one of the most important.

The problem statement is the key to your analysis because it frames the problem at hand. Indeed, some policy battles are won or lost simply by how the problem statement is crafted. For example, consider the different questions asked in these problem statements:

Problem Statement 1:

What type of tax credit, if any, should the president include in the next budget proposal?

Problem Statement 2:

What type and size of health insurance tax credit should the president include in the next budget proposal?

The first problem statement asks what type of tax credit, if any, should be considered. One possible answer to that question is that no tax credit of any kind should be considered. Another answer could involve a tax credit, but not one related to health insurance. The second problem statement suggests that the option of not proposing a health insurance tax credit is unacceptable. Instead, the second problem statement lends itself to an analysis of identifying the pros and cons of various health insurance tax credit options. In other words, one option that may be considered based on the first problem statement (no tax credit) is excluded based on the second problem statement.

Consider another example:

Problem Statement 1:

Should the governor's top priorities include initiating a new state program to reduce the number of uninsured residents?

Problem Statement 2:

Should the governor's priority of reducing the number of uninsured residents be accomplished by relying on currently existing programs?

Again, the first problem statement asks *whether* providing a new health care program for the uninsured should be at the top of the governor's agenda. It is possible that the answer is "No, other priorities such as education and transportation should take priority." The second problem statement starts with the governor committed to reducing the number of uninsured and asks how to best accomplish that goal. These may sound like similar questions, but they lead to very different analyses and (most likely) different recommendations.

It is possible that your client's values will be evident from the way the problem statement is phrased. For instance, in the most recent example the second policy statement clearly reflects the governor's desire to reduce the number of uninsured. Consider another example. You have been asked to write a policy analysis about the merits of importing low-cost prescription drugs from Canada. How might the problem statement differ if your client is a pharmaceutical lobbying group, on the one hand, and an elder rights association on the other? Here are two possible problem statements.

Acceptable problem statement for the pharmaceutical lobbying firm:

How can this firm help improve medical care quality in the United States by reducing the importation of dangerous prescription drugs from Canada?

Acceptable problem statement for the elder rights association:

How can this association help seniors obtain low-priced prescription drugs from Canada?

The vast differences in these problem statements reflect differing viewpoints regarding the importation of prescription drugs. A pharmaceutical lobbying firm is more likely to be concerned about reduced profits for its drug company clients and therefore would want to deter or restrict importation, which could lead to more competition in the market. One way to accomplish that goal is to phrase the issue as a safety/quality of care concern. An elder rights association is more likely to be concerned with high-priced prescription drugs in the U.S. and would therefore want to promote drug importation. One way to accomplish that goal is to phrase the issue as one of cost reduction.

It is also possible to write solid, yet neutral problem statements. From the immediate example above, analysts for both groups could use the following problem statement:

What action should [the client] take in response to recent congressional proposals relating to importing prescription drugs from Canada?

A neutral statement is not necessarily better or worse than a value-driven statement. The value-driven statement provides additional information about the direction of the policy analysis and clearly limits some of the options that might otherwise be considered. A neutral statement is often broader, leaving more options on the table at the outset. Yet, even if a neutral statement is used, the options the analyst considers and the recommendation the analyst makes will still be constrained by the client's values and needs.

Because it is possible to create numerous problem statements for any issue, how do you develop the best one? Follow these guidelines.

Make the Problem Statement Analytically Manageable

Acceptable problem statements can be broad or narrow. One is not better than the other; they suit different purposes. Policy analyses with broad problem statements may require more diverse information in terms of background (discussed in the next section) and may consider a wider range of issues in the paper's landscape section (discussed later in this chapter). Also, the recommendations may promote "big picture" changes instead of specific and tailored ideas. Narrower problem statements may require less extensive background and landscape information, but they may not capture big picture, systemic concerns relating to the problem under consideration.

Reflect on the following examples. They both may be acceptable problem statements, depending on the needs of your client.

A broad problem statement:

What action should the U.S. Department of Health and Human Services take to avoid another flu vaccine shortage?

A narrow problem statement:

How can the U.S. Department of Health and Human Services create incentives for additional manufacturers to supply flu vaccine to the United States?

The first problem statement could result in a variety of recommendations, such as improving surveillance to lower the incidence of flu in the future, developing new vaccines that have longer-lasting immunity, finding ways to entice additional manufacturers to provide supplies to the U.S., and others. It is a broad problem statement that will lead to an analysis that could recommend a wide variety of actions. The second problem statement focuses on one particular way to decrease a flu vaccine shortage—increasing the number of suppliers.

Although the analysis will also provide a number of options, all of the options will address the specific issue of increasing suppliers. Again, there is no single right or wrong problem statement. Whether it is more useful to have a broad or narrow problem statement will depend on the needs and concerns of your client.

However, it is possible to make a problem statement so vague that it will be impossible to write a sound policy analysis. Unfortunately, there is no easy way to differentiate an acceptably broad problem statement from an unmanageably vague one when you begin your analysis. You will know your problem statement is too vague, however, if you find it impossible to write a *complete and concise* policy analysis. Your paper will require too much information in the background and landscape sections if you draft an overly vague problem statement. In addition, you will find that you cannot devise a coherent series of options addressing the problem because the problem statement is too broadly defined. Instead of a concise and useful policy analysis, you will end up with a lengthy and unfocused paper.

If you believe your problem statement may be so vague that it is analytically unmanageable, ask yourself if you are addressing one specific problem that may be countered with a few specific options. If you are having trouble narrowing your problem statement, you can try including limitations based on geography (e.g., refer to a particular state or city), time (e.g., focus on the next year or over the next five years), or numerical boundaries (e.g., use a goal of reducing a figure by a certain percentage or a budget by a specific dollar amount). Consider this example:

An unmanageably vague problem statement:

What is the best use of Centers for Disease Control and Prevention's resources to improve the health status of our citizens?

This problem statement is not analytically manageable. It is extremely broad and unfocused. Using this problem statement, your analysis could address any health issue, such as access to care problems, the need to improve vaccination rates, racial disparities in health care, or many others. The list is endless and your policy analysis will be as well.

A manageable problem statement:

What preventive health issue should be the top priority for the Centers for Disease Control and Prevention next year?

This problem statement is analytically manageable. It is focused on preventive measures specifically and is limited to determining the top priority. In addition, the problem is focused on what can be done in the upcoming year. The second problem statement allows for a much more concise and directed policy analysis.

Do Not Include the Recommendation in Your Problem Statement

Another pitfall in writing problem statements is crafting a problem in a way that suggests a particular solution to the issue. A problem statement should define a specific problem; it should not indicate how that problem should be solved. If the answer is preordained, why bother with the analysis? When drafting your problem statement, ask yourself if you can imagine three, four, or five potentially viable options to address the problem. If you cannot, then you have not defined the problem well.

For example, assume you've been asked to address reducing medical malpractice insurance premiums. Here is a problem statement that leads the reader to one conclusion:

To what extent should jury awards be limited in malpractice cases in order to reduce malpractice premiums?

This problem statement leads to one very specific solution (limiting jury awards) as a way to counter a broad problem (reducing malpractice premiums). The only question presented by this problem statement is what the award limit should be. It does not provide a range of options for reducing malpractice premiums (one of which may be limiting jury awards) for your client to consider. (Of course, if you were specifically asked to address how to limit jury awards in malpractice cases, this would be an appropriate problem statement.) A better problem statement would be:

What action should be taken to stem the rise in malpractice premiums nationwide?

This problem statement lends itself to an analysis that considers several options. Possible alternatives include limiting jury awards, enacting regulations that limit the amount insurance companies can increase premiums each year, and a host of other options. The problem statement also narrows the focus of the analysis to national solutions.

Once you have written your concise and precise problem statement, you have set the framework for your analysis. Every other section of the analysis should relate directly to the problem statement. Remember that writing a policy analysis is an iterative process; you must review, revise, and tighten the information and arguments throughout the writing process. As you review the other components of your policy analysis, it may become evident that what you thought was the best problem statement can be further improved. There is nothing wrong with revising your problem statement as you craft your analysis, as long as you remain true to your client's values and power.

The Background Section

The first substantive information your analysis provides is in the background section. The background informs the reader why the particular problem has been chosen for analysis. This section should make clear why the issue is important and needs to be addressed now. In addition to providing general information about the topic, your background and landscape (discussed next) sections provide the information necessary to assess the options you lay out.

Much of the information in the background will be relevant regardless of who assigned the analysis. However, because the background provides information necessary to understand the problem, it is essential to understand the knowledge level of your client when constructing the background. For example, assume you are writing an analysis relating to state preparedness planning for smallpox vaccination in the event of a bioterror attack. Regardless of your client, your background would likely include information about why a smallpox attack is a threat, including (but not limited to):

- Reference to the September 11, 2001, attacks on the World Trade Center and subsequent events
- The belief that although smallpox has been eradicated as a natural disease, it is likely that samples of the virus still exist
- Reference to any information provided by the federal government or other sources relating to the possibility of a bioterror attack

If your client does not have knowledge relating to smallpox, you would also include details about smallpox transmission, the effects of the disease, the vaccination procedure, and the risks associated with vaccination.

In addition, your background should include whatever factual information is necessary to fully assess the options discussed. Remember, your client needs a complete picture, not just the information that supports the recommended action or your client's viewpoint. By the time the reader reaches your paper's options section, all of the information necessary to evaluate the options should have been presented in your background or landscape.

For example, assume one of your options for the smallpox vaccination state preparedness analysis is immediate compulsory vaccination of all first responders and establishment of a protocol for vaccinating the remaining population if there is a smallpox outbreak. In that case, your background (and possibly the landscape) should provide information regarding who first responders are, where they are located, how many there are, legal issues relating to compulsory vaccination, and so on.

Because the background section is an informational—not analytical—part of the analysis, the material provided in it should be mostly factual. The tone of the background is not partisan or argumentative. It should simply state the necessary information.

The Landscape Section

Together, the background and landscape sections frame the context of the analysis for your client. Whereas the background provides factual information to assist the client in understanding what the problem is and why it is being addressed, the landscape provides the overall context for the analysis by identifying key stakeholders and the factors that must be considered when analyzing the problem. In the following discussion, you will read about numerous types of people, groups, and issues that might be included in a landscape. These examples are meant to provide suggestions and provoke thought about what should be included in an analysis. It would be impossible to include everything discussed below in any single landscape section. It is the job of the policy analyst to choose among these options—to be able to identify whose views and which factors are the most salient ones in creating a complete landscape.

Identifying Key Stakeholders

Up to this point, the policy analysis discussion has focused on just one stakeholder—the client that asked for the policy analysis. The landscape brings in other stakeholders who have an interest in the issue. Although it is often impossible to include every possible stakeholder in a single analysis, it is necessary to identify the key stakeholders whose positions and concerns must be understood before a well-informed decision can be made.

How do you identify the key stakeholders particular to your issue? Unfortunately, there is no magic formula. The best approach is through research and thinking. Also, bear in mind that the stakeholders and issues discussed in the landscape must relate to your overall policy analysis. Your options must address the problem identified initially, and all of the information necessary to assess the options must be presented in the background and landscape. As you learn about the problem to be analyzed and think about options for addressing the problem, it should become apparent which stakeholders have a significant interest in the issue.

For example, assume your analysis relates to proposed legislation regulating pharmacists and pharmaceuticals.

Who are possible key stakeholders regarding this issue? They may include:

- Democratic and Republican politicians (you might need to distinguish among those in Congress, state legislatures, and governors)
- Pharmaceutical industry
- Health insurance industry
- American Association of Retired Persons (AARP) and other elder rights groups
- Advocacy groups for the disabled
- Pharmacists' lobby
- Foreign pharmaceutical companies
- Internet-based pharmaceutical companies

Can you think of others?

Which of these stakeholders *must* be included in an analysis depends on the exact problem being analyzed. For example, assume you are writing an analysis about requirements relating to how pharmacists inform consumers about their medications. If your problem dealt with face-to-face encounters only, Internet-based pharmaceutical companies would not be a key stakeholder. Alternatively, if the problem definition dealt with purchasing limitations over the Internet, Internet-based pharmaceutical companies must be included in the analysis. If your client is a politician in Florida, elder rights groups should be included in the analysis because there is a large and influential elderly population in Florida. If your client is someone running for public office in a county where the health insurance industry is a major employer, the views of those companies would be essential to include. In other words, although it is possible to make a generic list of the types of individuals and groups that could be included, the specific list for any policy analysis will depend on the client for whom the analysis is being written and the specific problem being addressed.

Identifying Key Factors

Once you have settled on a list of key stakeholders, it is necessary to analyze their position on the issue at the center of the analysis. Earlier, we described the landscape as the portion of the analysis that provides the overall context of the issue. The "overall context" refers to the mix of factors that are relevant when any decision is being made. These factors are used to analyze stakeholder positions. Although there is not one comprehensive list of context factors and not all factors are relevant to all analyses, the list in Box 10-1 includes some common factors that could be discussed.

This list of factors is by no means exhaustive, but rather is intended to provide a sense of the types of questions that are often relevant to understanding the context of a problem. Just

Box 10-1   Possible Factors to Include in a Landscape Section

Political Factors
- What is the political salience of the issue?
- Is this a front-burner issue?
- Is this a controversial issue?
- Do key constituents, opponents, interest groups, etc. have an opinion about the issue? Who is likely to support or oppose change?
- Is there bipartisan support for the issue?
- Is there a reason to act now?
- Is there a reason to delay action?

Social Factors
- Who is affected by this problem?
- According to the client who assigned the analysis, are influential or valued people or groups affected by this problem?
- Is there a fairness concern relating to this issue?

Economic Factors
- What is the economic impact of addressing and of not addressing this problem?
- Are various people or groups impacted differently?
- Are there competing demands for resources that relate to this issue?
- What is the economic situation of the state or nation? How does this affect the politics relating to this issue?

Practical Factors
- Is it realistic to try to solve this problem?
- Would it be more practical to solve this problem later?
- Are other people in a better position to solve this problem?
- What do we know about solutions that do or do not work?
- If this problem cannot be solved, is it still necessary (politically, socially) to act in some way to address the problem?

Legal Factors
- Are there legal restrictions affecting this problem?
- Are there legal requirements that impact the analysis?
- Is new legislative authority necessary to solve the problem?
- Is there legal uncertainty relating to this problem?
- Is future litigation a concern if action is taken?

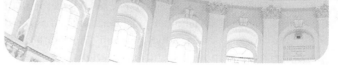

as it would be impossible to discuss every stakeholder who might be connected to the problem, it would be impossible to include in a concise analysis of all the issues raised by the five factors listed in Box 10-1. It is the policy analyst's job to be able to identify not only which key stakeholders must be included, but also which key factors must be discussed.

Consider again the example relating to limiting prescription drug purchases made over the Internet. Some key factors probably would include:

- *Political factor:* Who supports or opposes the limitation and how influential are they?
- *Economic factor:* Would it be costly to implement this limitation or costly to key constituents who may need more prescription drugs than allowed by the limit? Would it provide an economic benefit to some stakeholders?
- *Practical factor:* Is it possible to implement and enforce a restricted purchasing system over the Internet?
- *Legal factor:* Are there legal barriers to limiting Internet prescription drug purchases?

For each factor, the analysis should discuss relevant views of the stakeholders you included in your analysis. For example, when discussing economic factors, the analysis might explain that Internet-based pharmaceutical companies would experience a loss of revenue; some consumers would pay more for prescription drugs if they needed more than the limited amount; and storefront pharmaceutical companies would make money because consumers probably would have to fill more of their orders in person. Depending on the political situation, the analysis might explain that the client's most influential constituents are elderly people who use many prescription drugs and are likely to oppose any restriction, or that storefront pharmaceutical companies are large campaign contributors and would support a restriction.

Writing Structure

The landscape may be organized by stakeholder or by factor. In other words, it is acceptable to identify stakeholder #1 and then describe that stakeholder's views based on various factors, and then identify stakeholder #2 and describe that stakeholder's views, and so on. Alternatively, the landscape could be structured based on the factors described in Table 10-1. Within that structure, the landscape would address one set of factors (e.g., economic), then another set (e.g., social), and so on. Some stakeholders may not have relevant views for all of the factors, but each stakeholder must be addressed as often as necessary to convey their policy position. For example, the economic factors section would identify various stakeholders and their views based on economic concerns. It would include

information such as "Canadian companies would oppose regulating Internet pharmacies because it would increase the cost of doing business with Americans, while U.S. storefront pharmacists would support regulating Internet pharmacies because it may increase prices for their competitors' products."

When you discuss a particular view, it is important to identify which stakeholders hold that view. At the same time, do not insert opinions unattached to individuals or groups. For example, it would not be helpful to write, "Some oppose legislation regulating Internet pharmacies." Such a statement does not identify *who* opposes the legislation or *why* they oppose the legislation. If your client is going to be able to assess the political, practical, and ethical feasibility of taking a particular action, she needs to understand where the various groups stand and why they hold those views. Thus, a more helpful sentence would be: "RxData, a large software company that assists Internet pharmacies and who is a major employer in your congressional district, opposes legislation regulating Internet pharmacies because it will add costs to its business and may result in future employee layoffs." That sentence tells your client who is opposed to the legislation, why they are opposed to it, and why they are a key stakeholder.

The tone of the landscape should be neutral and objective. The landscape is not an argumentative section to persuade the reader that one view is better than another. Its purpose is to identify all of the key stakeholders and their concerns so the decision maker is well-informed before assessing options.

The Options Section

Once your client finishes reading the background and landscape sections, he should have a thorough understanding of the policy problem and the overall context in which a decision will be made. The time has come for him to consider what action to take. This is where your paper's options section comes in, providing three to five alternatives for your client to consider. This section is more than a recitation of various choices; it provides an analysis of each option by stating the positive and negative aspects of pursuing each path.

Identifying Options

The first step to writing your options section is to identify the various options you could analyze. Although you may develop a new option not previously considered by others, it is likely that you will find numerous possibilities that others have already suggested. Some places to find already-considered options include:

- Media
- Scholarly articles
- Interest group recommendations

- Think tanks/experts in the field
- Congressional testimony
- Legislation (passed or proposed)
- Agency reports

Another approach to developing options is to consider several major actions that policymakers often take to deal with a policy problem. For example, look at the following list of possible actions that, depending on the circumstances, could be added, eliminated, or altered by a policymaker in response to a policy problem:

- Taxes
- Subsidies
- Laws
- Regulations
- Programs
- Government organizations
- Information

Once you have compiled a list of options, how do you choose the best three to five options to include in the analysis? As always, the guiding principle underlying your decision is to base your decision on your client's values and powers. You should not suggest an option that clearly violates your client's values because your client will not seriously consider that option. For example, if your client has rejected spending new state money to solve a problem, you should not include an option that would cost the state money (or if you did, you would need to be clear about how these funds would be offset). Also, it is important to remember the extent of your client's power. For example, an analyst might recommend that a member of Congress introduce or sponsor a bill, or that an interest group submit a comment as part of the public notice and comment period before a regulation is finalized. On the other hand, an analyst should not recommend that a member of Congress force a state to pass a particular law because that action is not within Congress's power—the responsibility of passing state laws falls to state legislatures. Similarly, an interest group cannot issue an Executive Order or force an administrative agency to craft a regulation in a particular way. In other words, any option you include must be within the ability of your client to undertake.

In addition, you will probably want to include in your analysis any major proposals that are currently being considered. You may also choose to include proposals backed by key allies and constituents. Even if your client does not act on these proposals, it is important to be able to explain why "mainstream" options are being rejected. Also, it is often, but not always, appropriate to consider the status quo (the "do nothing" approach) as an option. Even when considering the do nothing tactic, it is necessary to evaluate the pros and cons of this op-

tion. In addition, your options should be different enough from one another to give your client a real choice. And one final rule to follow: Whichever alternative you ultimately recommend must be analyzed in the options section of your analysis.

All of the options included in the analysis must directly address the problem identified in your problem statement. For example, if your problem statement involved ways to reduce the number of uninsured individuals, an option that promotes increasing access to care for insured residents would be inappropriate because it does not directly address the problem. Indeed, everything in your analysis must flow from your problem statement, from what is included in the background and the issues discussed in your landscape, to the alternatives suggested in the options section, and (as discussed later) your final recommendation.

Assessing Your Options

Your options analysis must include a discussion of the pros (what is useful about an option) as well as the cons (what is problematic about an option) of each option. Although policymakers often seek a "silver bullet" that solves a problem without any negative effects, it is highly unlikely that such an option exists. As a result, an analysis must include the positive and negative aspects of an option. Also, all options must be analyzed equally. Do not provide more analysis for the option you decide to recommend even though it is your preferred option. Your client can make a fully informed decision only if you analyze what is both good and bad about each proposal.

In order to draft your pros and cons, you must identify the appropriate criteria for the analysis of the pros and cons and apply each criterion to all of the options. Many possible criteria could be used, so it is necessary to pick the ones that best fit your client's values and that address the key issues relating to the policy problem. Sometimes your client will provide you with criteria; other times you must deduce the correct criteria based on what you know about your client and the problem. Generally you should choose between three and five criteria for your analysis of the pros and cons. Typically, fewer than three will not allow for a full analysis, and more than five are difficult to assess in a relatively short analysis.

Your choice of criteria should reflect the concerns discussed in the landscape, where you identified the key factors relating to the problem. For example, if economic burden was an important aspect of the issue being considered, costs should be one of the criteria used to analyze the options. If the need for quick action was an important aspect of the issue, timeliness and administrative ease might be important criteria to consider. In general, cost and political feasibility are usually important criteria to include in your analysis. However, the specific

Box 10-2
Sample Options Criteria

Cost: How much does this option cost? (You may have to break this down: How much does it cost the federal government, state government, individuals, etc.)

Cost-benefit: How much "bang for the buck" does this option provide?

Political feasibility: Is this option politically viable?

Legality: Is this option legal? If so, are there any restrictions?

Administrative ease: Does this option have steep implementation hurdles?

Fairness: Are people impacted by this option treated fairly/equally?

Timeliness: Can this option be implemented in an appropriate or useful amount of time?

Targeted impact: Does this option target the population/issue involved?

criteria that are best for your analysis will depend on your client, the specific problem statement being addressed, and the landscape of the issue. Box 10-2 provides some criteria that could be considered when analyzing options. Can you think of others?

Writing Structure

When structuring your options section, you may find it helpful to use headings or bullets delineating each option. Your headings should clearly label each option. Also, it is generally useful to separate out the options by paragraph instead of having a continuous page or two assessing all of the options. The first sentence or two of each options paragraph should be a clear description of that option so the client understands what is being proposed; then assess the pros and cons of the option based on the criteria you identified. You should explicitly state the criteria prior to your options description.

For example, assume you are writing a policy analysis for the secretary of the Department of Health and Human Services about how to reduce the number of uninsured individuals. After drafting the necessary background and landscape information, you decided to assess the following options: 1) expanding existing public programs, 2) providing grants to states, and 3) providing tax credits to individuals. You decide the best criteria to use are cost to the federal government, political feasibility, and decreasing the number of unin-

sured. In your options section, you would have three different parts—one for each option—assessing the pros and cons based on the criteria you chose. Although the structure of the analysis may vary, you might have a paragraph looking something like this:

Option 1: Expand Public Programs. This option refers to an expansion of Medicaid to include mandatory coverage of childless adults up to 200% of the Federal Poverty Limit, and an increase in SCHIP eligibility to include children up to 300% of poverty. The most significant advantage of this option is that it will greatly decrease the number of uninsured individuals, more so than any other option presented. However, these gains may be ineffective because the provider community is likely to refuse additional Medicaid and SCHIP patients unless reimbursement rates are increased. The political feasibility of this option is extremely low because the current administration and Congress oppose expanding entitlement programs, which includes Medicaid. Another disadvantage is the very high cost to the federal government in a time where domestic spending is being drastically reduced due to high deficits and other burdens.

You would write a similar analysis for each of the options under consideration.

Side-by-Side Tables

You may choose to assess your options with the help of a side-by-side table. This table may be descriptive or analytic. A descriptive table would provide a description of each option but not provide any analysis. An analytic table would assess the options based on the criteria chosen. In either case, the table should be appropriately labeled and easy to read. As a general matter, a side-by-side table should supplement, not replace, your textual analysis because it is difficult to provide sufficient information within the space provided by a table. However, a table is a useful visual aid that may enhance the reader's understanding of your options and overall analysis. Tables 10-1 and 10-2 provide examples of side-by-sides.

As you can see from both tables, additional information is necessary for a complete analysis. In the text of your options section you would need to provide a more complete explanation of each option. It is difficult (but not impossible) to provide sufficient depth of analysis in a chart without creating a busy, difficult-to-read table.

Although the second table uses the terms low, medium, and high to assess the options, other terms or symbols (e.g., +, -)

TABLE 10-1   A Descriptive Side-by-Side Table

Reducing Number of Uninsured: Options Description

	Expand Public Programs	Grants to States	Tax Credits
General description	Expand Medicaid and SCHIP	Federal government provides funds to states to reduce uninsured	Federal government provides tax credits to individuals
Populations affected	Uninsured childless adults under 200% FPL, children under 300% FPL	Uninsured state residents, specific groups to be determined by state	Individuals earning less than $40,000 annually
Estimated reduction in uninsured	10 million	5 million	2 million
Payer	Federal and state	Federal	Federal
Optional or mandatory	Mixed	Optional	Optional

TABLE 10-2   An Analytic Side-by-Side Table

Reducing Number of Uninsured: Options Assessment

Options Criteria	Expand Public Programs	Grants to States	Tax Credits
Cost to federal government	High	Medium	Low
Political feasibility	Low	Medium	High
Reduce number of uninsured	High	Medium	Low

may be used. In addition, you may choose to include phrases instead of single words or symbols. Whatever choice you make, be sure that it is clear which assessment is positive and which is negative. When necessary, provide a legend explaining your terms. Also, some people prefer to use numerical assessments (e.g., 1 = low, 2 = medium, 3 = high). Although debates exist regarding the value of this type of quantitative assessment in a side-by-side chart, we strongly discourage it. Policy analysis is both an art and a science, and using a numerically based table can obscure that balance. An attempt to use quantitative measures may lead readers to assume a simple summation will suffice—just add up the columns and choose the best one. Overall, reducing the analysis to numerical labels hides the value judgments that are part of every analysis, fails to address whether certain criteria should be weighted more than others, and makes the optimal solution appear more certain than it probably is.

The Recommendation Section

The time has finally arrived in your policy analysis to make a recommendation. You should choose *one* of your options as your recommendation. Although it is possible to make more than one recommendation or a hybrid recommendation of multiple options, we discourage those approaches. Making multiple recommendations might make it necessary for your client to conduct further analysis to choose among the options. And making a hybrid recommendation (a combination of two or more options) is not appropriate unless the hybrid option was analyzed separately as a single option. In general, it is the analyst's job to organize and clarify the issues and place them in the context of the client's views and power. Ultimately, this should result in one path that you believe best suits your client.

The recommendation section should begin by clearly identifying which option is favored and why this option is

Box 10-3   Checklist for Writing a Policy Analysis

1. **Problem Statement**
   - Is my problem statement one sentence in the form of a question?
   - Can I identify the focus of my problem statement?
   - Can I identify several options for solving the problem?

2. **Background**
   - Does my background include all necessary factual information?
   - Have I eliminated information that is not directly relevant to the analysis?
   - Is the tone of my background appropriate?

3. **Landscape**
   - Does the landscape identify all of the key stakeholders?
   - Are the stakeholders' views described clearly and accurately?
   - Is the structure of the landscape consistent and easy to follow?
   - Is the tone of the landscape appropriate?
   - Does the reader have all the information necessary to assess the options?

4. **Options**
   - Do my options directly address the issue identified in the problem statement?
   - Do I assess the pros and cons of each option?
   - Did I apply all of the criteria to each options assessment?
   - Are the options sufficiently different from each other to give the client a real choice?
   - Are all of the options within the power of my client?

5. **Recommendation**
   - Is my recommendation one of the options assessed?
   - Did I recommend only one of my options?
   - Did I explain why this recommendation is the best option, despite its flaws?

preferred over the other ones. As mentioned in the options section, every alternative will have pros and cons. The recommendation section does not simply repeat the analysis in the options section. Instead, this portion of the analysis must explain why, despite the drawbacks, this is the best action to take based on your client's values and power. In addition, the recommendation section also identifies what, if any, actions may be taken to mitigate or overcome the negative aspects of your recommendation.

CONCLUSION

You now have a basic understanding of what policy analysis is and an introduction to the tools necessary to analyze a policy problem. Additionally, thinking through the process just described should train you to evaluate your options when *you* become the decision maker. The checklist in Box 10-3 provides examples of what should be included in each section of a written policy analysis.

REFERENCES

1. Patton CV, Sawicki DS. *Basic Methods of Policy Analysis and Planning*, 2nd ed. Englewood Cliffs, N.J.: Prentice Hall; 1993.

2. Stone D. *Policy Paradox: The Art of Political Decision Making*. New York: W.W. Norton; 2002.

3. Kingdon J. *Agendas, Alternatives, and Public Policies*, 2nd ed. New York: Addison-Wesley Educational Publishers; 1995.

4. Cohen M, March J, Olsen J. A garbage can model of organizational choice. *Admin Sci Q.* 1972;17:1-25.

5. Weissert CS, Weissert WG. *Governing Health: The Politics of Health Policy*, 2nd ed. Baltimore, Md.: Johns Hopkins University Press; 2002.

ENDNOTE

a. Kingdon's model is a revision of the "garbage can" model proposed by Michael Cohen, James March, and Jonathan Olsen.[4] The garbage can model consists of four unrelated streams (problems, solutions, participants, and choice opportunities), and the outcomes are determined by the mix of the streams and how the mix is processed.

Index

Page numbers followed by *f* denote figures; those followed by *t* denote tables

A